UNDERSTANDING MEDICAL TERMS

SECOND EDITION

UNDERSTANDING MEDICAL TERMS

A Guide for Pharmacy Practice

Walter F. Stanaszek, Ph.D. R.Ph.
Health Care Consultants, Inc.
Pharmacy Practice and Education
Norman, Oklahoma

Mary J. Stanaszek, R.R.A.
Health Care Consultants, Inc.
Health Care Information
Norman, Oklahoma

Robert J. Holt, M.A., R.Ph.
Health Care Consultants, Inc.
Community Pharmacy and Administration
Oklahoma City, Oklahoma

Steven Strauss, Ph.D., R.Ph.
Professor of Pharmacy Administration
Arnold & Marie Schwartz College of Pharmacy and Health Sciences
Long Island University
Brooklyn, New York

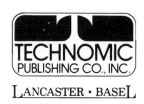

TECHNOMIC
PUBLISHING CO., INC.

LANCASTER · BASEL

Understanding Medical Terms
a**TECHNOMIC** publication

Technomic Publishing Company, Inc.
851 New Holland Avenue, Box 3535
Lancaster, Pennsylvania 17604 U.S.A.

Printed in the United States of America
10   9   8   7   6   5   4   3   2

Main entry under title:
    Understanding Medical Terms: A Guide for Pharmacy Practice, Second Edition

A Technomic Publishing Company book
Bibliography: p. 401
Includes index p. 403

Library of Congress Catalog Card No. 98-85738
ISBN No. 1-56676-595-1

CONTENTS

PREFACE TO THE SECOND EDITION

The need for a thorough understanding of medical terminology has not diminished in the least for pharmacists and other health care practitioners in the five years between the publication of the first edition of this book and this second edition. If anything, it has become greater. The pharmacy profession has further solidified its clinical role in patient care, and pharmacists are more entrenched than ever before in the role of counselor and advisor to both patients and practitioners alike. For more than a few pharmacists, what not long ago was an occasional question from a physician about appropriate drug therapy has become regular consultation concerning the interaction of drugs with the patient, his life, and the many other therapies he may be facing. Pharmacy chains, which not long ago installed glass walls to separate the pharmacist from customers, have asked technicians to count pills while pharmacists are in continuous contact with the patient.

Such practice changes have increased the demand for clinical knowledge among pharmacists, including a knowledge of medical terminology, and those demands have been passed on to the authors in preparation of the second edition of this book. While the role of the text is still to help pharmacists be more effective interpreters and counselors, some changes have been made in response to reader requests.

The most obvious changes were designed to make the book more useful as a reference when a specific need arises. It is still intended as a study tool, to be read from beginning to end in an organized learning sequence, but many readers found the need to return to these pages repeatedly over time to better understand terminology encountered in their daily professional lives. A complete index has been added, quickly allowing readers to find the discussion of medical terms they do not understand; many of the tables have been expanded to put more information at the readers' fingertips; and a table of common abbreviations has been added to each therapeutic chapter to give readers a more manageable amount of information at a time.

Otherwise, the text was expanded to include more recent terminology and more thorough explanations of medical terms. Medical practice and the entire health care system have changed, and the system terminology has changed with it. The National Institutes of Health has instituted an Office of Alternative Medicine, and the terminology of many alternative medical approaches is now included in this book. In short, the text is more complete for today's practitioner.

Many of the features of the first edition still remain. Although abbreviations are included in each chapter, the entire list is still included as Appendix A, allowing quick reference for unknown abbreviations. The text is still divided into two parts: the first four chapters cover the basis of medical terminology and provide an understanding of the components from which terms are formed; the second part examines more specific terminology as it relates to therapeutic categories. The figures are still included, simplifying anatomic terminology. And each chapter still includes a glossary with the definitions of major terms in the therapeutic category and a pronouncing glossary to aid in oral communication.

The philosophy underlying this book also has not changed. The text is still a learning tool for both practitioners and students. A continuing education manual is still available to help practitioners earn the appropriate credit for their study; self-tests are still included for each chapter, although they are now grouped together in Appendix B; the diagrams and the text are designed for clarity of understanding, rather than merely to compress the greatest mass of information into the smallest amount of space. In short, the authors have tried to make this book better serve the readers' needs. It is our sincere hope that you will think we succeeded.

PREFACE TO THE FIRST EDITION

The study of medical terminology is integral to any study of the medical system. Like any other field, medicine has its own special language, and an understanding of the language is necessary for an understanding of the discipline. Knowledge of medical language identifies those who belong in the inner sanctum, the brotherhood of those trained in the medical arts. It serves to admit those with the knowledge and exclude those who do not possess it. In this way, medical terminology provides an air of mystery and a cloak of authority for those in the health professions. Secondly, this ''hidden'' language protects the medical community from the public by denying the patient an understanding of his condition and treatment. Diagnoses, procedures, and treatment modalities are referred to by esoteric names that the patient does not understand, perhaps helping physicians and other health professionals exercise authority over the patient. Although medical terminology may serve these functions, the patient does not necessarily benefit.

The most legitimate function of any lexicon should be to provide clarity and specificity to communication. Medical terminology serves that purpose. Since medical terms do not vary in meaning from one generation to another or from one community to another, they are extremely precise in their definitions and allow those in the health care community to converse with each other with exactitude. This exactitude, however, is lost to those who do not speak the language. Therefore, it is essential for those within the health care community, including pharmacists, to master the language of the discipline if they are to take part in medical decision-making processes.

Generally, pharmacists have a good understanding of the medical terminology they frequently encounter. As students progress in pharmacy school, their knowledge of terms is expanded by the study of anatomy, physiology, pathology, pharmacology, and therapeutics, as well as by their internships. This book can help pharmacy students systematize such knowledge and refine their communication skills. Thus, this book is intended in part for pharmacy students. By the time they graduate, however, most students have a broad base of understanding for common medical terminology. So why should a practicing pharmacist need a book like this?

Most pharmacists are unique in their communities. In the community practice setting, pharmacists constitute the initial access to the health care system for a large number of patients. In the hospital, pharmacists often counsel patients about medications and other therapies, and they turn their patients over to community practitioners after discharge for further counseling. Indeed, the typical pharmacist interacts with more patients in a given day than any other health care professional. Pharmacists are often asked by patients to make sense of ''medical jargon'' to help them understand the frightening system in which they are trapped.

Additionally, the pharmacist must interact with the other health care providers. Clarifying orders, verifying medical necessity, evaluating the appropriate drug therapy in relation to other therapies and the patient's medical condition, reviewing records for quality assurance or drug use evaluation programs, and providing information on a wide range of health issues are all part of the pharmacist's basic role. To effectively communicate with physicians, nurses, technicians, therapists, and others in health care requires an unwavering ability to deal with the language of the profession.

So of all the health professionals, pharmacists are perhaps in the greatest need of a clear understanding of medical terminology and an ability to "translate" it into lay language. As simple translators, pharmacists need to know not only the specific term for a diagnosis, but also how to express that meaning in terms the patient will understand.

Much more important, though, is the ability to serve as "interpreter" for patients and the health care community. While a translator converts one language to another, an interpreter must provide a broader understanding. The pharmacist, therefore, must not only translate a term from English to "medical" and back again, but he or she should catch the nuances of each language and interpret the context as well as the definition. Some patients may use medical terminology to "sound scientific" and hide their fear; the pharmacist should be able to discern such usage and reassure these patients. Other patients may know the literal definition of a term without understanding how it applies to them; the pharmacist then must clarify the explanation so the patient truly understands.

But becoming an interpreter is not the only reason a pharmacist might need to study medical terminology. A basic problem is that pharmacy education has changed drastically over the last few decades. The educational system in the 1950s and 1960s included more of the medical sciences than ever before that time, but much less emphasis was placed on therapeutics and pathophysiology than in later years. Pharmacists who graduated in those decades were not exposed to the same terminology as their younger colleagues. The emphasis on clinical knowledge during the 1980s and into the 1990s expanded that base significantly, but it was still incomplete. After all, the five or six years required to become a pharmacist is hardly sufficient time to learn all one needs to know about the pharmaceutical sciences, much less the rest of the medical sciences. Programs incorporating a strong therapeutic base still can only cover the most common diseases and procedures; there simply is not enough time to learn it all.

So those pharmacists who have been out of school for some time may now be discovering a weakness in medical terminology. Even those whose practices have focused on the dispensing functions are finding that they are no longer insulated from the patient or the rest of the health care community. Practice is changing; patients are changing; indeed, the entire health care system is changing. And a grasp of medical terminology is one of the tools pharmacists need if they are to change with it.

Objectives

The role of this text, then, is to provide the practicing pharmacist (or pharmacy student, with a little guidance) a sufficient basis in medical terminology so that he or she is able to understand most of the medical terms encountered in practice. To do that, the book approaches terminology through a study of the parts of words—the prefixes, roots, and suffixes that create the meanings attributed to the total term.

Pharmacists and pharmacy students should approach this book as a study tool. It is organized in a learning sequence and can be read from beginning to end by those wanting a full understanding of the terminology involved. Or the individual therapeutic chapters can be studied separately for those wishing to refine their knowledge in a specific area. Either way, however, readers should begin their study with the first five chapters, which form the base for the rest of the book. By the time the reader has completed this text, he or she should be able to do the following:

- Identify common prefixes, roots, and suffixes used in medical terms and provide their definitions.
- Identify the prefixes, roots, and suffixes in each of a list of selected medical terms and define each term from the meaning of its components.
- Describe the role of prefixes, roots, and suffixes used in medical terms and how selected ones alter the definition of the term.
- Explain how combining forms differ from roots and how they are used in forming medical terms.
- Provide the appropriate medical term for each of a list of definitions by synthesizing the terms from the appropriate components.
- Describe how the definition of each term in a selected list is derived from the various possible combinations of components.
- Describe the anatomical composition of each of the discussed organ systems and explain how the relevant medical terms are developed.
- List the major procedures and therapeutic modalities used in the treatment of selected diseases for each organ system or therapeutic category covered.

A secondary role of this book is for continuing pharmaceutical education. It was written as an educational tool for pharmacists, as well as for pharmacy students. Its intent in part, therefore, is to make pharmacists more effective in practice by helping them deal more effectively with patients and other health care providers. Thus, by its very nature it was designed to be a continuing education tool. Part of any education is self-assessment as the student progresses, and self-study questions are found in Appendix A. Separately from the book, readers may also receive a larger examination covering the material in larger sections. That examination is designed to provide continuing pharmaceutical education credit for those successfully completing the text. For information concerning such credit, readers are directed to the separate continuing education component.

Because this book is intended for both pharmacy students and pharmacists, it contains a wide range of medical terms that are encountered in pharmacy practice. Some terms, however, are specifically excluded. For example, brand and generic drug names are generally omitted, as are chemical terms. Those in or preparing for the pharmacy profession are recognized as society's drug experts; their entire training is directed toward that end. Gaps that may occur in their knowledge of medical terms are likely to be in areas other than drugs and chemicals.

Also omitted is a thorough discussion of medical therapeutics. Although most of the chapters in Part II are organized by body systems or therapeutic categories, the focus is on terminology. Numerous other texts are available for those who wish to study anatomy, physiology, biochemistry, pharmacotherapy, medical therapeutics, or other approaches to the science of health care. Admittedly, terminology is integral to such studies, and this book may serve as the base on which the reader can build. But the intent herein is to help the reader learn the basic skills in communicating about patients, diseases, and therapies—not the skills used in treating disease.

Whatever reasons the reader has for studying medical terminology, the authors have endeavored to make that study both interesting and useful. We exhort you to apply diligence and attention to be successful.

PART I

THE BASIS OF
MEDICAL TERMINOLOGY

CHAPTER 1

Fundamentals of Medical Terms

Introduction

Like every other specialized discipline, the practice of medicine has evolved its own language over the years, using terminology not found in the general vocabulary. An understanding of medical terminology requires two basic elements: (1) some knowledge of the body structure and functions and (2) familiarity with meanings of the prefixes, suffixes, and roots comprising medical terms.

Most medical terms are composed of roots or stems derived from Greek or Latin and used in combination with prefixes and suffixes. These language sources are used interchangeably, such as in the term *appendicitis* containing the Latin *appendix* and the Greek suffix *-itis*. Terms derived from Greek and Latin have the advantage of being precise and unchanging. They have the same meaning in all countries; therefore, medical terminology is a universal language.

The fundamental method for building a medical vocabulary consists of analyzing a word by identifying its root, suffix, and prefix. Most medical terms are derivative; that is, they consist of a combination of two or more roots or word elements rather than a single Greek or Latin word. The identification of a term through structural analysis involves determining the meaning of each of its components that will either reveal the exact definition of the word or convey its applied meaning.

> Example: *myopathy* = *myo* (root meaning "muscle")
> + *pathy* (suffix meaning "disease")

Some words are comprised of more than one root, each of which retains its basic meaning. Such words, referred to as compounds, are very commonly found in medical terminology.

> Example: *osteoarthritis* = inflammation of the bone joints
> *osteo,* = meaning bone (root)
> *arthro,* = meaning joint (root)
> *itis,* = meaning inflammation (suffix)

For some medical terms, both the Greek and Latin spellings have been adopted as acceptable forms, so the spelling of a root can vary from one term to another. It is imperative, therefore, that a medical dictionary be consulted to determine the correct spelling of unfamiliar words. Because an incorrect spelling can convey an inaccurate impression, diagnosis, condition, or procedure, phonetic spelling has no place in the medical field.

As spelling of a root can vary, so too can pronunciation. Pronunciation of medical terms can be difficult initially, since no rigid rules can be followed. In addition, some words may be acceptably pronounced in more than one way. Common usage prevails; discrepancies in pronouncing medical terms will be found even in the same location.

> Example: *ab do" men*   or *ab" do men*
> *lab" o ra tory* or *la bor" a tory*
> *du" o de' num* or *du od' e num*
> *bar bit" u rate* or *bar" bi tu' rate*

. Although the pronunciations of a few key terms are provided in each chapter to help the reader grasp the basics of the spoken terms, pronunciation keys are not included for every term presented. After all, these pronunciations are available in all of the standard medical dictionaries, and every effort was made to keep this text to manageable proportions for the reader. Those pronunciations of which the reader is unsure should be determined from a medical dictionary. Repeated spoken use of the terms is the most helpful tool in acquiring mastery of expression.

The point of studying suffixes, roots, and prefixes is to refine the ability to analyze unknown words and derive an accurate meaning. How to go about that may initially seem backwards, but the definition of a term or its applied meaning can usually best be determined by beginning the analysis with the suffix and proceeding to the root and then the prefix. The reason is that the suffix often gives the general context, part of speech, or activity involved; the root then may determine the part of the body, the basic action, or other specific application or meaning. The prefix usually provides restriction or modification of the understanding derived from the suffixes and roots.

Suffixes

True suffixes consist of one or more syllables added to root words to modify the meaning and/or to indicate the part of speech—that the completed word is either a preposition or an adverb. Many endings, however, are nouns or adjectives added to a root to form a compound word. Such nouns and adjectives are not true suffixes; they are combinations of true suffixes and roots and may be referred to as combining forms or pseudosuffixes.

> Example: *-gloss*   (tongue)   Root
> *-al*   (related to)   True suffix
> *-glossal* (related to the tongue) Pseudosuffix

These compound endings may then be added to other prefixes or roots, as in the word *hypoglossal*. Because words are built of prefixes, roots, and suffixes, reasons arise to include multiple restrictions or modifications on the root, so a single word may contain more than one suffix at a time.

Table 1.1—Suffixes: Commonly Used Word Endings

Suffix	Meaning	Example	Suffix	Meaning	Example
-able	ability	palat*able*	-eal	of that kind,	poplit*eal*
-ible		flex*ible*	-eous	pertaining	calcan*eous*
-ile		fra*gile*		to	
			-ose		adip*ose*
-ac	related to,	cardi*ac*	-ous		mucin*ous*
-al	concerning,	abdomin*al*			
-an	pertaining	ovari*an*	-esis	condition,	pare*sis*
	to		-ia	state	dysplas*ia*
-ar		ocul*ar*	-iasis		cholelith*iasis*
-ary		papill*ary*	-id		flacc*id*
-ic		pyogen*ic*	-ism		catabol*ism*
-ical		pract*ical*	-ity		hyperacid*ity*
-ory		sens*ory*	-osis		diverticul*osis*
-tic		orthodon*tic*	-tia		prociden*tia*
			-tion		malabsorp*tion*
-ate	action	puls*ate*	-y		gou*ty*
-esis		enur*esis*			
-ure		meas*ure*	-cle	small	corpus*cle*
			-cule		mole*cule*
-form	resem-	veri*form*	-culum		tuber*culum*
	blance,		-culus		duct*ulus*
-oid	like	fibr*oid*	-et		pip*et*
			-ium		endocard*ium*
-e	agent	lactagogu*e*	-ole		arteri*ole*
-er		inhal*er*	-olum		horde*olum*
-ician		phy*sician*	-olus		bol*us*
-ist		urolog*ist*			
-or		levat*or*	-ious	capable of,	infect*ious*
				causing	

Table 1.2—Suffixes: Symptomatic and Miscellaneous

Suffix	Meaning	Example	Suffix	Meaning	Example
-agogue	producer, leader	sial*agogue*	-atresia	abnormal closure	proct*atresia*
-agra	attack, seizure	pod*agra*	-cele	hernia, swelling	hydro*cele*
-algia	pain	neur*algia*	-chesia	discharge	uro*chesia*
			-chezia	of foreign	hemato*chezia*
-aphia	touch	ambly*aphia*		substance	
-ase	enzyme	lip*ase*	-cide	destroy, kill	germi*cide*

Suffix	Meaning	Example	Suffix	Meaning	Example
-cleisis	closure	entero*cleisis*	-logy	science/ study of	cardio*logy*
-didymus -dymus	cojoined twin	atlo*didymus* triopo*dymus*	-lysis	dissolving, reduction	hemo*lysis*
-dynia	pain	pleuro*dynia*	-mentia	mind	de*mentia*
-ectasis	expansion, dilatation	angi*ectasis*	-metry -meter	measure/ instrument	opto*metry* cranio*meter*
-ema	swelling, distention	emphys*ema*	-nomy	law	tax*onomy*
-emia	blood	septic*emia*	-ol	alcohol, phenol	ethan*ol*
-ferent	bear, carry	ef*ferent*	-oma	tumor	carcin*oma*
-ferous	to bear, pro- duce	ossi*ferous*	-opia	slight defect	ambly*opia*
-fuge	expel, drive away	centri*fuge*	-opsia	condition of vision	xanth*opsia*
-genic	producing, origination	broncho*genic*	-ose	sugar	gluc*ose*
-iasis	presence/ formation of	nephrolith*iasis*	-osis	abnormal condition	dermat*osis*
-id	secondary lesion	tubercul*id*	-pagus	to fasten to- gether	diplo*pagus*
-ide	a binary compound	chlor*ide*	-pathy	disease	myelo*pathy*
-ine	a nitroge- nous compound	morph*ine*	-penia	lack, defi- ciency	leuko*penia*
-ite	division	metabol*ite*	-phagia	to eat, swal- low	dys*phagia*
-itis	inflammation	arthr*itis*	-phasia	speech	dys*phasia*
-lemma	sheath, en- velope	neuri*lemma*	-philia	to love, to crave	hemo*philia*
			-phobia	to fear	photo*phobia*

Suffix	Meaning	Example	Suffix	Meaning	Example
-plasia	develop-ment	hyper*plasia*	-stasis	at a stand-still	hemo*stasis*
-plegia	paralysis	hemi*plegia*	-staxis	hemorrhage	epi*staxis*
-pnea	breathing	dys*pnea*	-taxis	involuntary response to stimuli	rheo*taxis*
-poiesis	make, pro-duce	hemo*poiesis*			
-ptosis	to fall	blepharo*ptosis*	-thyma	condition of mind	cyclo*thymic*
-rrhagia	excessive discharge	meno*rrhagia*	-tome	cutting in-strument	osteo*tome*
-rrhea	flow	leuko*rrhea*	-tonia	stretching, causing ten-sion	hyper*tonia*
-rrhexis	rupture	cardio*rrhexis*			
-scope	instrument for viewing	broncho*scope*	-ule	small	tub*ule*
-spasm	involuntary contraction	entero*spasm*	-uria	condition of the urine	glycos*uria*
-stalsis	constriction	peri*stalsis*	-vert	turn	div*ert*
			-vorous	to eat	herbi*vorous*

Table 1.3—Suffixes: Surgical/Diagnostic Procedures

Suffix	Meaning	Example	Suffix	Meaning	Example
-centesis	puncture, aspiration	thora*centesis*	-ostomy	form an opening	col*ostomy*
-clasis	fracture	osteo*clasis*	-otomy	incision into	lapar*otomy*
-desis	fusion	arthro*desis*	-pexy	fixation, suspension	hystero*pexy*
-ectomy	excision	gastr*ectomy*			
-lysis	freeing	entero*lysis*	-plasty	repair	blepharo*plasty*
-ography	process	roentgen*ography*	-rrhaphy	suture	hernio*rrhaphy*
-oscopy	look within	cyst*oscopy*	-tripsy	crushing, friction	litho*tripsy*

Table 1.1 includes some commonly used word endings, along with their meanings and examples of their use in medical terms. Tables 1.2 and 1.3 list suffix endings denoting physiology, symptoms, and procedures. A study of true suffixes apart from their association with specific use—as, for example, those dealing with diagnostic terms (Chapter 3)—is difficult and necessitates repetition. For this reason, all of the true suffixes are introduced in this chapter and then presented again in specific areas to reinforce their common usage. Their sheer number makes learning these suffixes a daunting task, but careful review and repetition of these suffixes in a large number of terms simplifies the problem. In addition, the tables are useful for reference long after their original study.

Roots

The word *root* or *stem* is the fundamental or elementary part of the word that conveys its primary notion or significance. Modification of the basic meaning is then made by the addition of prefixes, suffixes, or other roots. The root should not be confused with a prefix or suffix, regardless of the position of the root within a word. Prefixes come at the beginning and suffixes at the end of a word, but a root can appear anywhere, including before or after another root. The roots (since there may be more than one) give the word its primary meaning; prefixes or suffixes, however, serve to modify that meaning. Those roots used in medical terminology generally indicate an organ or part of the body.

The term *combining forms* is often encountered in the study of medical terminology. A combining form of a root is created by the addition of a vowel, usually *o*, to the word root. This is done primarily for ease in pronunciation. These are, therefore, convenience forms and do not influence the meaning of a word root.

Example: (Combining Form)   *gastro-*
             (Root)   *gastr-*
             (Medical Terms)   *gastr(o)*dynia
                                  *gastr*algia
                                  *gastr*itis

Some roots end in vowels, so frequently there is no need to add a vowel to these roots to create a combining form. Further, the addition of a vowel would place two vowels in succession. Thus, a vowel is usually not added if the word root ends in a vowel and two vowels would be in sequence.

Example: *celio-*   (Root meaning abdomen)
             -oma   (Suffix meaning tumor)
             celioma   (tumor of the abdomen)

A medical dictionary should be consulted whenever correct spelling is in question.

Most of the medical terms in this text are categorized by body system or other therapeutic category in Part II. The list in Table 1.4, however, contains many commonly used roots or combining forms that do not readily fall into the body system classifications or that apply to more than one. Since the meaning of a word can be determined by

Table 1.4—Roots: Combining Forms, Miscellaneous

Root	Meaning	Example	Root	Meaning	Example
abdomin-	abdomen	*abdomin*al	clin-	bedside	*clin*ical
actino-	ray, radiated structure	*actino*genic	coleo-	sheath	*coleo*cele
adipo-	fat	*adipo*se	crymo- cryo-	cold	*crymo*philic *cryo*extraction
aer-	air, gas	*aer*ogram	crypt-	hidden	*crypt*ogenic
alge-	pain	*algo*spasm	cycl-	round, re-curring	*cycl*otropia
alveo-	hollow	*alveo*lus	cyt-	cell	*cyt*ology
ambulo-	walk about	*ambul*atory	desm-	fibrous con-nection	*desm*odynia
aneu-rysmo-	widening	*aneurysmo*rrha-phy	ergo-	work	*ergo*phobia
ankyl-	crooked, at-tached	*ankyl*osis	eury-	broad	*eury*cephalic
astro-	star	*astro*cyte	febri-	fever	*febri*le
auto-	self	*auto*clasis	gero-	aged	*gero*ntology
blast-	bud, germ	*blast*ocyte	glio-	glue	*glio*ma
blenno-	mucus	*blenno*rrhea	glyco-	sugar, sweet	*glyco*suria
bucc-	cheek	*bucc*inator	gony-	knee	*gony*ocele
calori-	heat	*calori*genic	gust-	taste	*gust*ation
celio- coeli-	abdomen	*celio*ma *coeli*oma	helio-	sun	*helio*therapy
cervico-	neck	*cervico*brachial	hidro-	sweat	*hidro*sis
chir-	hand	*chir*omegaly	histo-	tissue	*histo*logy
chron-	time	*chron*ograph	hydro-	water	*hydro*cele
clas-	smash, break	osteo*clas*is	hypno-	sleep	*hypno*tic

Root	Meaning	Example	Root	Meaning	Example
iatro-	medicine, physician	*iatro*genic	not-	the back	*not*algia
ictero-	jaundice	*ictero*genic	oligo-	few, little	*olig*uria
iso-	equal	*iso*tonic	omo-	shoulder	*omo*dynia
kinesio-	movement	*kinesio*logy	omphalo-	umbilicus	*omphalo*tomy
lapar-	loin, flank	*lapar*otomy	oneir-	dream	*oneir*ism
lepto-	slender, thin	*lepto*dermic	oxy-	sharp, keen	*oxy*cephalic
lip-	fat	*lip*oma	pachy-	thick	*pachy*onchia
litho-	stone	*litho*genesis	paleo-	old	*paleo*genetic
lyso-	dissolving	*lyso*genic	pan-	all	*pan*arthritis
macro-	large, long	*macro*nychia	papillo- papulo-	pustule	*papill*oma *papulo*squamous
mal-	ill, bad, poor	*mal*absorption	patho-	disease	*patho*logy
megalo-	large	*megalo*cyte	pedia-	child	*pedia*trics
mero-	part	*mero*tomy	pedo-	foot	*pedo*graph
micro-	small	*micro*gram	pero-	deformed	*pero*brachius
mio-	less, smaller	*mio*sis	phago-	devour, eat	*phago*cyte
morpho-	form	a*morpho*us	phanero-	appear, visible	*phaner*osis
muco-	mucus	*muco*purulent	photo-	light	*photo*phobia
myco-	fungi	*myco*logy	phren-	mind, diaphragm	*phren*ic
myx-	mucus	*myx*edema	phthisio-	wasting, atrophy	*phthisio*logy
necro-	death	*necro*sis	phyco-	seaweed	*phyco*bilins
nocto- nycto-	night	*nocto*uria *nycto*philia	physio-	nature	*physio*logy
noso-	disease	*noso*poietic	phyt-	plant	hemato*phyte*

Root	Meaning	Example	Root	Meaning	Example
platy-	flat, broad	*platy*podia	stereo-	solid, three dimensional	*stereo*scope
pod-	foot	*pod*iatrist			
			stetho-	chest	*stetho*scope
pros-	forward, anterior	*pros*ademic	sthen-	strength	myas*then*ia
prosop-	face	*prosop*oneuralgia	strepto-	twisted, curved	*strepto*bacillus
psychr-	cold	*psychr*algia			
			thanat-	death	*thanat*ology
puri-	pus	*puri*lent	theco-	sheath	*theco*dont
pyo-		*pyo*genic			
pyro-	fever, heat	*pyro*genic	thermo-	heat	*thermo*meter
radio-	ray	*radio*therapy	thrombo-	clot	*thrombo*cyte
schisto-	split, divide	*schisto*celia	tome-	cutting instrument	micro*tome*
scirrh-	hard	*scirrh*osity			
scler-		*scler*oderma	top-	place, topical	*top*ectomy
sit-	food	*sit*ophobia	topo-		*topo*graphy
somni-	sleep	in*somni*a	trachelo-	neck	*trachelo*dynia
sphygmo-	pulse	*sphygmo*manometer	ul-	scar, gingiva	*ul*orrhagia
splanchn-	viscera	*splanchn*ic	vermi-	worm	*vermi*fuge
staphylo-	grapelike cluster	*staphylo*toxin	viscer-	organ	*viscer*a
			vita-	life	*vita*min
stear-	fat	*stear*rhea	xeno-	strange, foreign	*xeno*phthalmia
steat-		*steat*olysis			
steno-	narrow, contracted	*steno*sis	zoo-	animal	*zoo*logy

knowledge of its basic parts, these examples should illustrate the value of learning root words as a basis for understanding medical terminology.

Prefixes

Prefixes are the most frequently used elements in the formation of medical terms. Most prefixes are commonly used in everyday language and are not unique to medical terminology, so those wanting to learn or improve their mastery of medical terminology have a sound basis on which to build.

Prefixes may be adjectives, adverbs, or prepositions that are used to indicate various relationships or conditions of the root word. Most prefixes have a final vowel that is deleted if the following root or stem begins with a vowel.

Since prefixes originate from both Latin and Greek, two different prefixes may have the same meaning. For example, the prefixes *poster-* and *retro-* both indicate "behind," as in the terms *posterior* and *retrograde*. Conversely, multiple meanings may be associated with a single prefix because of multiple sources for the prefix; *meta-*, for example, can mean both "over" and "after change."

True prefixes are distinguished from roots in that they serve only to modify the meaning of the root and have no significance alone. Roots that are used at the beginning of words are not considered to be true prefixes.

Example:	Prefixes	Roots
	*hyper*trophy	*hepato*megaly
	*brady*cardia	*osteo*myelitis

The prefixes listed in Tables 1.5 through 1.8 have been grouped according to the type of relationship or conditions that they identify. The examples serve to illustrate how prefixes are joined to root words.

Body as a Whole

Medical terms describing position or direction relative to the body are expressed in terms of the "anatomical position": the human body standing erect, arms at the sides and the palms of the hands turned forward. This reflects the **anterior** (*anter/o*) or front side, also called the ventral or belly side. The combining form for **posterior** is *poster/ o,* meaning "back"; **dorsal** (*dors/o*) also refers to the back side of an organism. The combining form for the side is *later/o.* **Unilateral** (*uni* = one) would denote one side, while **bilateral** (*bi* = two) means two or both sides. **Medial** pertains to the middle. Other combining forms referring to locations on the body include *super-*, meaning superior (e.g., superficial); *dist-*, meaning far or distant (e.g., distal); *proxim-*, meaning near (e.g., proximal); *caudo-*, meaning tail or lower part (e.g., caudal); and *cephal-*, meaning head (e.g., cephalad).

The abdomen is divided into nine anatomic regions. The right and left **hypochondriac** regions are those lying beneath (hypo-) the ribs, although the term also describes a person who is overly concerned with health and may imagine illness (named for the region of the body that was thought to be the seat of the disease). Between the hypochondria is

Table 1.5—Prefixes: Location, Direction, Tendency

Prefix	Meaning	Example	Prefix	Meaning	Example
a- an-	without, not	*aphasia* *anemia*	sym- syn-	together, with	*symphysis* *synarthrosis*
ab- apo- de-	away from	*abductor* *apophysis* *decapitate*	dextro-	to the right	*dextroversion*
			di- dis-	apart from	*diastemia* *dissect*
ad-	to, toward, near	*adnexia*	dia- per- trans-	through, across	*diaphragm* *perforate* *transection*
ambi-	both	*ambidextrous*			
amphi- ampho-		*amphibious* *amphoterism*	dorsi- dorso-	back	*dorsiflexion* *dorsolateral*
ana-	up, apart, across, back, again, ex- cessive	*anacatharsis* *anastasis*	e- ec- ex-	out from	*enucleate* *ectoblast* *exacerbation*
			ecto- exo- extra- extro-	outside	*ectoderm* *exogenous* *extracellular* *extrovert*
ante- fore- pre- pro-	before, forward	*antepartum* *forehead* *prenatal* *procidentia*			
			em- en- im- in-	in	*empyema* *enarthrosis* *impaction* *inflammation*
anter-	in front of	*anterograde*			
anti-	against, op- posite	*antitoxin*	endo- ento- intra-	within	*endocardium* *entocele* *intraocular*
contra- counter- ob-		*contraceptive* *counterirritant* *obdormition*			
			epi-	upon, over	*epigastric*
cata- kata-	down, according to	*catatonic* *katathermometer*	eso-	inward	*esotropia*
circum- peri-	around, about	*circumflex* *pericarditis*	extra- hyper- per-	more, excessive	*extraocular* *hypertrophy* *pertussis*
co-	together, with	*coarctation*			
com- con-		*commissure* *conductor*	pleo- super-	more, excessive	*pleomorphic* *supernumerary*

Prefix	Meaning	Example	Prefix	Meaning	Example
gen-	producing, coming to be	*gen*etics	medi- mes- mid-	in the middle	*medi*al *mes*ocephalic *mid*brain
homo-	same	*homo*geneous	meta-	over, after, change	*meta*stasis
hyper-	above, over	*hyper*trophy			
hypo- infra- sub-	below, under, beneath, less, deficient	*hypo*tension *infra*orbital *sub*cutaneous	opistho- poster-	behind, backward	*opistho*tic *poster*omedian
			para-	beside, near	*para*centesis
			post-	after, behind	*post*partum
im- in- ir- non- un-	not	*im*miscible *in*articulate *ir*reducible *non*toxic *un*conscious	primi- prot-	first	*primi*para *prot*oderm
			re-	again	*re*habilitation
inter-	between	*inter*costal	retro-	backward, behind	*retro*grade
intro-	into	*intro*version	super- supra- ultra-	above, excessive	*super*natant *supra*renal *ultra*sonic
ipsi- iso-	same, equal	*ipsi*lateral *iso*metric			
			tel- tele- telo-	end, distance	*tele*diastolic *tele*opsia *telo*phase
juxta-	near	*juxta*position			
latero-	to the side	*latero*flexion	trans-	across, through	*trans*plant
levo-	to the left	*levo*version			
sinistro-	to the left	*sinistro*cardia	ventro-	anterior	*ventro*fixation

the **epigastric** (*epi* = upon, *gastr* = stomach) region. The right and left **lumbar** regions are separated by the **umbilical** (naval) region. Below are the **hypogastric** and left and right **inguinal** or iliac regions. Areas in the abdominal cavity are also divided by quadrants, designated as right upper quadrant (**RUQ**), left upper quadrant (**LUQ**), right lower quadrant (**RLQ**), and left lower quadrant (**LLQ**).

The body has two principal body cavities designated as the **ventral** (front) and **dorsal** (back). The smaller dorsal cavity contains the cranial and spinal cavities. The ventral cavity contains the thoracic (chest) cavity, separated from the abdominal cavity by the **diaphragm.** Lowest is the pelvic cavity. The serous membrane lining these two (abdominopelvic) cavities is called the **peritoneum.** Organs within the cavities are sometimes referred to as **viscera.**

Table 1.6—Prefixes: Size, Condition, State

Prefix	Meaning	Example	Prefix	Meaning	Example
allo-	not normal	*allo*tropic	ischio-	suppress, restrain	*isch*uria
ambly-	dim, dull	*ambly*opia	leio-	smooth	*leio*myoma
			malaco-	soft	*malac*ia
aniso-	unequal, dissimilar	*aniso*cyosis	medulo-	marrow	*medullo*blastoma
atel-	imperfect	*atel*ectasis	mis-	bad, wrong, improper	*mis*carriage
atreto-	lack of opening	*atreto*cystia	mogi-	painful, difficult	*mogi*phonia
bio-	relation to, life	*bio*logy	myel-	marrow	*myel*oma
brachy- brevi-	short	*brachy*cephalic *brevi*collis	neutro-	neither	*neutro*phil
			poikilo-	varied	*poikilo*derma
brady-	slow	*brady*cardia	poly-	many, much	*poly*uria
caco-	bad, ill	*caco*genic	presby-	old	*presby*opia
cry-	cold	*cryo*surgery	proto-	first, original	*proto*vertebra
dolicho-	long	*dolicho*sigmoid	pseudo-	false	*pseudo*pregnancy
dys-	difficult, painful	*dys*pnea	sclero-	hard	*sclero*sis
eu-	well, easily, good	*eu*phoria	scoli-	curved, crooked	*scoli*osis
haplo-	single, simple	*haplo*id	tachy-	fast	*tachy*cardia
heter-	different, other	*heter*ochylia	torsi-	twist	*torsi*on
			trachy-	rough	*trachy*phonia
holo-	entire	*holo*graphy	varico-	twisted, swollen	*varico*se
homeo- homo-	like, similar	*homeo*stasis *homo*geneous	xero-	dry	*xero*cheilia

Table 1.7—Prefixes: Number, Measurement

Prefix	Meaning	Example	Prefix	Meaning	Example
mono- uni-	one	*mono*cyte *uni*lateral	deca-	ten	*deca*meter
			micro-	one one- millionth	*micro*gram
bi- bin- di- diplo- dis-	two, twice	*bi*furcation *bin*aural *di*cephalus *diplo*coccus *dis*mutase	milli-	one one- thousandth	*milli*liter
			centi-	one one- hundredth	*centi*meter
ter- tri-	three, third	*ter*tiary *tri*ceps	deci-	one tenth	*deci*gram
quad- tetra-	four	*quad*ruplet *tetra*plegia	hecto-	hundred	*hecto*liter
penta- quinqu- quinti-	five	*penta*valent *quinqu*evalent *quinti*para	kilo-	thousand	*kilo*gram
hex- sex-	six	*hex*asaccharide *sex*tuplet	demi- hemi- semi-	half	*demi*lune *hemi*cardia *semi*conscious
hept- sept-	seven	*hept*achromic *septi*para	ambi- amphi- ampho-	both	*ambi*dextrous *amphi*bious *ampho*teric
octa-	eight	*octa*gonal	multi- poly-	many	*multi*para *poly*chromatic
nona-	nine	*nona*n			

Table 1.8—Prefixes: Color

Prefix	Meaning	Example	Prefix	Meaning	Example
chroma-	color	*chroma*tography	ciner- glauc- polio-	gray	*ciner*itious *glauc*oma *polio*myelitis
alb- albumin- leuk-	white	*alb*inuria *albumin*uretic *leuk*emia	cirrh- flav- lute- xanth-	yellow	*cirrh*osis *flavo*protein *lute*in *xanth*oma
amaur-	dark	*amaur*osis			
chlor- verdin-	green	*chlor*anemia *verdo*hemoglobin			

Prefix	Meaning	Example	Prefix	Meaning	Example
cyano-	blue	*cyano*mycosis	melan- nigro-	black	*melan*oma *nigro*sine
erythr- rube-	red	*erythr*ocyte *rube*lla	purpur-	purple	*purpur*a

Glossary

anterior—front; ventral

caudal—pertaining to the tail

cephalic—cranial; referring to the region of the head

diaphragm—muscle separating the thoracic and abdominal cavities

distal—far from the beginning or attachment of a structure

dorsal—posterior; back

epigastric—region above the stomach

hypochondriac—two upper regions of the body, located below the cartilage of the ribs

hypogastric—referring to the lower middle region of the body

inguinal—regions near the groin, also known as the iliac regions located near the upper hip bone

lateral—pertaining to the side

LLQ—region of the body containing the left ovary, fallopian tube, and ureter and part of the intestines

lumbar—regions of the body near the waist

LUQ—region of the body containing the stomach, spleen, and parts of the liver, pancreas, and intestines

medial—pertaining to the middle plane of the body

peritoneum—membrane that surrounds the organs in the abdominopelvic region of the body

posterior—back; dorsal

proximal—near the beginning or attachment of a structure

RLQ—region of the body containing the appendix, right ovary, fallopian tube, ureter, and part of the intestines

RUQ—region of the body containing the gallbladder and parts of the liver, pancreas, and intestines

superficial—on or near the surface

umbilical—region of the navel or umbilicus

ventral—anterior; front

CHAPTER 2

The Health Care System Structure

Medical Specialties

The study and practice of medicine is generally structured on the basis of the various specialties designated within the health care field. As will be noted from the listing of medical specialties in Table 2.1, most end with the suffix-*logy,* meaning "the study or science of" the specialty. Likewise, the individuals who practice in these fields are denoted by the suffix-*ist* or-*logist* meaning "one who" and "one who studies." For example, given that the root word for heart is *cardio,* a cardiologist is one who practices (studies) in the field on cardiology, treatment of heart disease.

Historically, these specialties and subspecialties developed from general practice. As diagnosis and treatment became more complicated and the knowledge base related to each area grew, some practitioners progressively limited their practices to specific areas. Each specialty began regulating itself through "specialty board certification," and eventually many came under the general jurisdiction of the American Medical Association **(AMA),** which still endorses these certifying boards, although each is self-governing. More than fifty specialties and subspecialties now require specified postgraduate training and examination. Although privately governed, specialty certification is recognized by the federal government as a criterion for reimbursement and participation in various public programs.

Health Care Organizations

Health care delivery systems encompass a number of terms that should be familiar to the pharmacist. The entire system has undergone numerous changes in the last two decades and is still in a continuing state of flux. Those terms that applied earlier are being replaced or expanded at an astonishing rate, and pharmacists who work within the system can easily become confused by the plethora of terms for health care delivery systems, financial arrangements, or care providers.

The most noticeable changes have been in the financial arrangements of health care providers. Prospective reimbursement of medical services based on projected cost for a patient category replaced the traditional Medicare retrospective reimbursement system that had paid providers on the basis of the services rendered. Diagnosis-related groups (DRGs) of disorders in major diagnostic categories (MDCs) determine the reimbursement a hospital receives for treating an individual patient. Determinations are made by the Health Care Financing Administration (HCFA), rather than the provider, theoretically leading to increased efficiency in the provision of health care.

Table 2.1—Medical/Dental Specialties

Abdominal Surgery	Hematology	Pain Medicine
Addiction Medicine	Infectious Disease	Pathology
Allergy and Immunology	Internal Medicine	Pediatrics
Anesthesiology	Nephrology	Pedodontics
Cardiology	Neurology	Periodontics
Chiropody	Neurosurgery	Physical Medicine and
Chiropractic	Obstetrics and	Rehabilitation
Colon and Rectal Surgery	Gynecology	Plastic Surgery
Dermatology	Oncology	Prosthodontics
Emergency Medicine	Ophthalmology	Psychiatry
Endocrinology	Oral and Maxillofacial	Pulmonary Medicine
Endodontics	Surgery	Radiation Oncology
Epidemiology	Oral Pathology	Radiology
Family Medicine	Orthodontics	Rheumatology
Gastroenterology	Orthopedic Surgery	Surgery
General Surgery	Orthopedics	Thoracic Surgery
Genetics	Osteopathy	Urology
Geriatrics	Otolaryngology	

A variety of prospective payment systems were subsequently developed to increase financial efficiency and provide more effective managed care. Health maintenance organizations (HMOs) have become the standard form of reimbursement in many parts of the country. HMOs manage cost and care by controlling the entire health care delivery process. Preferred provider organizations (PPOs) furnish a viable alternative in other areas by offering different levels of reimbursement or coverage for providers who contract with the group. Primary care physicians (PPPs) coordinate basic services and referrals within the organizations. A health systems agency (HSA) is a nonprofit organization mandated by the federal government to regulate development of health services and facilities within a particular location. Independent practice arrangements (IPAs) formed an alternative for those health care providers who wished to remain independent and self-employed.

Another major influence in health care financing is Medicaid, the major welfare program for health care in most states. As the largest payer of long-term care claims, Medicaid, along with Medicare, sets many of the regulations covering extended care facilities (ECFs) such as quality assurance (QA) programs.

Other agencies also enforce quality measures. In addition to Medicare regulations, most hospitals are accredited by the Joint Commission on Accreditation of Healthcare Organizations (JCAHO), which issues extensive standards and interpretive guidelines affecting quality of services. In hospitals, pharmacists have long performed drug utilization review (DUR) or drug regimen review (DRR) functions, partly in response to JCAHO initiatives. DUR encompasses a retrospective evaluation of prescribing and drug administration practices in the institution. Drug use evaluation (DUE) is becoming more valuable, which is often either concurrent or prospective. Both DUR and DUE are also playing a role in the ambulatory setting, especially in managed care programs.

A host of federal government agencies is involved in the delivery or regulation of health care. The central authority on the national level is vested in the Department of

Table 2.2—Abbreviations Associated with Health Care Professions

CMA	certified medical assistant	NNP	neonatal nurse practitioner
CMHN	community mental health nurse	NP	nurse practitioner
		OB	obstetrician
CNS	clinical nurse specialist	OT	occupational therapist
CST	certified surgical technologist	PA	physician assistant
DC	doctor of chiropractic	PCA	patient care assistant/aide
DDS	doctor of dental surgery	PDN	private duty nurse
DO	doctor of osteopathy	PHN	public health nurse
DPM	doctor of podiatric medicine	PNP	pediatric nurse practitioner
EENT	eye, ear, nose and throat specialist	PNS	practical nursing student
		PSW	psychiatric social worker
EMT	emergency medical technician	PT	physical therapist
		PTA	physical therapy assistant
ENT	ear, nose and throat specialist	RD	registered dietitian
		RDH	registered dental hygienist
FACP	Fellow of the American College of Physicians	RDMS	registered diagnostic medical sonographer
FACS	Fellow of the American College of Surgeons	RN	registered nurse
		RPA	registered dental hygienist
HCA	health care aide	RPh	registered pharmacist
IMG	internal medicine group (practice)	RPT	registered physical therapist
		RRA	registered record administrator
JMS	junior medical student		
LPN	licensed practical nurse	RSO	radiation safety officer
LVN	licensed vocational nurse	RT	radiologic technologist; respiratory therapist
MD	medical doctor		
ME	medical examiner	SMR	senior medical resident
MICN	mobile intensive care nurse	SMS	senior medical student
MRA	medical record administrator	SN	student nurse
MS	medical student	SP	speech pathologist
MSC	medical social consultant	SW	social worker
MT	medical technologist		
NA	nurse assistant; nurse anesthetist		

Health and Human Services (DHHS), which is responsible for the nation's massive programs of social security and public assistance. Administration and financing of health programs within the DHHS are primarily under the jurisdiction of the Social Security Administration (for Medicare) and the Health Care Financing Administration (HCFA). Direct provision of health care, however, generally falls to the U.S. Public Health Service and its subdivisions such as the Indian Health Service. Also within the DHHS is included the National Institutes of Health (NIH) that funds and conducts much of the health-related research in the United States.

Several specific health programs are administered by other federal agencies. The main responsibility for protecting the health of workers at their place of employment rests with the Occupational Safety and Health Administration (OSHA) within the Department of Labor. As all pharmacists are aware, regulation of controlled substances rests with the Drug Enforcement Administration (DEA) within the Department of Justice, which also provides health facilities in federal prisons. These facilities are staffed by personnel from the Public Health Service (PHS). Health care for military personnel is provided and

Table 2.3—Abbreviations Associated with Health Care Systems

AACP	American Association of Colleges of Pharmacy	**CDC**	Centers for Disease Control
AAFP	American Academy of Family Physicians	**CHAMPUS**	Civilian Health and Medical Program of the Uniformed Services
AAMA	American Association of Medical Assistants	**DEA**	Drug Enforcement Administration
AAP	American Academy of Pediatrics	**DHHS**	Department of Health and Human Services
AAPA	American Academy of Physician Assistants	**DRG**	diagnosis-related group
ACA	American College of Apothecaries	**DRR**	drug regimen review
		DUE	drug use evaluation
ACS	American Cancer Society; American College of Surgeons	**DUR**	drug utilization review
		ECF	extended care facility
		HAS	health systems agency
ADA	American Dental Association; American Diabetes Association	**HCFA**	Health Care Financing Administration
		HMO	health maintenance organization
AHA	American Heart Association; American Hospital Association	**IPA**	independent practice arrangement
AMA	American Medical Association	**JCAHO**	Joint Commission on Accreditation of Healthcare Organizations
ANA	American Nurses Association; American Neurologic Association	**MDC**	major diagnostic category
		NIH	National Institutes of Health
AOA	American Optometric Association	**OSHA**	Occupational Safety and Health Administration
APhA	American Pharmaceutical Association	**PHS**	Public Health Service
APHA	American Public Health Association	**PPO**	preferred provider organization
		PPP	primary care physician
ASCP	American Society of Clinical Pathologists; American Society of Clinical Pharmacists	**QA**	quality assurance
		VNA	Visiting Nurses Association

administered by the Department of Defense and for dependents by CHAMPUS (Civilian Health and Medical Program of the Uniformed Services). The same role for military veterans is performed by the Department of Veterans Affairs, formerly known as the Veterans Administration (VA).

Tables 2.2 and 2.3 list abbreviations associated with health care professions and health care systems, respectively.

Glossary

abdominal surgery—medical specialty dealing with procedures involving the abdominal cavity

addiction medicine—medical specialty dealing with diagnosis and treatment of habitual psychological and physiological dependence on a substance or practice

allergy and immunology—medical specialty concerned with diagnosis and treatment of disorders involving immunity, sensitivity, and allergies

anesthesiology—study of anesthesia and anesthetics

cardiology—medical specialty dealing with diagnosis and treatment of heart disease

chiropody—podiatry; medical specialty concerned with the diagnosis and treatment of diseases, injuries, and defects of the foot

chiropractic—science that utilizes the recuperative powers of the body and the relationship between its functions and the musculoskeletal system in restoration and maintenance of health

colon and rectal surgery—medical specialty dealing with procedures involving the lower intestinal tract

dermatology—medical specialty dealing with diagnosis and treatment of disorders of the skin

emergency medicine—medical specialty dealing with provision of critical immediate care

endocrinology—medical specialty dealing with diagnosis and treatment of disorders of the endocrine glands

endodontics—dental specialty dealing with treatment of diseased tooth pulp

epidemiology—study of the prevalence and spread of disease within a community

family medicine—medical specialty concerned with providing continuous, comprehensive care to all age groups

gastroenterology—medical specialty concerned with diagnosis and treatment of disorders of the stomach and intestines

general surgery—medical specialty dealing with treatment of disease, injury, or deformity by operation or manipulation

genetics—branch of science that deals with heredity

geriatrics—medical specialty dealing with diagnosis and treatment of diseases associated with aging

gynecology—medical specialty dealing with diagnosis and treatment of the genital tract in females

hematology—medical specialty concerned with diagnosis and treatment of disorders of the blood and blood-forming tissues

infectious disease—medical specialty concerned with diagnosis and treatment of diseases caused by microorganisms

internal medicine—medical specialty dealing with diagnosis and nonsurgical treatment of diseases

nephrology—medical specialty concerned with diagnosis and treatment of disorders of the kidney

neurology—medical specialty dealing with diagnosis and treatment of disorders of the nervous system

neurosurgery—surgical specialty dealing with surgical procedures of the nervous system

obstetrics—medical specialty dealing with management of pregnancy, labor, and the puerperium

oncology—medical specialty dealing with the properties and features of neoplasms and their treatment

ophthalmology—medical specialty dealing with diagnosis and treatment of disorders of the eye

oral pathology—dental specialty involved in the study and identification of oral diseases

oral surgery—branch of dentistry concerned with diagnosis and treatment of diseases, injuries, and deformities of the oral and maxillofacial region

orthodontics—dental specialty dealing with correction of malformations of growth as they affect the oral structures

orthopedic surgery—surgical specialty dealing with operative procedures involving the musculoskeletal system

orthopedics—medical specialty dealing with diagnosis and treatment of disorders of the bones, muscles, and joints

osteopathy—use of diagnostic and therapeutic measures of ordinary medicine in addition to manipulative measures

otolaryngology—medical specialty dealing with diagnosis and treatment of disorders of the ears and throat

pain medicine—medical specialty dealing with the management of pain

pathology—medical specialty dealing with diagnosis by study of nature, causes, and effects of disease

pediatrics—medical specialty concerned with the diseases of children

pedodontics—dental specialty treating children

periodontics—dental specialty dealing with treatment of diseases of the gums and supporting structures

physical medicine and rehabilitation—study and treatment of disease primarily by mechanical and other physical methods

plastic and reconstructive surgery—surgical specialty concerned with restoration, construction, reconstruction, or improvement in the shape and appearance of body structures

prosthodontics—dental specialty involved in care of patients needing dentures

psychiatry—medical specialty dealing with diagnosis and treatment of mental disorders

pulmonary medicine—medical specialty dealing with diagnosis and treatment of disorders of the respiratory system

radiation oncology—medical specialty dealing with treatment of neoplasms by radiant energy

radiology—science concerned with radiant energy and actions of rays proceeding from X rays, radium, and other radioactive substances

rheumatology—medical specialty dealing with diagnosis and treatment of arthritis and rheumatic diseases

surgery—specialty dealing with treatment by manual and operative procedures

thoracic surgery—surgical specialty involving procedures of the chest cavity

urology—medical specialty dealing with diagnosis and treatment of the urinary tract in both males and females and the genital organs in the male

CHAPTER 3

Translating the Medical Record

Medical terminology is sometimes viewed as those words encountered in an anatomy and physiology class, plus the terms describing the components of the health system. If that were the case, most of the terminology a health care provider would need could be developed from the roots, prefixes, and suffixes found in Chapter 1 along with a smattering of the therapeutic terminology found in Part II. Such a view is based on the faulty assumption that terminology is equivalent to "the naming of parts." In reality, medical terminology is the entire language through which members of the health care system communicate about their activities, patients, procedures, diagnoses, and myriad other concerns.

That communication is carried out among providers, between providers and patients, and between providers and society as a whole. As a result, pharmacists must understand medical terminology on many different levels. One area that cannot be ignored is the medical record, a document found in one form or another in essentially every hospital, physician's office, long-term care facility, and pharmacy. The medical record is an important focus of terminology because (1) medical terminology is highly concentrated in its pages to efficiently use the document to record as much medical information as possible in a limited space, and (2) the record relies heavily on uniform organization and content to decrease misinterpretation.

The information contained in the pages of the medical record covers all aspects of patient care and the patient's interaction with the health system, so it is quite extensive. Further, the information appears in the same order and the same format in the records of all patients of a given institution; therefore, part of learning terminology is learning how things are organized in the record. Billing from all institutions must be handled similarly by different payers, various providers all refer to the same record, and a single record may be used in many contexts; providers must learn to record their findings and conclusions in a uniform manner so others can decipher them with minimal confusion. Thus, medical terminology is as much a form of coding and cataloging as it is a form of naming.

Provision of Patient Services

The American Medical Association (**AMA**) categorizes services provided by physicians according to Evaluation and Management (**E/M**) coding. These are divided into broad categories such as office visits, hospital visits, and consultations. Standardized definitions are used to minimize potential for different interpretations and to maximize consistency of reporting by physicians in various specialties. The terms discussed below are encountered in all medical records; therefore, they should be familiar to the pharmacist.

A **new patient** is one who has not received professional services from the physician or specialty group within the past three years. An **established patient** is one who has received services within that length of time. **Chief complaint (CC)** is a brief statement of symptoms, problems, diagnosis, or factors that have precipitated the encounter. **Concurrent care** refers to provision of similar services to the same patient by more than one physician on the same day. **Counseling** indicates discussion with the patient and/or family member regarding diagnostic results, impressions, recommendations, prognosis, risks and benefits of treatment options, instructions for treatment and/or follow-up, and/or education.

When a health care provider first encounters a patient, a basic activity is often taking the patient's history. **Family History (FH)** is a review of health status or cause of death of parents, siblings, and children; specific diseases related to problems identified; and hereditary diseases or risk factors of family members. **History of present illness (HPI)** is a chronological description of the present illness, including descriptors of location, severity, context, and associated signs and symptoms specifically related to the presenting problem. **Past history** includes significant information regarding prior illnesses and injuries, surgery, and hospitalizations; current medication regimen; allergies; and immunization and dietary status. **Social history** is an age-appropriate review of marital status and/or living arrangements; current employment and occupational history; level of education; use of drugs, alcohol, and tobacco; sexual history; and other relevant social factors.

Review of Symptoms (ROS) refers to an inventory of body systems obtained through questioning directed toward identifying signs and symptoms that the patient has experienced. For coding and classification purposes, the body areas recognized are head, neck, chest, abdomen, genitalia, groin, buttocks, back, and extremities. The organ systems denoted are eyes, ears, nose, mouth, and throat; cardiovascular; respiratory; gastrointestinal; genitourinary; musculoskeletal; skin; neurologic; psychiatric; and hematologic/lymphatic/immunologic.

Physical Assessment

Initial physical assessment of a patient generally follows the format outlined above. Medical terms encountered within each of these areas are numerous and varied and are generally presented in the relevant chapter in Part II pertaining to the specific body system being addressed. Perhaps one of the most useful tools in approaching the medical record is to become familiar with the various abbreviations commonly utilized in reference to patient evaluation and monitoring. Many of these are presented in Table 3.1. A sample of root words pertaining to symptoms or disorders is given in the Pronouncing Glossary. Also helpful is a review of the various suffix endings that refer to various conditions or general context.

Diagnostic Testing

Laboratory tests include evaluation of parameters such as blood, urine, stool, cerebrospinal fluid, tissues, and organisms found in the body. Eponyms associated with diagnostic testing are listed in Table 3.2; abbreviations commonly encountered are included in Table 3.3.

Table 3.1—Abbreviations Associated with Patient Assessment

A	alive; ambulatory; assessment	BRP	bathroom privileges
A & P	auscultation and percussion; anterior and posterior; assessment and plans	BS	blood sugar; bowel/breath sounds; bedside; before sleep
AAN	attending's admission notes	BSA	body surface area
AAOx3	awake and oriented to time, place, and person	BSC	bedside commode
		BUE	both upper extremities
AAOx4	awake and oriented to person, place, time, and date	CB	code blue; chair and bed
		CBR	complete bed rest
		CC	chief complaint; critical condition
ABR	auditory brain stem response; absolute bed rest	CCE	clubbing, cyanosis, and edema
ABS	at bedside	CCMSU	clean catch midstream urine
ACI	aftercare instructions	CDB	cough, deep breathe
ADT	anticipate discharge tomorrow	CF	Caucasian female
AFVSS	afebrile, vital signs stable	CH	child; chronic; chest
ALS	advanced life support	CHD	childhood diseases
AMA	against medical advice	CL	critical list
Amb	ambulate, ambulatory	CM	Caucasian male
A & O	alert and oriented	CMSUA	clean midstream urinalysis
AOB	alcohol on breath	C/O	complains of
AOC	area of concern	COD	cause of death
AP	anterior-posterior; abdominal-peritoneal; apical pulse	CPM	continue present management
A & R	advised and released	CPR	cardiopulmonary resuscitation
ASA I	healthy patient with localized pathological process	CR	complete remission
		CRT	cathode ray tube
ASA II	patient with mild to moderate systemic disease	CSM	circulation, sensation, movement
ASA III	patient with severe systemic disease limiting activity but not incapacitating	CTB	ceased to breathe
		CT & DB	cough, turn, and deep breathe
ASA IV	patient with incapacitating systemic disease	CTD	chest tube drainage
		CTP	comprehensive treatment plan
ASA V	moribund patient not expected to live	CU	cause unknown
ASC	altered state of consciousness	CUD	cause undetermined
		CV	cardiovascular
ATC	around the clock	CVS	clean voided specimen
ATLS	advanced trauma life support	CWMS	color, warmth, movement, sensation
AVSS	afebrile, vital signs stable	CXR	chest X ray
A & W	alive and well	DA	direct admission
BB	bed bath	DAT	diet as tolerated
BF	black female	DB & C	deep breathing and coughing
BFP	biologic false positive	DC	discontinue; discharge
BLE	both lower extremities	DD	differential diagnosis; dry dressing
BLESS	bath, laxative, enema, shampoo, and shower	D & D	diarrhea and dehydration
BLS	basic life support	DH	developmental history
BM	black male; bowel movement	DHS	duration of hospital stay
BMI	body mass index	DNI	do not intubate
BO	body odor	DNKA	did not keep appointment
BP	blood pressure; bed pan	DNR	do not resuscitate
BR	bathroom; bedrest		

DOA	dead on arrival; date of admission
DOB	date of birth
DS	discharge summary
DT	discharge tomorrow
DTV	due to void
DU	diagnosis undetermined
Dx	diagnosis
E	Eedema
EBL	estimated blood loss
ECR	emergency chemical restraint
EENT	eyes, ears, nose, throat
EHB	elevate head of bed
EMR	emergency mechanical restraint; empty, measure, and record
ENT	ear, nose, and throat
EOA	examine, opinion, and advice
FB	finger breadth
FBW	fasting blood work
FC	fever, chills; Foley catheter
FCSNVD	fever, chills, sweating, nausea, vomiting, diarrhea
FF	force fluids
FH	family history
FMH	family medical history
FOB	foot of bed; father of baby
FOC	father of child
FOD	free of disease
FOOB	fell out of bed
FP	family planning; family practice; flat plate; false positive
FTP	failure to progress
FTT	failure to thrive
F/U	follow-up
FUN	follow-up note
FUO	fever of undetermined/ unknown origin
GA	general appearance; gestational age
GHQ	general health questionnaire
GI	gastrointestinal
GSE	grip strong and equal
GU	genitourinary
HAT	head, arms, and trunk
HB	hold breakfast
HBBW	hold breakfast blood work
HC	home care; house call
HCM	health care maintenance
HEENT	head, eyes, ears, nose, throat
HHC	home health care
H & N	head and neck
HNV	has not voided
H/O	history of
HOB	head of bed
HOB UPSOB	head of bed up for shortness of breath

H & P	history and physical
HPI	history of present illness
HV	has voided
Hx	history
IAN	intern admission note
I & O	intake and output
IOC	intern on call
IOV	initial office visit
IPPA	inspection, palpation, percussion, auscultation
ITP	interim treatment plan
KJ	knee jerk
KVO	keep vein open
L	lumbar; lingual
LA	left arm
LB	low back; left buttock; large bowel; left breast
LE	lower extremities; left eye
LF	left foot
LKKS	liver, kidneys, spleen
LKS	liver, kidneys, spleen
LL	left leg, lower lip
LLE	left lower extremity
LLQ	left lower quadrant
LLT	left lateral thigh
LOC	loss/level of consciousness; level of care
LUE	left upper extremity
LUQ	left upper quadrant
L & W	living and well
MAE	moves all extremities
MAEEW	moves all extremities equally well
MCC	midstream clean-catch
MCCU	midstream clean-catch urine
MDS	minimum data set
MDTP	multidisciplinary treatment plan
MH	marital/menstrual history; mental health
M & M	morbidity and mortality
MOD	medical officer of the day
MOF	multiple organ failure
MS	musculoskeletal
MSU	midstream urine
NAD	no acute/apparent distress; nothing abnormal detected; no appreciable disease
NBM	no/normal bowel movement; nothing by mouth
NBS	normal bowel sound; no bacteria seen
NCD	normal childhood diseases; not considered disabling
NCPR	no cardiopulmonary resuscitation
ND	normal development; not done/diagnosed
NED	no evidence of disease

NKA	no known allergies	REMS	rapid eye movement sleep
NKDA	no known drug allergies	RHB	raise head of bed
NKMA	no known medication allergies	RL	right leg, right lung
NOOB	not out of bed	RLE	right lower extremity
NPO	nothing by mouth	RLQ	right lower quadrant
NREM	non-rapid eye movement	RO	rule out; routine order
NREMS	non-rapid eye movement sleep	RRE	round, regular, and equal
NSA	no significant abnormality	RRRN	round, regular, react normally
NSC	no significant change	RUE	right upper extremity
NTP	normal temperature and pressure	RUQ	right upper quadrant
N & V	nausea and vomiting	ROS	review of symptoms
NVD	nausea, vomiting, and diarrhea	S	subjective findings
NYD	not yet diagnosed	SBR	strict bedrest
O & A	observation and assessment	SCB	strictly confined to bed
OH	occupational history	SER	somatosensory-evoked response
OOB	out of bed	SH	social history
OOBBRP	out of bed with bathroom privileges	SOAP	subjective, objective, assessment, and plan
OP	outpatient; operation	SOB	shortness of breath
P & A	percussion and auscultation	SR	system review
PERL	pupils equal, reactive to light	S & S	signs and symptoms
PERRLA	pupils equal, round, regular, accommodate to light	Sx	symptoms
PH	past history; public health	TBA	to be admitted; to be absorbed
PI	present illness	TBR	total bed rest
PMH	past medical history	TCDB	turn, cough, and deep breathe
PO	postoperative; phone order	TPR	temperature, pulse, respirations
POC	postoperative care	UCD	usual childhood diseases
POD 1	postoperative day one	UE	upper extremity
POMR	problem-oriented medical record	ULN	upper limits of normal
PRRE	pupils round, regular, equal	ULQ	upper left quadrant
PS I	healthy patient with localized pathological process	V	vomiting
		VER	visual evoked response
PS II	patient with mild to moderate systemic disease	VS	vital signs
		VSS	vital signs stable
PS III	patient with severe systemic disease limiting activity, but not incapacitating	WDWN-BF	well-developed, well-nourished black female
		WDWN-BM	well-developed, well-nourished black male
PS IV	patient with incapacitating systemic disease	WDWN-WF	well-developed, well-nourished white female
PS V	moribund patient not expected to live	WDWN-WM	well-developed, well-nourished white male
Pt	patient	WF	white female
PTA	prior to admission; pretreatment anxiety	WM	white male
		WN	well nourished
PVD	patient very disturbed	WNL	within normal limits
Px	physical exam; prognosis	X3	orientation as to person, place, and time
RALT	routine admission laboratory tests	X & D	examination and diagnosis
RAP	resident assessment protocol	YACP	young adult chronic patient
REM	rapid eye movement	YLC	youngest living child

Table 3.2—Eponyms Utilized in Diagnostic Terminology

Argyll Robertson pupil	does not respond to light, but reacts to accommodation; seen in syphilis, encephalopathy, and diabetes
Ashby techniques	nonradioisotope techniques for determining red cell volume and red cell life span by injecting red cells of a different blood type into the recipient
Babinski sign/test/reflex	test for pyramidal tract disturbance where stroking the lateral aspect of the sole of the foot normally produces plantar flexion of the great toe
Barany test	caloric test of semicircular canal
Beck triad	low arterial pressure, high venous pressure, and absent apex beat; cardiac tamponade
Beevor sign	upward displacement of umbilicus due to paralysis of lower rectus abdominis
Bekhterev-Mendel reflex	tapping the dorsum of the foot normally causes extension of the 2nd and 5th toes; flexion indicates a pyramidal lesion
Bence-Jones protein	abnormal protein found in the urine of patients with multiple myeloma; consists of monoclonal light chains of the gamma globulin molecules
Benedict solution	copper sulfate solution used to test for glycosuria
Bing sign	extension of the great toe following a pricking of the dorsum of the toe or foot with a pin, seen in pyramidal tract lesions
Blumberg sign	rebound tenderness indicating peritoneal inflammation
Cheyne-Stokes breathing/respiration	recurrent episodes of hyperpnea followed by apnea seen in elderly patients with cardiovascular disease and cardiac failure

Table 3.3—Abbreviations Associated with Diagnostic Tests

Abbreviation	Meaning	Type of Test*
ACT	automated coagulation time	B
ADH	antidiuretic hormone	Ch
ALP	alkaline phosphatase	Ch
APTT	activated partial thromboplastin time	B
ASO	antistreptolysin O titer	I
BAC	blood alcohol content	Ch
BUN	blood urea nitrogen	U
C & S	culture and sensitivity	M
CAT	computerized axial tomography	O
CBC	complete blood count	B
CF	complement fixation	I
CK	creatine kinase	Ch
CMV	cytomegalovirus	M
CPK	creatinine phosphokinase	Ch
CSF	cerebrospinal fluid	C
CT	Coombs test	B
CT	computerized tomography	O
Diff	differential	B
DST	dexamethasone suppression test	Ch
EBV	Epstein-Barr virus	M
ECG, EKG	electrocardiogram	O
ECHO	echocardiogram	O
EEG	electroencephalogram	O
EGD	esophagogastroduodenoscopy	E
EIA	enzyme immunoassay	I
ELISA	enzyme-linked immunosorbent assay	I,M
ERCP	endoscopic retrograde cholangiopancreatography	E
ESR	erythrocyte sedimentation rate	B
FBG	fasting blood glucose	Ch
FBS	fasting blood sugar	Ch
FSH	follicle stimulating hormone	U
FTA	fluorescent treponemal antibody tests	B
GTT	glucose tolerance test	Ch
HA	hemagglutination assay	I
Hb	hemoglobin	B
HBV	hepatitis B virus	I
HCT	hematocrit	B
HCV	hepatitis C virus	I
HDL	high-density lipoproteins	Ch
HDV	hepatitis D virus	I
HEV	hepatitis E virus	I
HIV	human immunodeficiency virus	M
HSV	herpes simplex virus	I
ICP	intracranial pressure	C

Abbreviation	Meaning	Type of Test*
IFA	indirect fluorescent antibody	I
IFE or **IEP**	immunofixation electrophoresis	I
IHA	immune hemagglutination assay	I
IPG	impedance plethysmography	O
ISO	alkaline phosphatase enzymes	Ch
LDH	lactic dehydrogenase	Ch
LDL	low-density lipoprotein	Ch
LH	luteinizing hormone	U
MAI	mycobacterium avium-intracellulare	M
MCHC	mean corpuscular hemoglobin concentration	B
MCV	mean corpuscular cell volume	B
MHA-TP	microhemagglutination assay for Treponema pallidum antibodies	I
MRI	magnetic resonance imaging	R
PAP	prostatic acid phosphatase	Ch
PCR-DNA	polymerase chain reaction	M
PCV	packed cell volume	B
PET	positron emission tomography	N
PKU	phenylketonuria	U
PMNS	polymorphonuclear neutrophils	B
PPBS	postprandial blood sugar	Ch
PPLO	pleuropneumonia-like organisms	M
PRA	plasma renin angiotensin	Ch
PSA	prostate-specific antigen	Ch
PT	prothrombin time	B
PTT	partial thromboplastin time	B
RA factor	rheumatoid arthritis factor	I
RAI	radioactive iodine uptake	N
RBC	red blood cell count	B
RIA	radioimmunoassay	N
RID	radial immunodiffusion	N
RPR	rapid plasma reagin	I
SAE	signal-averaged electrocardiogram	O
SED	sedimentation rate	B
SG	specific gravity	U
SGPT	serum glutamic pyruvic transaminase	Ch
SPECT	single-photon emission computerized tomography	N
SPEP	serum protein electrophoresis	I
STS	serologic test for syphilis	I
T3	triiodothyronine	Ch
T4	thyroxine	Ch
TBG	thyroxine binding globulin	B
TCT	thrombin clotting	B
TEE	transesophageal echocardiography	O
TIBC	total iron binding capacity	B
TRH	thyrotropin-releasing hormone	Ch

Abbreviation	Meaning	Type of Test*
TSH	thyroid stimulating hormone	N
TT	thrombin time	B
UPEP	urine protein electrophoresis	I
VDRL	Venereal Disease Research Laboratory	B
VLDL	very low density lipoprotein	Ch
WBC	white blood cell count	B

*B = blood   C = cerebrospinal fluid   U = urine
Ch = chemistry   M = microbiologic   I = immunodiagnostic
N = nuclear medicine   E = endosopic   R = radiologic
O = other

Blood studies assess disorders of cell production (**hematopoiesis**), synthesis, and function. Examination of the blood and bone marrow are the primary means of determining blood disorders. **Venipuncture** is used to procure larger samples of blood for testing. Bone marrow specimens are obtained through needle biopsy or aspiration. A **hemogram** includes platelet count, white blood cell count (**WBC**), red blood cell count (**RBC**), hematocrit (**Hct**), and indices. A complete blood count (**CBC**) includes a hemogram plus differential count.

Blood chemistry studies include assessment of **electrolytes** (potassium, magnesium, sodium); glucose (insulin, **FBS**); hormones (progesterone, cortisol); enzymes (**CPK**, amylase, lipase); lipoproteins (cholesterol); thyroid function (thyroxine); and metabolic end products (creatinine, uric acid). Automated instrumentation allows for a wide variety of chemical tests to be performed on a single blood sample.

Urinalysis (UA) is performed to detect abnormalities of kidney function or metabolic end products. It can assess color, odor, turbidity, specific gravity, pH, glucose (**glucosuria, glycosuria**), ketones (**ketonuria**), blood (**hematuria**), protein (**proteinuria**), bilirubin, urobilirubin, nitrate and leukocyte esterase, and other abnormalities seen in microscopic analysis. These abnormalities may include bacteria, casts, epithelial cells, fat bodies, and red or white blood cells.

Stool analysis involves tests on the **feces** (plural of the Latin *Faex* for dregs) for the presence of blood (e.g., **melena**), bile, or parasites. Stool can also be examined by chromatographic analysis for the presence of gallstones (cholelithiasis).

Cerebrospinal fluid (**CSF**) is obtained by lumbar puncture, which involves insertion of a spinal needle between the fourth and fifth lumbar vertebrae (lower bones of the spine) into the space surrounding the spinal cord. A **manometer** is then attached to record the opening CSF pressure. This may reflect an increased intracranial pressure (**ICP**). The fluid may show xanthochromia (*xanth* = yellow, *chrom* = color), denoting some type of infection or possible drug interference.

Microbiologic studies are intended to detect the presence of disease-causing organisms termed **pathogens.** Specimens may be obtained from any site harboring the organisms: blood; urine; sputum; feces; discharges from wounds, eyes, ears, or genitals; or cerebral spinal fluid. **Bacteriologic** studies attempt to identify a specific organism; antibiotic sensitivity studies then determine the response of that organism to different classes and types of antibiotics. This procedure is generally referred to as a culture and sensitivity (**C &**

S). Categories of laboratory tests used for diagnosis of infectious diseases include smears and stains, animal inoculation, tissue biopsy, serologic testing, and skin testing.

Immunodiagnostic or **serodiagnostic** tests study antigen–antibody reactions for diagnosis of infectious disease, autoimmune disorders, neoplastic disease, and immune allergies. They also test for blood grouping and typing, tissue and graft transplant matching, and cellular immunology. Serologic testing, also termed **microbial immunology,** evaluates antigens of bacteria, viruses, fungi, and parasites. Terms related to these procedures include polymerase chain reaction **(PCR),** rate nephelometry, flow cytometry, complement fixation **(CF),** and enzyme immunoassay **(EIA).** Serologic tests for syphilis **(STS)** include fluorescent treponemal antibody absorption **(FTA-ABS),** rapid plasma reagin **(RPR),** Venereal Disease Research Laboratory **(VDRL),** and microhemagglutination assay for *Treponema pallidum* antibodies **(MHA-TP).**

Radiology, the use of **X rays,** is sometimes called **roentgenography.** Use of these rays is commonly employed in diagnosis, as well as treatment, of disease. Detection of dental cavities (caries), abnormalities in various organs such as the chest, and trauma to bones are examples.

Tomography or sectional roentgenography is a technique of obtaining a series of X-ray pictures revealing a specific layer of the body. Computerized tomography, commonly referred to as **CT** or **CAT** scans, ionize X rays through the body at several angles. These X rays are detected upon absorption and relayed to a computer for analysis that subsequently projects a composite picture of the organ being surveyed. This procedure, sometimes using dye called a **contrast medium,** can detect abnormalities in various organs of the body. For example, the digestive system may be analyzed using barium sulfate for a barium swallow (upper GI series), small bowel series, or barium enema. Similarly, iodine compounds are utilized in procedures involving the bile ducts **(cholangiography),** blood vessels **(arteriography),** bronchi **(bronchography),** or gallbladder **(cholecystography).** Other terms likely to be encountered with this area of diagnosis include **fluoroscopy, xeroradiography,** and magnetic resonance imaging **(MRI).**

Nuclear studies utilize radionuclide imaging to allow visualization of organs and regions that cannot be seen on X-ray film. Computerized radiation detection equipment such as scintillation detectors to locate gamma rays is used. **Radiopharmaceuticals (radioisotopes, radionuclides)** disperse throughout an area to show differences between normal and diseased tissue. Also, very small amounts of radioactive substances may be administered to a patient so that body fluids and glands can be examined for concentration of radioactivity. Examples of this are scans of the heart, bones, brain, liver/spleen, and lung, as well as the Schilling test and radioactive iodine uptake **(RAI).** Positron emission **tomography (PET),** known as pet scans, combines use of positron-emitting **isotopes** and emission-computed tomography to measure tissue function in a given region of the body. A **SPECT** technique, single-photon emission computed tomography, provides a three-dimensional image from a multiple view composite.

Ultrasonography (*-graphy,* meaning "a recording") is a means of visualizing soft tissue structures of the body by recording the reflection of ultrasonic waves directly into the tissues. A microphone-like device called a transducer is moved over a specific body part to produce the display **(sonogram)** shown on a cathode ray tube **(CRT)** or high resolution video monitor. The Doppler method allows for detailed visualization of anatomy and flow of blood vessels. Ultrasound studies are most often done to evaluate fetal health; to characterize soft tissue organs such as the liver, gallbladder, or kidneys; and to screen for masses of the male reproductive organs. Heart sonograms evaluate cardiac

Table 3.4—Abbreviations Denoting Locations Within the Health Care Facility/System

A & D	Admitting and Discharge		**NBN**	newborn nursery
A & I	Allergy and Immunology		**NCC**	neonatal care center
ASC	ambulatory surgery center		**NICU**	neonatal/neurosurgical
CCRU	Critical Care Recovery Unit			intensive care unit
CCU	coronary care unit		**NTC**	neurotrauma center
CDC	Centers for Disease Control;		**OB**	obstetrics
	cancer detection center		**OCU**	observation care unit
CICU	cardiac intensive care unit		**OHRR**	open heart recovery room
CMHC	community mental health		**OME**	Office of the Medical
	center			Examiner
CORF	comprehensive outpatient		**OPC**	outpatient clinic
	rehabilitation facility		**OPD**	outpatient department
CPC	cerebral palsy clinic		**OR**	operating room
CS	Central Supply		**OT**	occupational therapy
CSU	cardiac surveillance unit;		**PARU**	postanesthetic recovery unit
	cardiovascular surgical unit		**PCCU**	postcoronary care unit
DHHS	Department of Health and		**PCU**	progressive care unit
	Human Services		**Peds**	Pediatrics
DIC	Drug Information Center		**PER**	pediatric emergency room
EMS	emergency medical services		**PICU**	pediatric intensive care unit
ER	emergency room		**RICU**	respiratory intensive care unit
GMC	general medicine clinic		**R-S ICU**	respiratory-surgery intensive
ICCU	intensive coronary care unit			care unit
ICF	intensive care facility;		**SHS**	student health service
	intermediate care facility		**SICU**	surgical intensive care unit
ICU	intensive care unit		**SS**	Social Services
IICU	infant intensive care unit		**STU**	shock trauma unit
LCH	local city hospital		**VAH**	Veterans Administration
LTCF	long-term care facility			Hospital
MICU	medical/mobile intensive care		**VAMC**	Veterans Administration
	unit			Medical Center
MR	medical record department		**VH**	Veterans Hospital
MSS	minor surgery suite			

structure and blood flow (**echocardiography**); breast sonograms differentiate cysts from solid lesions and assist with aspirations and biopsies. Head and neck sonograms evaluate pathology in the cerebral, carotid, and vertebral arteries; differentiate masses in the thyroid and parathyroid glands; and assist in removal of foreign bodies from the eye.

Endoscopy (-*oscopy,* meaning "examination of") is a general term denoting examination of body organs or cavities by means of an **endoscope.** These fiberoptic instruments allow for direct visual examination of internal body structures by means of a lighted lens attached to a tube. The most commonly performed of these involve the joints (**arthroscopy**), lungs (**bronchoscopy**), intestines (**colonoscopy, sigmoidoscopy**), stomach (**gastroscopy**), or other combinations (esophagogastroduodenoscopy [**EGD**], endoscopic retrograde cholangiopancreatography [**ERCP**], or proctosigmoidoscopy).

An **electrocardiogram (ECG, EKG)** is the graphic recording *(-gram)* of the electrical currents that initiate contractions of the heart *(-cardio)*. Other terms associated with more specific diagnostic procedures involving the heart and circulatory system include signal-averaged electrocardiogram **(SAE)**, transesophageal echocardiography **(TEE)**, impedance plethysmography **(IPG)**, and phonocardiography.

Other special diagnostic studies include the **electroencephalogram (EEG)**, which measures and records electrical impulses from the cortex of the brain. This is used for several purposes, such as to assist in diagnosing epilepsy, narcolepsy, and Alzheimer's disease. It is used to evaluate brain tumors, abscesses, subdural hematomas, cerebral infarcts, and intracranial hemorrhages. This procedure is also used to determine electrocerebral silence or "brain death." Terms associated with EEG include auditory brain stem response **(ABR)**, visual-evoked response **(VER)**, and somatosensory-evoked response **(SER)**. EEG recording techniques are used in combination with computer data processing to evaluate electrophysiologic integrity of these pathways.

Medical Services

Other definitions pertinent to procedural coding of health care services include those describing and cataloging medical services. **Consultation,** for example, is a service provided by a health care professional whose opinion or advice regarding evaluation and/or management of a specific problem is requested by another health care professional. **Emergency** services are those provided in an organized facility for the provision of unscheduled episodic services to patients who present for immediate medical attention.

Critical care services involve care of the unstable critically ill or injured patient who requires constant medical attendance. Such services are most often provided to patients with central nervous system failure; circulatory failure; shock-type conditions; renal, hepatic, or respiratory failure; overwhelming infection; or postoperative complications. **Neonatal intensive care** includes management, monitoring and treatment of critically ill neonates, including nutritional maintenance, metabolic and hematologic maintenance, pharmacologic control of the circulatory system, and even the administrative roles of supervision of cognitive and procedural activities of the health care team. These services are provided in a neonatal intensive care unit **(NICU)**.

Nursing facility services are provided in nursing facilities, intermediate care facilities **(ICFs)** or long-term care facilities **(LTCFs).** Terms likely to be encountered in these settings include a resident assessment instrument **(RAI)**, minimum data set **(MDS),** and resident assessment protocol **(RAP)**.

Table 3.4 lists a number of abbreviations commonly used to denote locations of various health care services.

Pronouncing Glossary

Root	Meaning	Example	Pronunciation
adipo-	fat	adipose	AD e pos
alge-	pain	neuralgia	nur AL ji ah
ambulo-	walk about	ambulatory	AM bu la tor ee
ankyl-	crooked, attached	ankylosis	ANG ki LO sis
crymo-	cold	crymodynia	kri mo DIN I ah
cryo-		cryogenic	kri o JEN ik
febri-	fever	febrile	FEB ril
gero-	aged	gerontology	JER on TOL o ji
hidro-	sweat	hidrosis	hi DRO sis
ictero-	jaundice	icterogenic	IK ter o JEN ik
lepto-	slender, thin	leptodermic	LEP to DER mik
litho-	stone	lithogenesis	lith o JEN e sis
mal-	ill, bad, poor	malabsorption	mal ab SORP shun
malaco-	soft	malacotomy	MAL a KOT o mi
necro-	death	necrosis	ne KRO sis
oligo-	few, little	oliguria	OL i GU ri ah
patho-	disease	pathology	pa THOL o ji
pedia-	child	pediatrics	PE di AT riks
puri-	pus	purulent	PU ru lent
pyo-		pyogenic	PI o JEN ik
scirrh-	hard	scirrhous	SKIR us
scler-		scleroderma	skler o DER mah
steno-	narrow, contracted	stenosis	ste NO sis
strepto-	twisted, curved	streptococcus	STREP to KOK us

Glossary

bacteriologic—pertaining to diagnosis of the presence and identification of bacteria in the body

casts—material that includes various elements of blood resulting from bleeding in the kidney or lung

complement fixation—serologic test for viral antibodies

culture—growing of microorganisms on living tissue cells on a special medium that will support the growth of a given material

cytometry—the counting of blood cells

echocardiography—the ultrasonic record of the size, motion, and composition of various cardiac structures

endoscopy—instrumental examination of the interior of a canal or hollow organ

flow cytometry—test to determine antibody–antigen reactions using a laser beam

fluoroscopy—provision of X-ray recordings on a fluorescent screen

glucosuria—glycosuria; the urinary excretion of glucose, especially in large quantities

hematopoiesis—hemopoiesis; process of formation and development of blood cells

hematuria—any condition in which the urine contains blood or red blood cells

hemogram—findings of a thorough examination of the blood

immunodiagnosis—the process of determining specified immunologic characteristics of individuals or of cells, serum, or other biologic specimens

ketonuria—enhanced urinary excretion of ketone bodies

lipoproteins—compounds containing lipids (''fats'') and proteins

magnetic resonance imaging—nuclear magnetic resonance; use of a magnetic field and radio waves to form images of the body

manometer—instrument for indicating the pressure of gases or tension of the blood

melena—presence of blood in the stools

nephelometry rate—test to determine antigen-antibody reactions by scattering a light beam through a solution

pathogen—any virus, microorganism, or other substance causing disease

PET—technique that produces a cross sectional image of the distribution of radioactivity in a region of the body

phonocardiography—recording of the heart sounds with an instrument utilizing a microphone, amplifier, and filter

plethysmography—measuring and recording changes in volume of an organ or other part of the body

polymerase chain reaction—test to determine antigen–antibody reactions by amplifying low levels of specific DNA sequences

proteinuria—presence in the urine of large amounts of protein

radioimmunoassay—procedure utilizing radioactive chemicals and antibiotics to detect the presence of drugs and hormones in a blood specimen

radiography—roentgenography; examination of any part of the body for diagnostic purposes by means of roentgen rays (X rays)

radioisotope—an unstable isotope that decays to a stable state by emitting radiation

radiopharmaceutical—radioactive chemical or drug used as a diagnostic or therapeutic agent

serologic testing—method for analyzing blood specimens for antigen–antibody reactions

smear—specimen preparation by spreading a small quantity of the material across a glass slide

sonogram—image produced by ultrasound

SPECT—single-photon emission computed tomography, provides a three-dimensional image from a multiple view composite.

stain—salts composed of positive and negative ions used on smears for assistance in studying an organism

tomography—sectional roentgenography; movement of the X-ray tube during exposure to produce a sharper image of the selected plane as compared to the others

ultrasound—referring to measurement of deep structures in the body by measuring the reflection or transmission of high frequency or ultrasonic waves

venipuncture—the puncture of a vein, usually to draw blood or inject a solution

xeroradiography—the making of a radiogram utilizing a specially coated charged plate developed with dry powder rather than liquid chemical

CHAPTER 4

Abbreviations, Eponyms, and Lay Terms

Abbreviations

Evaluating the components of medical terms to derive a definition is not always sufficient. Medicine, like every other field, uses a host of abbreviations to "simplify" the communication process. Although the sheer number of abbreviations in common use precludes simplicity—rather, they often add to confusion—their very existence and common usage require that pharmacists be familiar with many of them.

Abbreviations are used as shortened forms of disease names, diagnostic procedures, anatomical terms, quantities, routes of administration, and practically anything else that may appear in medical terminology. Thousands of abbreviations are used with at least a modicum of regularity, so no one should be expected to remember them all. In fact, volumes have been published that merely list medical abbreviations and their meanings, yet none of these lists is complete. The key for a practitioner is to know those abbreviations that are likely to be encountered in practice and to be able to find those others that arise unexpectedly.

As structured in the previous chapters, abbreviations relating to the specific topic will be presented throughout the text. A comprehensive listing can be found in Appendix A. It may be useful to review the list as a reminder of those abbreviations that have been forgotten; more importantly, however, the list can be utilized for future reference.

Eponyms

Specific diseases, syndromes, or conditions are sometimes indicated by the name of a person, usually the individual who first identified the disorder, as a "shortcut" in terminology similar to an abbreviation or acronym. These *eponyms,* as they are called, are found throughout the medical literature and sometimes are much more familiar than the medical term for the same condition. While these are not scientific terms, familiarity with those encountered most frequently is helpful in a study of medical terminology and often necessary in the clinical setting. Some conditions are most widely known by the eponym in both medical and lay circles (e.g., Alzheimer's disease); others are more commonly known by the medical term, and the eponym is rarely used (for example, the term *leprosy* appears more frequently than Hansen's disease).

Table 4.1 presents a selected list of some eponyms. A standard medical dictionary or

Table 4.1—Eponyms

Ackerman tumor	verrucous carcinoma of the larynx
Addison's disease	chronic adrenocortical insufficiency (caused by atrophy or destruction of the adrenal glands)
Adson syndrome	compression of the brachial plexus leading to sensory disturbance of the upper extremity; also known as Naffziger syndrome
Albright syndrome	hereditary osteodystrophy-pseudohypoparathyroidism; also polycystic fibrous dysplasia
Alport syndrome	hereditary nephritis with nerve deafness and occasional platelet defect and cataract
Alzheimer's disease	dementia presenilis (a general mental deterioration)
Andersen's disease	type 4 glycogenosis (a glycogen storage disease)
Argyll Robertson pupil	does not respond to light, but reacts to accommodation; seen in syphilis, encephalopathy, and diabetes
Arnold Pick syndrome	a perceptive blindness with central atrophy where patient cannot fix reflexively on objects within the gaze
Arthus phenomenon	inflammation resulting from antigen–antibody (IgE) combining in tissues with resultant local reaction and damage
Aschoff nodules	granuloma specific for rheumatic fever
Ashby technique	nonradioisotope technique for determining red cell volume and red cell life span by injecting red cells of a different blood type into the recipient

Babinski sign/test/reflex	test for pyramidal tract disturbance where stroking the lateral aspect of the sole of the foot normally produces plantar flexion of the great toe
Baker cyst	enlargement of the popliteal bursa or herniation of the synovial membrane of the knee joint often associated with degenerative disease of the knee
Bamberger disease	saltatory spasm; polyserositis
Barany syndrome	unilateral headache in the back of the head with recurrent deafness, vertigo, tinnitus, and abnormal pointing test, corrected by stimulating nystagmus
Barany test	caloric test of semicircular canal
Barlow disease	infantile scurvy
Barraquer-Simons disease	progressive lipodystrophy
Barrett ulcer	esophageal ulcer
Barrett's syndrome	chronic peptic ulcer of the lower esophagus
Basedow disease	thyrotoxicosis
Basedow syndrome	myeloneuropathy, not due to vitamin B_{12} deficiency
Beck triad	low arterial pressure, high venous pressure, and absent apex beat; cardiac tamponade
Beevor sign	upward displacement of umbilicus due to paralysis of lower rectus abdominis
Bekhterev-Mendel reflex	tapping the dorsum of the foot normally causes extension of the second and fifth toes; flexion indicates a pyramidal lesion
Bell's palsy	paralysis of the facial muscles supplied by the seventh cranial nerve

Bence-Jones protein	abnormal protein found in the urine of patients with multiple myeloma; consists of monoclonal light chains of the gamma globulin molecules
Benedict solution	copper sulfate solution used to test for glycosuria
Bennett fracture	fracture of the base of the first metacarpal
Berger disease	glomerulonephritis with mesangial IgA deposition
Bernard syndrome	see Horner syndrome
Besnier-Boeck disease	sarcoidosis
Bing sign	extension of the great toe following a pricking of the dorsum of the toe or foot with a pin, seen in pyramidal tract lesions
Blumberg sign	rebound tenderness indicating peritoneal inflammation
Bouchard nodes	seen in gout and osteoarthritis in the proximal interphalangeal joints
Bright's disease	used to denote kidney disease; actually nephritis with albuminuria and edema
Buerger's disease	thromboangiitis obliterans (inflammation of the wall and connective tissue surrounding medium-sized arteries and veins)
Burnett's syndrome	milk-alkali syndrome (a chronic kidney disorder)
Calve disease	osteochondrosis of the vertebrae
Cannon syndrome	increase in adrenaline secretion during emotional stress, resulting in palpitations and sweating
Caplan's syndrome	progressive massive necrosis of the lung, seen with rheumatoid arthritis

Charcot's triad	intention tremor, nystagmus, and scanning speech seen in brain stem involvement in multiple sclerosis
Charcot-Marie-Tooth disease	peroneal muscular atrophy (of the leg muscles near the fibula)
Christensen-Krabbe disease	progressive cerebral poliodystrophy
Christmas disease	hemophilia B; sex-linked recessive hereditary bleeding disorder
Colles' fracture	fracture of the lower end of the radius with displacement of the bone
Concato's disease	polyserositis
Conn's syndrome	primary aldosteronism (over-secretion of the hormone)
Costen syndrome	dental malocclusion with associated neurologic headache
Creutzfeldt-Jakob disease	"mad cow" disease; spastic pseudo-sclerosis with spinal degeneration
Crohn's disease	regional enteritis (inflammation of the intestine)
Cushing's syndrome	pituitary basophilism (disorder of basophilic blood cells)
DaCosta syndrome	circulatory neurasthenia
Darling disease	histoplasmosis
DeQuervain's disease	subacute thyroiditis
Deutschländer's disease	tumor of metatarsal bone
Diamond-Blackfan syndrome	congenital hypoplastic anemia characterized by progressive anemia with sparing of white cells and platelets
Di Guglielmo's disease	acute or chronic erythroleukemia
Down's syndrome	mongolism

Dressler's syndrome	complications developing several days to weeks following a myocardial infarction; postmyocardial infarction syndrome
Dubin-Johnson syndrome	chronic idiopathic jaundice
Duchenne's syndrome	anterior spinal paralysis with neuritis
Duhring's disease	dermatitis herpetiformis
Dupuytren's disease	plantar fibromatosis (abnormal growth of fibrous tissue on the sole of the foot)
Eales disease	recurrent retinal and vitreous hemorrhage of unknown etiology
Ebstein's disease	congenital heart disorder with tricuspid valve displacement into the right ventricle
Ehlers-Danlos syndrome	hyperelasticity of the skin, easy bruising, and joint extensibility usually due to faulty collagen synthesis
Engelmann disease	progressive diaphyseal dysplasia
Epstein's disease	diphtheroid; an infection suggesting diphtheria
Epstein syndrome	nephrotic syndrome; edema, proteinuria, hypoalbuminemia, and hyperlipidemia
Epstein-Barr virus	a herpetovirus found in lymphoma and mononucleosis
Erb's palsy	progressive bulbar paralysis involving the muscles of the upper arm
Erb-Charcot disease	spastic diplegia (paralysis of corresponding parts on both sides of the body)
Erb-Goldflam disease	myasthenia gravis
Ewing's sarcoma	a malignant tumor of the bone marrow seen in children

Fanconi's syndrome	renal tubular dysfunction
Farber disease	disseminated lipogranulomatosis giving nodular plaques in the skin
Felty's syndrome	rheumatoid arthritis with splenomegaly and leukopenia
Filatov disease	infectious mononucleosis
Fisher syndrome	ophthalmoplegia, ataxia, and loss of tendon reflexes
Foix-Alajouanine syndrome	subacute necrotizing myelopathy, often associated with thrombophlebitis or vascular malformation of the spinal cord
Folling's disease	phenylketonuria
Forbes disease	type 3 glycogenosis; a glycogen storage disease
Friedreich disease	paramyoclonus multiplex
Fröhlich syndrome	adiposogenital dystrophy; pituitary tumor with obesity and sexual infantilism
Gamstorp disease	periodic paralysis, usually with hyperkalemia
Gardner syndrome	variant of congenital polyposis of the colon
Gasser syndrome	acute transient aplasia of erythropoietic tissue in young children; also acute hemolytic uremic (HUR) syndrome in children
Gehrig disease	amyotrophic lateral sclerosis
Gélineau disease	narcolepsy
Gerhardt disease	erythromelalgia
Gerhardt syndrome	bilateral abductor paralysis of the larynx

Gierke's disease	type 1 glycogenosis; a glycogen storage disorder
Goldflam disease	myasthenia gravis (a chronic, progressive muscular weakness)
Goodpasture syndrome	acute glomerulonephritis with hemoptysis, intrapulmonary hemorrhage, and anemia
Grave's disease	toxic goiter; hyperthyroidism
Guillain-Barré syndrome	acute idiopathic polyneuritis (simultaneous inflammation of a large number of the spinal nerves)
Gull disease	myxedema; hypothyroidism
Hamman-Rich syndrome	idiopathic diffuse interstitial pulmonary fibrosis
Hammond disease	congenital athetosis
Hansen's disease	leprosy (a chronic granulomatous infection of the skin)
Harley disease	paroxysmal hemoglobinuria
Hashimoto's disease	lymphadenoid goiter; thyroiditis
Hirschsprung disease	dilation of the colon causing obstruction at the rectum with resultant constipation and growth retardation
Hodgkin's disease	anemia lymphatica; also a term for lymphoma
Hoppe-Goldflam disease	myasthenia gravis
Huchard disease	essential hypertension
Jakob-Creutzfeldt disease	progressive encephalopathy believed caused by a slow virus
Kahler disease	multiple myeloma
Kasabach-Merritt syndrome	hemangioma-thrombocytopenia syndrome

Kawasaki syndrome	febrile illness of unknown etiology occurring mainly in children under five years
Kimmelstiel-Wilson disease	glomerulosclerosis (scarring within the kidney glomeruli)
Klein-Levin syndrome	periodic attacks of sleep and hunger with amnesia for periods of the attacks, related to narcolepsy
Kohler disease	aseptic necrosis of the navicular bone
Larsen-Johansson disease	osteochondrosis involving the apex of the patella
Legg-Calve-Perthes disease	epiphyseal aseptic necrosis of the upper end of the femur
Legionnaire's disease	*Legionella pneumophila* infection
Little disease	spastic paraplegia
Lyme disease	*L. borreliosis* (inflammatory disorder transmitted by the tick)
Mallory-Weiss syndrome	hematemesis due to a tear in the esophagus following forceful vomiting
Marie-Strümpell disease	ankylosing spondylitis (arthritis of the spine)
McArdle's disease	type 5 glycogenosis; accumulation of glycogen in muscle
Meniere's disease	endolymphatic hydrops (excessive accumulation of fluid in the inner ear)
Meyer's disease	adenoids (chronic inflammation of the pharyngeal tonsil)
Monge disease	mountain sickness
Morgagni's disease	also known as Stokes-Adams syndrome
Oguchi's disease	hereditary night blindness

Oppenheim-Ziehen disease	dystonia musculorum deformans
Ortner syndrome	left vocal cord paralysis associated with enlarged left atrium in mitral stenosis
Osler's disease	erythremia (increase in size of bone marrow and blood volume)
Osler-Vaquez' disease	erythremia; polycythemia rubra vera
Paget's disease	osteitis deformans (generalized skeletal disorder with thickening and softening of bone)
Parkinson's disease	shaking/trembling palsy
Pick's disease	multiple polyserositis (with ascites, hepatomegaly, peritonitis, and pleural effusion); also cerebral atrophy of frontal and temporal lobes resulting in senile dementia
Plummer's disease	hyperthyroidism with a nodular goiter
Pompe's disease	type 2 glycogenosis; accumulation of glycogen in heart, muscle, liver, and nervous system
Pott's disease	tuberculous spondylitis (inflammation of the vertebra)
Pott's fracture	fracture of the lower end of the fibula with outward displacement of the foot
Purtscher syndrome	sudden blindness following severe trauma or prolonged exposure with exhaustion and shock
Rasmussen's syndrome	a type of progressive encephalopathy seen in juveniles
Raynaud's disease	idiopathic, paroxysmal, bilateral cyanosis of the digits
Reye's syndrome	postinfectious syndrome of liver, kidney, and brain damage seen in children

Rokitansky disease	postnecrotic cirrhosis of the liver
Rust disease	tuberculous spondylitis of the cervical region
St. Giles disease	leprosy
St. Vitus' dance	ballism; ballismus (jerking or shaking movements)
St. Zachary disease	mutism
Sanders disease/syndrome	epidemic keratoconjunctivitis
Saunders disease	acute gastritis in infants due to excessive carbohydrate in the diet
Simmonds disease	hypopituitarism
Sjögren's syndrome	group of symptoms associated with rheumatoid arthritis seen in menopausal women
Steele-Richardson-Olszewski syndrome	progressive supranuclear paralysis
Stein-Leventhal syndrome	hirsutism, amenorrhea, enlarged polycystic ovary
Stevens-Johnson syndrome	erythema multiforme (acute skin eruptions, sometimes due to drug allergy)
Still's disease	juvenile-type rheumatoid arthritis
Stokes-Adams syndrome	slow or absent pulse, vertigo, syncope, and convulsions, usually as the result of heart block
Vaquez' disease	erythremia; polycythemia rubra vera
Vincent's disease	necrotizing ulcerative gingivitis (inflammation of the gums)
von Gierke's disease	type 1 glycogenosis; glycogen accumulation in liver and kidney

Wilks disease	subacute glomerulonephritis; subcutaneous tuberculosis
Zollinger-Ellison syndrome	peptic ulceration with gastric hypersecretion

Table 4.2—Lay Terms and Medical Terms

Lay Term	Medical Term	Lay Term	Medical Term
Adam's apple	prominentia laryngea	cataract	phacomalacia
afterbirth	placenta and membranes; secundines	change of life	menopause; climacteric
		charley horse	muscle contusion or overstrain
ankle bone	talus	chest	thorax (region)
appetite loss	anorexia		pectus (muscle)
armpit	axilla	chickenpox	varicella
athlete's foot	dermatomycosis; tinea pedis	clap	gonorrhea
		clubfoot	talipes equinovarus
bag of waters	amniotic sac		
bad breath	halitosis; ozostomia; stomatodysodia	cold in the head	coryza
		cold sore	herpes simplex
		collar bone	clavicle
bag of waters	amniotic sac	color blindness	achromatopsia
baldness	alopecia	consumption	tuberculosis
barber's itch	mentagra; sycosis	corn	clavus; hetoma
bedsore	decubitus ulcer	cross eye	esotropia
bed wetting	enuresis	crib death	sudden infant death syndrome
birth control	contraception		
birthmark	nevus	croup	laryngitis
black and blue spot	livedo	curvature of spine	scoliosis; lordosis; kyphosis
blackhead	comedo	cut	laceration
bleeding	hemorrhage	dandruff	dermatitis seborrheica
blood clot	embolus; hematoma; thrombus		
		double vision	amphodiplopia; diplopia; monodiplopia
blood poisoning	septicemia; toxemia		
blue, turning	cyanosis	drooping lids	blepharoptosis
boil	furuncle	earache	otalgia; otodynia; otoneuralgia
bowel	colon		
breast bone	sternum	eardrum	tympanic membrane
bruise	contusion		
bunion	hallux valgus	earwax	cerumen
calf	sura (region)	elbow	cubitus, ulna
	fibula (bone)	face lift	rhytidoplasty

Lay Term	Medical Term	Lay Term	Medical Term
farsightedness	hypermetropia	milk leg	plegmasia alba dolens
fever	pyrexia	miscarriage	abortion, sponta- neous
fever blister	herpes simplex		
fits	convulsions; sei- zures	moles	nevi
flat footed	pes planus	morning sickness	hyperemesis gravidarum
food poisoning	botulism		
freckle	ephelis; ephelides	mumps	epidemic parotitis
gas pain	tympanism; tym- panites	nearsightedness	myopia
		night blindness	nyctalopia
German measles	rubella	nosebleed	epistaxis
goiter	thyrocele	numbness	paresthesia
green sickness	chlorosis	parrot fever	psittacosis
hand	manus	pigeon breast	pectus carinatum
hangnail, infected	paronychia	piles	hemorrhoids
harelip	chiloschisis	pink eye	conjunctivitis
hay fever	allergic rhinitis; pollenosis; polli- nosis	prickly heat	miliaria
		rickets	rachitis
		ringing in the ear	tinnitus
head cold	coryza	ringworm	tinea
headache	cephalgia	running ear	otorrhea
heartburn	pyrosis	runny nose	rhinorrhea
heatstroke	siriasis; thermo- plegia	saddleback	lordosis
		St. Vitus dance	chorea; ballism
heel bone	calcaneus	scar	cicatrix
hiccup	singultus	shin bone	tibia
high blood pres- sure	hypertension	shingles	herpes zoster
		sleeping sickness	encephalitis
hip joint	articulatio coxae	sleepwalking	somnambulance
hives	urticaria	slimy	glairy
humpback	kyphosis	smallpox	variola
ingrown nail	unguis incarnatus	soft spot	fontanel; fonticu- lus
itching	pruritus		
jaw bone	mandible	spit	expectorate
kneecap	patella	spitting blood	hemoptysis
knock-knee	genu valgum; tibia valga	stirrup bone	stapes
		stomach ache	gastralgia; gastro- dynia
lead poisoning	plumbism		
lice	pediculosis	stroke	cerebrovascular accident
lisp	sigmatism		
lockjaw	tetanus	sty, stye	hordeolum
low blood	hypotension; ane- mia	thigh bone	femur
		tick fever	Rocky Mountain spotted fever
lues	syphilis		
lumbago	myositis; muscle overstrain	tongue tie	ankyloglossia
		toper's nose	rhinophyma

Lay Term	Medical Term	Lay Term	Medical Term
trench mouth	necrotizing ulcerative gingivitis	wheezes	asthma
		whiskey nose	rhinophyma
tumor	neoplasm	whooping cough	pertussis
vomit	emesis	windpipe	trachea
vomiting blood	hematemesis	womb	uterus
wart	verruca; verruga; thymion	wrist	carpus
		wryneck	torticollis; loxia
water on the brain	hydrocephalus	yellow skin	jaundice
web fingers	syndactylism		

Table 4.3—Lay Terms for Drugs

Lay Term	Drug	Lay Term	Drug
coke, dandruff of the gods, hubba, toot, blow, nose candy, snow, white, flake, snow dust, gold dust, green gold, her, she, *dama blanca,* white lady, happy trails, Jam, pimp's drug, Bernice, star-spangled powder, C, cadillac/champagne of drugs, leaf, freeze, happy dust, Peruvian lady	cocaine	smack, junk, white junk, TNT, crap, Rufus, Mexican Tar/brown, Persian Brown, dujie, horse, stuff, snow, Harry, H, Dava, black tar	diacetylmorphine (heroin)
		junk, smack, scag, H, hard stuff, black tar, Tootsie roll, China white	heroin
		China White, MPTP, MPPP, PEPAP	synthetic heroin
crack, rock, base, freebase	synthetic cocaine	cotton brothers	heroin + morphine
hot rocks	synthetic cocaine + tar heroin	speedball, goofball, dynamide, hot rocks	heroin + cocaine
space base	synthetic cocaine + PCP	poor man's speedball	heroin + amphetamine
liquid lady, speedball	cocaine + alcohol	atom bomb, dusting	heroin + marijuana

Lay Term	Drug	Lay Term	Drug
pot, mary jane, MJ, weed, grass, smoke, boo, puff, hagga, macohna, joint, wac	marijuana (cannabis)	mist, soma, sherman, super kool, peep, super grass, ozone	phencyclidine (PCP)
		Space Base	cocaine + PCP
hot rocks	marijuana and freebase	C & M	cocaine + morphine
hash	hashish	Champagne, caviar	cocaine + alcohol
acid, window panes, orange/ purple wedges sunshine, California sunshine, blotter acid, paper acid, microdots, purple haze, ghost, thawk, beast, blue/pink/ yellow drops, white lightening, yellow/blue/brown/ green caps	lysergic acid diethylamide (LSD)	big M, dreamer, Ms Emma, cube juice, hard stuff, hocus, unkie, white stuff, encel, morpho	morphine
		schoolboy, cough syrup, number 4s	codeine
		loads, hits, four doors	codeine + glutethimide
angel dust, dust, hog, PeaCe pill, crystal, crystal joints, killer weed, CJs, sheets, peace weed, elephant/monkey tranquilizer, TIC, embalming fluid, TAC, KJ, rocket fuel, fuel, cycline, zoom, supergrass, superjoint, superweed, good, LBJ, white powder, busy bee, green tea leaves, Aurora borealis, horse tracks, surfer, snorts, scuffle, cadillac,	phencyclidine (PCP)	Dolly, dolophine	methadone
		blues, blue morphan/morphine	oxymorphone
		T's and Blues, T's and B's, Tops and Bottoms, Teddies and Betties	pentazocine + tripelennamine
		Soup	pentazocine + diphenhydramine
		Tea and Crackers	pentazocine + methylphenidate
		Blue Velvet	paregoric/heroin/ morphine + tripelennamine

Lay Term	Drug	Lay Term	Drug
barbs, candy, goofballs, sleeping pills, downs, downers	barbiturates	meth, crank, crystal meth, whites, trucker's speed, cross-tops, beans, bennies, black beauties, white crosses, ice	amphetamines
Mickey Finn	chloral hydrate + alcohol		
reds, red devils, pinks, red birds	secobarbital	serenity, tranquillity, peace pill (STP)	4-methyl-2,5dimethoxyamphetamine
yellows, yellow jackets	pentobarbital	golden eagle, tile, LSD-25, psychodrine, MDA	4-bromo-2,5dimethoxyamphetamine
ludes, sopors, sopes, lemmons, 714s	methaqualone	Eve	MDEA (a synthetic amphetamine)
snappers, poppers	amyl nitrate aerosols	ADAM, ecstasy, the big E, XTC	3,4-methylenedioxyamphetamine
rush, locker room, super bullet, jacaroma	butyl nitrate aerosols	Love pill, speed for lovers, mellow drug of America (MDA)	methylenedioxyamphetamine
laughing gas	nitrous oxide		
Bennies, speed, uppers, pep pills, dexies, Hearts, crystal, speed,		T's and Blues	Talwin + pyribenzamine

medical textbook should be consulted if further definition and/or description of the terms is desired. Most are listed in such references under the heading "disease" or "syndrome."

Lay Terms

Knowledge of medical terminology is essential for communication within the health care system. However, the pharmacist, like other health care professionals, must also be able to effectively communicate with the patient. This often involves the ability to "translate" terms used by the patient to determine correlation with the correct medical term. For example, in describing the location of an injury, illness, or discomfort, the patient is much more likely to indicate the lay term "windpipe" rather than its medical equivalent "trachea." The list in Table 4.2 includes terms commonly encountered in referring to parts of the body. Similarly, reference to symptoms, disorders, and diseases are often made in the lay terms listed. The list is not meant to be complete; terms have been selected on the basis of their common usage and those most likely to be encountered in the practice setting.

Slang, or lay terms, for drugs are abundant, particularly with reference to illicit or recreational drug use. When questioned as to ingestion of a substance, the patient is likely to respond with one of the common terms. Since pharmacists often must deal with these terms, they have been included as a separate listing in Table 4.3, even though they are not part of traditional medical terminology.

PART II

THERAPEUTIC TERMINOLOGY

CHAPTER 5

The Cardiovascular System and Its Disorders

Terminology of the cardiovascular system has become increasingly more important for pharmacists in recent years. Thirty years ago, the public often thought of hypertension—if at all—only by the name "high blood pressure," and hypertension frequently went undiagnosed and untreated. Fifteen years ago, laymen were just beginning to hear about cholesterol, and serum lipid levels never entered the public consciousness; today, a large percentage of adult Americans have had serum cholesterol determinations, and many people know and understand the results of those tests. Pharmacists are dealing with a public with a mixed grasp of cardiovascular terminology, so they must be able to converse on all levels of sophistication.

Laymen frequently refer to the cardiovascular system as the "circulatory" system because its primary function is to circulate blood throughout the body, providing nutrients, oxygen, and numerous immune components to the tissues and removing the by-products of metabolism and other cellular activities. Although "circulatory" seems fairly descriptive, other body systems (e.g., the lymphatic system) also circulate components, limiting the specificity of the term. Since they must communicate with both other professionals and patients, pharmacists need all levels of terminology, from the exact terms used in the medical community to the less specific language of patients.

Anatomy and Physiology

Cardiovascular (CV) refers to the system that includes the heart and blood vessels and is associated with the spleen, liver, and bone marrow in the formation and replacement of blood cells. The system is functionally centered around the heart, the muscular organ that pumps blood through the rest of the system. The Greek word *kardia* is the source of the most common root referring to the heart. This root is usually anglicized to *cardi-* (or *cardio-* in its combining form) and is found in such terms as **cardiomyopathy** (disease [-*pathy*] of the muscle [*myo-*] of the heart [*cardio-*]), **cardiomegaly** (enlargement of the heart; *mega-* indicating large and the-*ly* suffix denoting a condition or disease), and **endocarditis** (inflammation [-*itis*] of both the heart's inner [*endo-*] layer and valves caused by a bacterial or fungal infection).

The root *cor-* also refers to the heart, as in **coronary thrombosis,** a blockage of a coronary artery by a blood clot. The root actually comes from the Latin word *corona*, which means crown; with only a little imagination, one can see in Figure 5.1 that the two coronary arteries sit atop the heart and circle it somewhat like a crown.

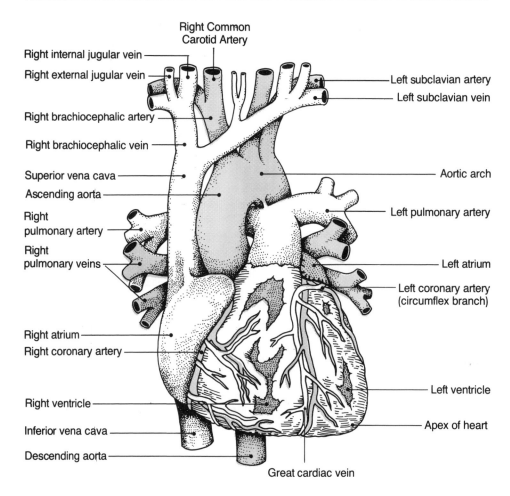

Right Common
Carotid Artery

Right internal jugular vein

Right external jugular vein

Right brachiocephalic artery

Right brachiocephalic vein

Superior vena cava

Ascending aorta

Right
pulmonary artery

Right
pulmonary veins

Right atrium

Right coronary artery

Right ventricle

Inferior vena cava

Descending aorta

Left subclavian artery

Left subclavian vein

Aortic arch

Left pulmonary artery

Left atrium

Left coronary artery
(circumflex branch)

Left ventricle

Apex of heart

Great cardiac vein

Figure 5.1—The Heart.
Anterior external view, showing surface features and great vessels.

    The heart is located in the center of the thorax as part of the **mediastinum,** the partition near the middle of the thorax, which contains the heart, large arteries, the great veins, and parts of several other systems (**trachea** and **bronchi** of the respiratory system and the **esophagus** of the digestive system, for example). The heart acts as a pump, using the contractile force of the **myocardium** to force blood from the left **ventricle** into the **aorta** and on to the systemic circulation.

    The heart beats or contracts with a wringing action that requires a freedom of movement within the crowded confines of the mediastinal partition. To separate the heart from its surrounding structures, the **pericardium** (*peri-*: around) forms an envelope around the heart. The pericardial cavity, which lies between the outer surface of the heart and the inner surface of the pericardium, is filled with pericardial fluid that lubricates the beating action.

    Blood vessels, the second major component of the system, are interconnecting tubular structures carrying blood throughout the body to acquire and supply nutrients to the cells;

remove by-products of cellular functions and deliver them to other organs for elimination; and transport hormones, antibodies, leukocytes, and numerous other regulatory and defensive components. **Vascular** simply indicates reference to vessels (*vas-* or *vaso-*: vessel or duct). Thus, an area such as the scalp, which has a large concentration of blood vessels, is said to be highly **vascularized,** the verb form of vascular. The same root appears in several terms describing actions of the blood vessels, such as **vasodilation, vasoconstriction,** and **vasospasm.** A second root, *angio-,* more frequently refers to diseases or procedures related to blood vessels. For example, **angiopathy** and **angiography** are, respectively, diseases (*-pathy*) and imaging (*-graphy*) of the blood vessels.

Other roots are more specific for the type of vessel. The root *arterio-* indicates arteries, as in **arteriosclerosis** (hardening [*-sclerosis*] of the arteries). Arteriosclerosis is the result of **atherosclerosis,** the formation of hard plaques (*athero-,* from atheroma, a grainy tumor) within the arteries, although the terms are often used interchangeably. **Veins** are referred to with the roots *veni-* and *phlebo-,* which is why a **phlebotomist** performs a **venipuncture** to draw blood from a vein. A dilated vein, however, is indicated by the root *varico-,* as in **varicosity** and **varicocele.**

The largest artery is the aorta, which emerges from the top of the heart as the ascending aorta (Figure 5.1), curves back over the heart in the aortic arch, and leads down through the thorax as the descending aorta. At the mid-abdominal level (near the upper portion of the hip bone known as the **ilium**), it splits into the two **common iliac arteries,** which supply the lower extremities and pelvis. Beginning at the heart with the coronary arteries and continuing along its entire length, the aorta gives rise to numerous other arteries supplying blood to various parts of the body.

Each organ or organ group has its own blood supply; like the coronary and iliac arteries, most are named for the structures they supply or near which they arise. The **mesenteric plexus,** for example, is a tangled network (*plexus*: Latin for ''braid'') of arteries supplying the mesentery and gastrointestinal tract that it supports; likewise, the **testicular** or **ovarian arteries** serve the reproductive glands. A pair of **renal arteries** arise from the sides of the abdominal aorta to supply the kidneys with nutrients and circulate the blood through the kidneys for excretion. Similarly, the **hepatic artery** serves the liver; it, however, traverses from the gastrointestinal tract directly to the liver, allowing hepatic metabolism of molecules absorbed from the gut before they reach the systemic circulation. Most of the major vessels pharmacists should recognize are named for the tissues they supply (e.g., **uterine artery**) or structures to which they are proximate (e.g., **femoral vein**). The **subclavian artery,** for example, lies below (*sub-*) the clavicle, while the anterior and posterior **tibial arteries** are the front and back branches of the artery which parallels the tibia in each leg.

The brain is supplied by both the subclavian arteries (which serve the neck and the thoracic wall as well as the base of the brain) and the **carotid arteries** (which extend upward to supply the remainder of the head and neck). On each side of the neck, the common carotid artery bifurcates, with the internal carotid artery as the primary supply to the brain and other intracranial and orbital structures; the external carotid artery serves other head and neck structures. At the point of bifurcation is the carotid sinus, a dilatation of the vessel equipped with nerve endings to respond to changes in blood pressure.

The arteries become thinner and simpler structures as they repeatedly branch within all parts of the body into microscopic **arterioles** (the diminutive form of ''arteries''), which finally branch into a network of **capillaries,** the endothelial tubes within the tissues. The transfer of oxygen, carbon dioxide, nutrients, hormones, and other substances

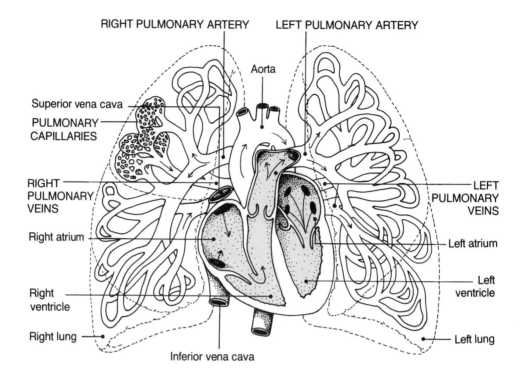

RIGHT PULMONARY ARTERY   LEFT PULMONARY ARTERY

Aorta

Superior vena cava
PULMONARY
CAPILLARIES

RIGHT
PULMONARY
VEINS

Right atrium

Right
ventricle

Right lung

LEFT
PULMONARY
VEINS

Left atrium

Left
ventricle

Left lung

Inferior vena cava

Figure 5.2—Pulmonary Circulation and Circulation Through the Heart.

takes place at the capillary level. Capillaries then converge to form **venules,** the beginnings of the venous system. The venules then further converge to form the veins returning blood to the **superior vena cava** and **inferior vena cava,** the great veins emptying into the right atrium.

In addition to the systemic circulation, which supplies the organs and tissues of the body, the pulmonary circulation allows exchange of carbon dioxide and oxygen to replenish the blood's oxygen supply and eliminate volatile waste. After the blood is pumped in turn from the right atrium and right ventricle, it passes through the pulmonary arteries, arterioles, and capillaries (Figure 5.2). The pulmonary venous circuit then returns the oxygenated blood back to the left atrium to enter the systemic circulation.

Roots derived from the major compartments of the heart are frequently incorporated into terms applied to the coronary anatomy. The structure that is the source of the impulses initiating coronary contraction, for example, is the **sinoatrial node,** a node or knot of conduction fiber located approximately between the **coronary sinus** and the atrium. Knowing that a sinus is simply a cavity could be enough for a person to discern that the coronary sinus is a cavity or broadening of the veins as they enter the heart; specifically, it is the junction of the two large veins (*vena* in Latin) that empty into the right atrium— the upper or superior vena cava and the lower or inferior vena cava. Other structures are similarly named for coronary compartments. The **atrioventricular notch,** for example, is the notch or indentation between the atrium and ventricle, and the **interatrial septum** is the septum or divider between (*inter-*) the two atria.

The pumping action of the heart is effected through sequential contractions of the atria and ventricles. Contraction is initiated in the sinoatrial node; the impulses then spread as an electrical wave over the surface of the cardiac muscles of the right atrium and the interatrial septum to the myocardium of the left atrium. The two atria contract almost in unison to force the blood through the openings between the atria and the ventricles, the **atrioventricular orifices.**

One-way valves fill the atrioventricular orifices to prevent ventricular contraction from simply forcing blood back into the atria. The **tricuspid valve** between the right atrium and ventricle is formed from three flaps or "cusps," and the **bicuspid valve** has two cusps to close the left atrioventricular orifice. The bicuspid valve is also referred to as the **mitral valve** because the cusps approximate the shape of a miter, a tall, ornamented cap worn by Roman catholic bishops.

The impulses from the right atrium gather at the atrioventricular node, which conducts them toward the right ventricle. Contraction in the ventricles begins in the interventricular septum, which shortens with the contraction. The impulse then stimulates contraction in the **apex** (which is formed from the tip of the left ventricle), moves up and around the heart in a wringing action, and terminates near the atrioventricular groove where the blood is leaving the ventricles.

An understanding of cardiovascular anatomy and normal physiology can lay an important foundation for understanding pathologies and how they might be treated. After all, most cardiovascular diseases arise from physiologic abnormalities in the arteries, veins, or heart itself, and the objective of many treatment modalities is restoration of normal function.

Therapeutics

Diseases

The most common cardiovascular disorder in humans is **hypertension,** an elevation in systolic blood pressure (measured at **systole,** the time of strongest contraction of the left ventricle), diastolic blood pressure (measured at **diastole**), or both. Arising from a variety of causes, hypertension is a significant risk factor for cardiovascular morbidity and mortality as well as other end organ damage.

Hypertension is frequently categorized by etiology. If it is not linked to a single identifiable etiology, it is classified as **primary** or **essential hypertension.** Individuals may be genetically predisposed to hypertension, but other factors influence one another and **blood pressure (BP).** Primary hypertension may result from a combination of genetic, **neurogenic** (produced [*genesis*] by the nervous system [*neuro-*]), environmental, humoral, vascular, and other factors, but the relative contribution of each cannot be determined. Although no pathologic changes occur early in primary hypertension and patients generally remain asymptomatic until complications develop, generalized **arteriolar sclerosis** ("hardening" of the arterioles) will ultimately occur, particularly in the kidneys. As the heart works harder against the higher pressure, **LVH** or **left ventricular hypertrophy** (hypertrophy is excess cell reproduction and growth) gradually develops and leads to ventricular dilation. Also, coronary, cerebral, aortic, renal, and peripheral atherosclerosis are more common and more severe in hypertensive patients. Further complications are numerous, including left ventricular heart failure, retinal hemorrhages, cerebral vascular insufficiency, and renal failure. Primary hypertension may produce a variety of clinical symptoms such as headache, dizziness, **epistaxis** (nosebleed), and nervousness as a result of complications.

Unlike primary hypertension, **secondary hypertension** is caused by or is "secondary" to some underlying pathology. Among the more common causes of secondary hypertension are any type of bilateral renal parenchymal disease or such potentially curable disorders as **Cushing's syndrome,** primary **aldosteronism, hyperthyroidism, coarctation** (stricture or contraction) of the aorta, or renal vascular disease. If the etiologic factors can be determined early enough, the hypertension is often reversible with surgery or other appropriate treatment of the underlying pathology. Once the secondary hypertension has progressed, however, correction of the abnormality usually does not result in normotensive blood pressure.

Whether primary or secondary, hypertension is also classified by severity. At the more severe end, **hypertensive crisis** is defined as a diastolic blood pressure >120 to 130 mm Hg and is further subdivided into **hypertensive emergency** (with end-organ damage) or **hypertensive urgency** (without end-organ damage). Hypertensive urgency with a higher diastolic pressure (>130 mm Hg) is referred to as accelerated hypertension, and reduction in blood pressure should be achieved within 24 hours in such urgencies. Diastolic pressure above 130 mm Hg with end-organ damage is classified as **malignant hypertension;** hypertensive emergency and malignant hypertension require rapid reduction in blood pressure.

Congestive heart failure (CHF) is a complex syndrome in which cardiac output is insufficient, resulting in decreased blood flow to the tissues and congestion in the pulmonary and/or systemic circulation. Decrease in the **ventricular filling pressure,** or **preload,** may be caused by a reduction in the atrial "kick" of blood into the ventricle at the end of diastole, as is seen in **atrial fibrillation** or any other condition in which the atrial pumping is ineffective. Such decreased preload may reduce cardiac output through the loss of maximal ventricular stretching. Conversely, an increase in preload, such as in patients with **venous congestion,** can decrease output if cardiac contractility is compromised. And increases in **afterload,** the pressure on the ventricle at the end of systole, also decrease output and cardiac efficiency.

Depending on the etiology, CHF may be primarily right- or left-sided, which refers to which side of the heart primarily is affected. Hypertension, **aortic valve disease, mitral regurgitation** (reflux of blood back through an improperly closing mitral valve), and **coronary artery disease** all can increase back pressure from the systemic circulation onto the left ventricle, so they characteristically lead to left ventricular failure. Left heart failure may produce **tachycardia** (rapid heart rate), fatigue and **dyspnea** (difficulty breathing) on exertion, and **pleural edema** from increased pulmonary venous pressure. Right ventricular failure, which is most commonly secondary to left ventricular failure, causes systemic venous hypertension and edema. Other etiologies include **mitral valve stenosis** (narrowing), primary pulmonary hypertension, **pulmonary stenosis,** multiple **pulmonary thrombosis** (presence of a thrombus or clot), or **tricuspid valve regurgitation.** Treatment of CHF often relies on diuretics and sodium restriction to reduce venous hypertension and digitalis preparations to increase cardiac contractility. Rest, oxygen, correction of arrhythmias, and elimination of any contributing factors are also essential to effective therapy.

Numerous cardiac **arrhythmias** may result from abnormalities in the conduction system of the heart, changes in vagal and other neural tone, other pathologies such as congestive heart failure, or the administration of a variety of drugs. Some, such as **sinus**

bradycardia (slow heart rate arising from the sinoatrial node) and **sinus tachycardia** (fast heart rate), are generally benign in the absence of other disease and may require no treatment besides correction of any underlying pathologies. Others, however, require direct treatment or are indicative of other pathology. **Premature ventricular contractions (PVCs)**—also called **ventricular premature beats (VPBs)**—are depolarizations of the ventricle before the next expected beat and may be precipitated by diseases causing myocardial inflammation, myocardial stretching as in CHF, or **ischemia** (insufficient blood flow) as in coronary artery disease, or even by excess digitalis.

Nomenclature of cardiac arrhythmias is generally descriptive of the origin of the impulse, the chamber affected, and/or the change in rate. For example, **paroxysmal supraventricular tachycardia** is a sudden (paroxysmal) increase in heart rate (tachycardia) caused by atrial reentry at the A-V node (supraventricular, which indicates a source in the node or atrium, both of which are "above" the ventricle). **Atrial ectopic tachycardia** is also from an atrial source, but the rapidly firing site of automaticity is in the atrial myocardium rather than the sinoatrial node (*ectopic* = away from the normal site). **Atrial flutter** and **atrial fibrillation** are often secondary to the same disorders, particularly arteriosclerotic heart disease and **rheumatic mitral valvular disease,** but they differ in rate. Both result from continuous electrical activity in the atrium, but fibrillation arises from chaotic reentry of impulses within the atrial myocardium while the continuous electrical activity in atrial flutter is organized into cyclic waves, producing an atrial rate between 240 and 400 beats per minute.

Ventricular fibrillation displays similar chaotic spread of impulses and rapid rate of contraction, but the impulses spread throughout the ventricular myocardium rather than the atrium. The most frequent cause is ventricular myocardial infarction. Because the fibrillating ventricle is unable to effectively pump blood, the arrhythmia is fatal if not immediately terminated. The abnormal rhythm can be converted to normal sinus rhythm with application of a direct electrical current, a procedure called **DC defibrillation.** The primary therapy is prevention, using antiarrhythmic medications to suppress PVCs and prevent ventricular fibrillation.

Other arrhythmias are referred to by their cause, as in **heart block,** which is any of a variety of blockages of the electrical conduction from the atrium to the ventricle or throughout the heart. Another is even named for the tracing produced by an electrocardiogram while the arrhythmia is occurring; **Torsades de Pointes** literally means "turning on points" and derives from the electrocardiogram tracing, which resembles a series of twists.

Examining the prefix and root of the term *arrhythmia* gives the meaning "without rhythm," which is fairly accurate for conditions such as atrial flutter and ventricular fibrillation. Other arrhythmias, however, are not actually without a rhythm; rather, the existing rhythm is simply irregular, too fast, too slow, or in some other way pathological. Thus, the term **dysrhythmia** (abnormal rhythm) is becoming more prevalent and may eventually supplant *arrhythmia* in the literature entirely.

The term *angina* describes a spasmodic, choking, or suffocative pain, and the term *pectoris* refers to the chest. The condition usually known as **angina pectoris** is actually a result of **myocardial ischemia** (insufficient blood flow to the myocardium, "ischemia" coming from the Greek words meaning "to suppress blood") caused by some fixed blockage such as atherosclerotic plaques or the dynamic blockage of coronary artery **vasospasm.** It is characterized by a sensation of **precordial** (in front of the heart) discomfort, pressure, or feeling of strangulation, just as its name implies. The only symptom may be a vague and barely troublesome ache, or the pain may rapidly escalate to an intense precordial crushing sensation. Although most patients experience pain that is limited to the precordial region, it may radiate to the left shoulder and down the arm; extend through the back; radiate into the neck, throat, and jaws; and occasionally extend down the right arm. Angina pectoris occurs when myocardial oxygen demand exceeds the ability of coronary arteries to provide oxygen, most frequently precipitated by exertion and relieved by rest or sublingual nitroglycerin. Extensive coronary atherosclerosis is almost always present, as is patchy **myocardial fibrosis** (formation of fibrous tissue in the myocardium). Such angina is sometimes referred to by the more specific name of **chronic stable exertional angina** because the blockage is fixed, exertion initiates symptoms, and progression is fairly slow.

Diagnosis of angina pectoris is clinically established from the symptoms, although it is usually confirmed by ischemic changes in **electrocardiogram (ECG,** also referred to as **EKG)** during an attack. The ECG tracings during an angina attack may display numerous changes that help in evaluating the cause of the pain, but the most notable is often a characteristic depression of the **S-T segment** of the tracing. Also helpful may be an **exercise tolerance test,** which uses exercise on a treadmill to determine the level of cardiac work, blood pressure, and heart rate required to induce angina.

Variant angina (Prinzmetal angina) is characterized by pain at rest and S-T segment elevation during an attack rather than depression; thus, it "varies" from typical angina pectoris. In some patients, variant angina seems to be related to occlusion of a single large vessel and vasospasm, although the condition is not always vasospastic or limited to involvement of a single vessel.

Nocturnal angina occurs at night when the patient is resting, although it is often preceded by a dream accompanied by extensive changes in blood pressure and respiration. Myocardial ischemia may also be "silent," have no symptoms (and therefore no angina), or only be detected secondarily during a routine ECG; it is then termed **silent myocardial ischemia.** At the other extreme is **unstable angina,** also called **preinfarction angina, crescendo angina,** or **angina at rest.** A medical emergency, unstable angina is a progressing or unremitting angina that often precedes a myocardial infarction (formation of an infarct, or necrotic area caused by lack of blood flow, often secondary to a thrombus or embolus).

Since the cause of angina pectoris is myocardial ischemia, coronary arteriography (imaging of the coronary arteries) may be useful in detecting specific areas of partial or total arterial occlusion, which may then be repaired surgically with a **coronary artery bypass graft (CABG)** or with **balloon angioplasty** ("repair of the artery"). Drug therapy usually includes beta-blockers, long-acting nitrates, or other agents for prophylaxis and/or nitroglycerin to relieve acute attacks.

Myocardial infarction (MI) produces pain that is similar to angina pectoris, but the pain is usually much more severe. An infarction results from a **thrombus** (blood clot) or **embolus** (clot or other plug) blocking an artery sufficiently to produce necrosis. An MI results if the occlusion is in a coronary artery, thus affecting the myocardium. The extent of necrosis and the patient's prognosis depend largely on which artery is involved, the extent of occlusion, and the presence of collateral circulation. In a large **transmural** infarct (full thickness—*transmural* literally means "through the wall"), a large area of myocardium may necrose; if 40% or more of the left ventricular mass is infarcted, the heart is usually unable to pump effectively, and the patient will die of cardiogenic shock.

Myocardial infarction may cause **cardiac arrest**—cessation of heart beat—which can in turn lead to **respiratory arrest.** Either of these conditions requires immediate **cardio-pulmonary resuscitation (CPR)** to restore respiration and heart beat. Treatment may also involve the emergency **thrombolysis** (dissolution [*lysis*] of a clot) with a variety of thrombolytic agents.

Thrombosis is also involved in a number of other disorders, generally named for the location of the clot or the ischemic tissues. **Deep vein thrombosis (DVT)** results from thrombus formation in the deep veins of the leg, resulting in swelling, discoloration, pain, and a number of other symptoms. Diagnosis can be aided with **venography,** radiographic imaging of the vein, and treatment usually includes oral anticoagulation therapy. Pulmonary embolism results from a clot or other plug in the pulmonary arteries, and stroke is ischemia or infarction of part of the brain. Thromboembolism can also be **cardiogenic**—caused by a cardiac event. For example, cardioversion for atrial fibrillation, whether by direct current or pharmacologic cardioversion, increases the short-term risk of thrombus formation and stroke, calling for anticoagulant therapy in many patients. Similarly, cardiac valve replacement increases the risk of thrombosis, although a **bioprosthetic** valve may produce less risk than a mechanical prosthetic valve.

All these thrombotic disorders are localized responses to endothelial damage or an altered surface in contact with blood components. A diffuse response to coagulation is more rare but can occur in response to malignancies, bacterial endotoxins, or other events resulting in thrombin in the systemic circulation. The resulting disorder is referred to as **disseminated intravascular coagulation (DIC).**

Shock arises from many causes, but the definitive clinical characteristic is profoundly reduced tissue perfusion. A complex syndrome, shock requires immediate treatment to restore hemodynamics to oxygenate the tissues and prevent damage and death. Although the clinical result is the same, the underlying cause is essential in providing proper treatment, which at least partly focuses on reversing the underlying pathology.

Hypovolemic shock is caused by a reduced blood volume, which may be **hemorrhagic** (caused by bleeding, whether external as in traumatic injury or internal such as from a perforated ulcer or a ruptured aneurysm) or **nonhemorrhagic.** Diarrhea, vomiting, unreplaced excess perspiration, or diabetes mellitus can cause severe dehydration, which can reduce blood volume sufficiently to result in nonhemorrhagic hypovolemic shock. Similarly, severe burns result in volume depletion, and ascites or any other conditions that sequester large volumes of fluid outside the vasculature will cause hypovolemia in the vessels and reduce tissue perfusion.

If cardiac function has an etiologic role in a shock state, it is known as **cardiogenic shock.** Myocardial infarction, cardiomyopathy, or decreased cardiac output can reduce the effectiveness of cardiac function sufficiently to cause shock. Physiologic disorders can also induce cardiogenic shock. For example, **pericardial tamponade,** mitral valve disorders, and aortic stenosis can reduce cardiac output to the point of inducing shock.

Septic shock results from a complex sepsis cascade related to a wide variety of infections. Difficult to treat, in part because of its complexity and in part because of limited treatment options for many of the involved factors, septic shock is often fatal. **Neurogenic shock** arises from a disorder of the nervous system, such as brain damage, which decreases cardiac function, vasodilation, or some other mechanism.

Pharmacists studying cardiovascular terminology should not ignore the disorders that seemed to come to the fore of American consciousness in the 1990s as a major risk factor in a large number of other cardiovascular disorders—**dyslipidemias.** Formerly, the term **hyperlipidemia** was the most commonly used since it describes an excess lipid

---

Table 5.1—Common Diseases of the Cardiovascular System

Cardiac:	aortic valve disease	Vascular:	angiopathy
	bacterial endocarditis		aortic aneurysm
	cardiac tumors		aortitis
	cardiomegaly		aortostenosis
	cardiomyopathy		arteriovenous fistula
	congenital heart disease		coronary artery disease
	ductus arteriosus		hemangioma
	megacardia		phlebolithiasis
	mitral regurgitation		varicocele
	myocarditis		varicose veins
	rheumatic valvular heart disease		vasospasm
			venous congestion
Pericardial:	cor pulmonale		venous thrombosis
	pericardial tamponade		
	pericarditis	Other:	orthostatic hypotension
			shock

---

level in the blood, which was the distinguishing characteristic of the entire group of disorders; then **hypercholesterolemia** became the more common term since cholesterol seemed to be the most significant chemical involved in the negative sequelae. Even the more specific term **hyperlipoproteinemia** has been used extensively since the excessive components are lipoproteins.

The most common term is now dyslipidemia because it describes the abnormal (*dys-*) level of lipid components in the blood. With this approach to the disorders, clinicians now consider the implications of the balance of total **triglycerides; very-low-density lipoprotein (VLDL), low-density lipoprotein (LDL),** and **high-density lipoprotein (HDL),** which are the lipoproteins that transport endogenous cholesterol; **chylomicrons,** which transport dietary cholesterol; and **cholesterol** itself. Thus, patients may have elevations of one or more components and decreases in others. Each of the classes of drugs alters different components in different ways, so the specific syndrome from which the patient suffers is essential in determining effective treatment.

Several other diseases of the cardiovascular system should be part of the pharmacist's basic vocabulary and are listed in Table 5.1. A clear understanding of these terms can provide the basis for understanding still other terms related to the cardiovascular system as they arise in consultations with other health professionals and with patients. Abbreviations commonly encountered in reference to the cardiovascular system are listed in Table 5.2.

Diagnosis

Numerous diagnostic procedures, ranging from simple **auscultation** to specialized invasive techniques, are used to detect cardiovascular diseases and abnormalities. The simplest classification of procedures begins with those that are noninvasive and require little

Table 5.2—Abbreviations Associated with the Cardiovascular System

A2	aortic second sound	**CA**	cardiac arrest; carotid/
AAA	abdominal aortic aneurysm/		coronary artery
	aneurysmectomy	**CAB**	coronary artery bypass
ABE	acute bacterial endocarditis	**CABG**	coronary artery bypass graft
ACLS	advanced cardiac life support	**CABS**	coronary artery bypass
ACV	atrial/carotid/ventricular		surgery
AES	anti-embolic stocking	**CAD**	coronary artery disease
AF	atrial fibrillation	**CAR**	cardiac ambulation routine
AFB	aorto-femoral bypass	**CCHD**	cyanotic congenital heart
AID	automatic implantable		disease
	defibrillator	**CCI**	chronic coronary insufficiency
ALMI	anterolateral myocardial	**CCU**	coronary care unit
	infarction	**CHB**	complete heart block
AMI	acute myocardial infarction	**CHD**	congenital heart disease
AOP	aortic pressure	**CHF**	congestive heart failure
APB	atrial premature beat	**CI**	cardiac index
APC	atrial premature contraction	**CICU**	cardiac intensive care unit
APD	atrial premature	**CLBBB**	complete left bundle branch
	depolarization		block
AR	aortic regurgitation	**CO**	cardiac output
A-R	apical-radial (pulse)	**CoA**	coarctation of the aorta
ARF	acute rheumatic fever	**COAD**	chronic obstructive arterial
AS	aortic stenosis;		disease
	arteriosclerosis	**COU**	cardiac observation unit
ASCVD	arteriosclerotic cardiovascular	**CPA**	cardiopulmonary arrest
	disease	**CPB**	cardiopulmonary bypass
ASD	atrial septal defect	**CPR**	cardiopulmonary resuscitation
ASH	asymmetric septal	**CR**	cardiorespiratory; cardiac
	hypertrophy		rehabilitation
ASHD	arteriosclerotic heart disease	**CRBBB**	complete right bundle branch
ASMI	anteroseptal myocardial		block
	infarction	**CS**	coronary sclerosis
ASO	arteriosclerosis obliterans	**CSE**	cross section
ASVD	arteriosclerotic vessel disease		echocardiography
AtFib	atrial fibrillation	**CSICU**	cardiac surgery intensive
AV	arteriovenous; atrioventricular		care unit
AVA	arteriovenous anastomosis	**CSU**	cardiac surveillance unit;
AVF	arteriovenous fistula		cardiovascular surgery unit
AVN	atrioventricular node;	**CV**	cardiovascular
	arteriovenous nicking	**CVP**	central venous pressure
AVR	aortic valve replacement	**CVRI**	coronary vascular resistance
AVS	atrioevenous shunt		index
AVT	atypical ventricular	**CVS**	cardiovascular system
	tachycardia	**DAH**	disordered action of the heart
AWI	anterior wall infarct	**DIC**	disseminated intravascular
BBB	bundle branch block		coagulation
BBBB	bilateral bundle branch block	**DVR**	double valve replacement
BCA	balloon catheter angioplasty;	**DVT**	deep vein thrombosis
	brachiocephalic artery	**EAT**	ectopic atrial tachycardia
BE	bacterial endocarditis	**ECC**	emergency cardiac care
BEC	bacterial endocarditis	**ECG**	electrocardiogram
BP	blood pressure	**ECHO**	echocardiogram
BPM	beats per minute	**EDM**	early diastolic murmur

EDV	end-diastolic volume	LVE	left ventricular enlargement
EH	essential hypertension; enlarged heart	LVEDP	left ventricular end diastolic pressure
EKG	electrocardiogram	LVEDV	left ventricular end diastolic volume
EMB	endomyocardial biopsy	LVEF	left ventricular ejection fraction
EPM	electronic pacemaker	LVF	left ventricular failure
HASHD	hypertensive arteriosclerotic heart disease	LVFP	left ventricular filling pressure
HB	heart block	LDH	left ventricular hypertrophy
HBP	high blood pressure	LVMM	left ventricular muscle mass
HCM	hypertropic cardiomyopathy	LVP	left ventricular pressure
HCVD	hypertensive cardiovascular disease	LVPW	left ventricular posterior wall
HF	heart failure	LVV	left ventricular volume
HHD	hypertensive heart disease	M	murmur
HLHS	hypoplastic left heart syndrome	MABP	mean arterial blood pressure
		MAP	mean arterial pressure
HLV	hypoplastic left ventricle	MDM	mid-diastolic murmur
HMI	healed myocardial infarction	MF	myocardial fibrosis
HOCM	hypertrophic obstructive cardiomyopathy	MI	myocardial infarction; mitral insufficiency
HR	heart rate	MR	mitral regurgitation
HSM	holosystolic murmur	MS	mitral stenosis
HT	hypertension	MVO$_2$	myocardial oxygen consumption
HTC	hypertensive crisis		
HTN	hypertension	MVP	mitral valve prolapse
HTVD	hypertensive vascular disease	MVR	mitral valve replacement/ regurgitation
IAA	interrupted aortic arch	MVS	mitral valve stenosis
IABP	intra-aortic balloon pump	NSR	normal sinus rhythm
IASD	interatrial septal defect	NSSTT	nonspecific ST and T wave
ICCU	intermediate coronary care unit	OCCC	open chest cardiac compression
ICD	instantaneous cardiac death	OCCM	open chest cardiac massage
IHD	ischemic heart disease	OHD	organic heart disease
IOH	idiopathic orthostatic hypotension	OMI	old myocardial infarct
		P2	pulmonic second heart sound
IRBBB	incomplete right bundle branch block	PAB	premature atrial beat
		PAC	premature atrial contraction
ISH	isolated systolic hypertension	PAF	paroxysmal atrial fibrillation
IVR	idioventricular rhythm	PAOP	pulmonary artery occlusion pressure
IVS	intraventricular septum		
IVSD	intraventricular septal defect	PAT	paroxysmal atrial tachycardia
LA	left atrium	PCCU	postcoronary care unit
LAE	left atrial enlargement	PDA	patent ductus arteriosus
LAH	left atrial hypertrophy	PMV	prolapse of mitral valve
LBBB	left bundle branch block	PMW	pacemaker wires
LBP	low blood pressure	PSVT	paroxysmal supraventricular tachycardia
LCA	left coronary artery		
LCX	left circumflex coronary artery	PTCA	percutaneous transluminal coronary angioplasty
LEA	normal arterial anatomy of the lower extremity	PVB	premature ventricular beat
LEV	normal venous anatomy of the lower extremity	PVC	premature ventricular contraction
LHF	left heart failure	PVP	peripheral venous pressure
LMCA	left main coronary artery	PVR	peripheral vascular resistance
LSM	late systolic murmur	PVT	paroxysmal ventricular tachycardia
LV	left ventricle		

QRS	principal deflection in an electrocardiogram		**SVRI**	systemic vascular resistance index
RA	right atrium		**SVT**	supraventricular tachycardia
RAC	right atrial catheter		**T1**	tricuspid first sound
RBBB	right bundle branch block		**TA**	tricuspid atresia
RBCD	right border cardiac dullness		**TAA**	thoracic aortic aneurysm
RBD	right border of dullness		**TAH**	total artificial heart
RCA	right coronary artery		**TAO**	thromboangiitis obliterans
RCD	relative cardiac dullness		**TAPVR**	total anomalous pulmonary venous return
RDVT	recurrent deep vein thrombosis		**TCABG**	triple coronary artery bypass graft
RHD	rheumatic heart disease		**TI**	tricuspid insufficiency
RHF	right heart failure		**TMI**	threatened myocardial infarction
RMCA	right main coronary artery		**TMP**	thallium myocardial perfusion
RRR	regular rhythm and rate			
RV	right ventricle		**TOF**	tetralogy of Fallot
RVE	right ventricular enlargement		**TPH**	thromboembolic pulmonary hypertension
RVET	right ventricular ejection time			
RVH	right ventricular hypertrophy		**TPM**	temporary pacemaker
RVR	rapid ventricular response		**TPVR**	total peripheral vascular resistance
S1	first heart sound			
S2	second heart sound		**TVP**	transvenous pacemaker
SA	sinoatrial		**UEA**	upper extremity arterial (study)
SAE	signal-averaged electrocardiogram			
			UEV	upper extremity venous (study)
SAH	systemic arterial hypertension			
SB	sinus bradycardia		**VAD**	vascular/venous access device
SBE	subacute bacterial endocarditis			
			VDH	valvular disease of the heart
SBP	systolic blood pressure		**VER**	ventricular escape rhythm
SCD	sudden cardiac death		**VF**	ventricular fibrillation
SDL	serum digoxin level		**VG**	ventricular gallop
SEM	systolic ejection murmur		**VPB**	ventricular premature beat
SEP	systolic ejection period		**VPC**	ventricular premature contractions
SM	systolic murmur			
SPVR	systemic peripheral vascular resistance		**VPD**	ventricular premature depolarization
ST	sinus tachycardia		**VR**	ventricular rhythm
SVPB	supraventricular premature beat		**VT**	ventricular tachycardia
			VTE	venous thromboembolism
SVR	supraventricular rhythm; systemic vascular resistance		**VWM**	ventricular wall motion

preparation of the patient. Techniques such as **phonocardiography** (recording heart sounds to localize a disorder) and **echocardiography** (imaging the heart using ultrasonic waves) are safe, cause no discomfort to the patient, and carry no risk, yet they extend the clinical information available for diagnosis. A second group, which includes treadmill stress testing, also uses noninvasive measures, but the patient requires preparation and is at some risk. Invasive techniques like **cardiac catheterization** are not routine extensions of the clinical examination and are reserved for problems that cannot be resolved without them.

Auscultation involves listening for sound within the body. It can be as simple as using a stethoscope to detect **Korotkoff sounds** (the sounds of blood flow through compressed veins when measuring blood pressure with a **sphygmomanometer**) or more complex such as listening to the heart with a stethoscope to detect unusual sounds and analyze the phases of the cardiac cycle. Variations in the four basic heart sounds, the presence of opening snaps from the valves, ejection sounds, systolic clicks of the mitral valve, or the more prolonged sounds of murmurs can aid the diagnosis of mitral valve disease, valvular regurgitation, and various cardiomyopathies. The use of microphones on the chest wall allows the graphic display of heart sounds and **phonocardiography** allows further refinement in determining the source of irregular heart sounds and isolating the focus of a disorder.

Electrocardiography (ECG) produces tracings of the electrical conduction within the heart by measuring electrical changes through several leads attached to the patient's chest. Specific abnormalities in the ECG tracing may assist in the diagnosis of cardiac arrhythmias, myocardial infarction, angina pectoris, and numerous other disorders. During a stress test, the patient is progressively exerted by increasing the incline and speed of a treadmill (or, less frequently, the speed and resistance of a bicycle) while an ECG reading is taken to determine the amount of work required to induce myocardial ischemia, angina, or other cardiac changes.

Noninvasive visualization of cardiac structures can be performed using pulse-reflected ultrasound to produce an echocardiogram, line tracings that indicate sound reflection by structures within the heart. Echocardiography allows evaluation of the systolic and diastolic internal dimensions of both ventricles and the left atrium and visualization of all four cardiac valves, making it useful in detecting mitral valve stenosis, **valvular vegetations** (growths on the valves), aortic stenosis, ventricular hypertrophy, atrial septal defect, and even left bundle branch block because of a characteristic abnormal septal motion. Structural abnormalities detected with echocardiography can be diagnostic for **hypertrophic subaortic stenosis,** congenital anomalies such as transposition of the great vessels, atrial tumors, and pericardial effusions.

Two-dimensional echocardiography (2-D echo) combines multiple scans into a "real-time" echocardiogram that can be recorded on videotape. The cross-sectional nature of the 2-D echo provides a realistic picture of the heart in motion, further enhancing the diagnostic utility of the technology. **Doppler ultrasound** incorporates one other mode, recording the velocity of moving echoes, usually moving columns of blood, which can be particularly useful in diagnosis of peripheral vascular disease.

Several radiographic procedures are also useful tools in the diagnosis of cardiovascular disease. **Plain chest roentgenography** uses frontal and lateral chest X rays primarily to evaluate the possibility of heart disease from heart size, heart shape, and lung vasculature. Plain chest roentgenograms can silhouette the cardiac chambers, although individual ventricular outlines cannot be discriminated; such chest films are helpful in diagnosis of atrial dilation secondary to fibrillation, for example, but less valuable for diseases like left ventricular hypertrophy. Images of the pulmonary vasculature, however, provide information about left ventricular function and other circulatory states.

Angiography employs a contrast medium injected into arteries, veins, or heart chambers to define anatomy, disease, or blood flow on a series of roentgenograms. Depending on the placement of the needle or catheter through which the dye is injected and the volume and rate of injection, angiograms can opacify chambers to detect cardiomegaly and space-occupying tumors, define valvular functioning to determine competence, demonstrate flow characteristics in vessels to allow diagnosis of aneurysms, atherosclerotic narrowing, infarctions, or numerous other disorders. Most angiograms include X rays taken six times per second, but the images are not visible as they are made since the film must be processed. Image intensification and amplification fluoroscopy, however, have made **cineangiography** (moving pictures of vessels) possible. Although resolution is lower than with still films, the motion better depicts many cardiac events.

Cardiac catheterization is a specialized technique whereby a flexible catheter is passed along veins or arteries into the heart to explore structures, measure pressures and blood-gasses, and inject radiopaque dyes for angiography. Relying on **fluoroscopy** with an image intensifier and a television system, catheterization allows the physician to use radiopaque catheters and dyes to measure septal defects, locate and quantify partial occlusions, isolate the sources of arrhythmias, and determine vascular function. Invasive and requiring specialized training, cardiac catheterization is usually reserved for problems that cannot be resolved without it.

Laboratory tests utilized to evaluate myocardial damage, such as from a myocardial infarction, include determination of **serum creatine phosphokinase (CPK)** and **lactic dehydrogenase (LDH),** both of which are released when muscle is damaged. CPK levels rise within 3–4 hours of an MI, but other muscle damage (such as an IM injection) will also elevate levels of the enzyme; isoenzyme studies can help distinguish the origin of elevated CPK. LDH also rises in response to numerous events, but **electrophoresis** can separate the isoenzymes to differentiate between myocarditis and congestive heart failure, for example.

Cardiopulmonary function can be evaluated by measuring blood gasses and pH, and direct measurements during cardiac catheterization can provide even more specific information. Among the determinations used are **arterial oxygen saturation (SaO_2), oxygen tension (PO_2), carbon dioxide tension (PCO_2),** and **pH.**

The elevated serum cholesterol and triglycerides found in hyperlipoproteinemias are associated with increased risk of atherosclerosis and are often a focus of treatment for patients with ischemic diseases. A hyperlipidemia is often present in patients with coronary artery disease and is probably contributory to the pathology, although it is not actually diagnostic of cardiovascular disease.

Surgical Procedures and Other Terms

Pharmacists frequently encounter a variety of other terms in relation to the cardiovascular system besides diseases and anatomy. Some relate to patient treatment areas of the hospital such as the **intensive care unit (ICU)** and **coronary care unit (CCU),** while others deal with surgical procedures.

Most of the surgical terms pose little problem for pharmacists who hear them frequently. As previously mentioned, a coronary artery bypass graft (CABG, sometimes pronounced ''cabbage'') may be helpful in relieving anginal symptoms in patients with coronary artery occlusions by dissecting a section of femoral or other vein from the leg and inserting it to direct blood flow around the occlusion. The surgical attachment between the bypass and the artery is called an **anastomosis.** Numerous other bypasses and arterial grafts are performed to circumvent an occlusion, aneurysm, or other arterial defect, and they are usually named for the artery being bypassed.

A CABG is a type of **thoracic** or **open-chest surgery** in that the sternum is split and the chest opened with a rib-spreader. The lay term **open-heart surgery,** however, refers to a surgical procedure requiring an incision into the heart. Open-heart surgery includes such procedures as cardiac valve replacements and repair of defects in the atrioventricular septum.

Pronouncing Glossary of Roots

Root	Meaning	Example	Pronunciation
angio-	vessel	angiopathy	an jee AH puh thee
arterio-	artery	arteriosclerosis	ar TEER ee oh skler OH sis
athero-	gruel	atheroma	a ther OH mah
atri-	atrium, cavity	atrium	A tree uhm
cardio-	heart	cardiomegaly	card ee oh MEG ah lee
hema- hemo- sangui-	blood	hemapoiesis hemophilia sanguirenal	heem ah POY ee sis heem oh FILL ee yah sang WE reeh nal
phlebo- veni-	vein	phlebolith venipuncture	FLEEB oh lith VANEE punk chur
sphygmo-	pulse	sphygmomanometer	sfig moh ma NAH me ter
varico-	dilated vein	varicocele	VAR ih koh seal
vaso-	vessel, duct	vasodilation	VASO die lay shun
ventriculo-	heart cavity	ventriculitis	vin TRIK u LIE tis

Glossary

aneurysm—dilation of an artery or presence of a blood-containing tumor connected directly to the opening of the artery

angina pectoris—severe constricting pain in the chest due to ischemia of the heart muscle

angiography—X-ray visualization of the blood vessels

angiopathy—general term for any disease of the blood vessels

angioplasty—reconstruction of a blood vessel

aorta—the main trunk of the arterial system, arising from the base of the left ventricle

aortitis—inflammation of the aorta

aortostenosis—narrowing of the aorta

aortography—radiographic visualization of the aorta and its branches

arrhythmia—an irregular heartbeat

arteriography—X-ray visualization of an artery after injection of a contrast medium

arteriole—a minute artery with a muscular wall

arteriosclerosis—hardening of the arteries

atherosclerosis—presence of fat deposits in the large and medium-sized arteries

artery—blood vessel that carries blood from the heart to various parts of the body

atrial fibrillation—rapid, irregular twitching of the cardiac muscular wall

atrioventricular—pertains to the atrium (pl. atria) and ventricle

auscultation—listening to the sounds made by the body structures to aid in diagnosis

bradycardia—abnormally slow heartbeat

capillaries—part of the circulatory system where exchange of substances takes place

cardiac catheterization—passage of a tubular instrument into the heart through an artery or vein

cardiogenic shock—a sudden physical disturbance resulting from decline in cardiac output

cardiomegaly—enlargement of the heart

cardiomyopathy—disease of the myocardium or heart muscle

cardiovascular—pertaining to the heart and blood vessels

carotid—pertaining to an artery in the neck region

congestive heart failure—a syndrome involving insufficient cardiac output with decreased blood flow to the tissues and congestion in the pulmonary and/or systemic circulation

cor pulmonale—enlargement of the right ventricle caused by disease of the lungs

coronary—usually used to denote the heart

coronary artery—division of the aorta that provides blood supply to the heart

diaphoresis—profuse sweating

diastole—the period of dilation of the heart cavities

ductus arteriosus—a vessel found in the fetus, which connects the left pulmonary artery with the descending aorta

dysrhythmia—irregularity in the rhythm of the heartbeat

echocardiography—ultrasonic recording of the size, motion, and composition of various cardiac structures

edema—swelling

electrocardiogram—ECG; EKG; a graphic record of the heart's action currents

embolism—blockage of an artery (blood clot)

endocarditis—inflammation of the inner layers of the heart

endocardium—the innermost layer of heart tissue

hemangioma—a congenital condition where growth of vascular tissue becomes a mass

hypertension—elevation of the blood pressure above the normal range

hypertrophy—general increase in bulk or size of a part or organ, not caused by tumor formation

iliac artery—one of two branches of the aorta that supply the lower extremities and pelvis

ischemia—lack of blood in an area of the body caused by mechanical obstruction of the blood supply

leukocyte—white blood cell

megacardia—cardiomegaly; enlargement of the heart

mitral regurgitation—dysfunction of the bicuspid valve of the heart

myocarditis—inflammation of the heart muscle

myocardium—the muscular wall of the heart

necrosis—pathologic death of one or more cells

orthostatic hypotension—a form of low blood pressure that occurs when standing

paroxysmal—occurring in short bursts

pericarditis—inflammation of the area surrounding the heart

pericardium—refers to the area surrounding the heart

phlebolithiasis—formation of stones in the vein

phlebotomist—one who draws blood

phlebotomy—incision into a vein for the purpose of drawing blood

phonocardiography—recording of heart sounds with an instrument using a microphone, amplifier, and filter

precordial—located in front of the heart

premature ventricular contractions—PVCs; type of irregularity in heartbeat

pulmonary circulation—provides for exchange of carbon dioxide and oxygen in blood

sinoatrial node—location on the right atrium where contractions of the heart originate

sinus—a channel for the passage of blood or lymph without the coats of an ordinary vessel

stenosis—narrowing of a lumen

stress test—diagnostic method to evaluate function of the heart via measurement of effects of physical exertion

subclavian—pertaining to the artery or vein beneath the clavicle or collarbone

Swan-Ganz catheterization—procedure directing a thin, flow-directed catheter using a balloon to carry it through the heart to a pulmonary artery

systole—the contraction of the heart

tachycardia—abnormally rapid heart beat

thrombosis—clotting within a blood vessel

tricuspid valve—closes the right atrioventricular opening

variant angina—Prinzmetal angina; type of angina characterized by pain at rest

varicosity—condition of having a dilated vein

varicocele—abnormal dilation of veins of the spermatic cord

varicose veins—characterized by dilation of veins, usually in the lower extremities

vascular—relating to or containing blood vessels

vasoconstriction—narrowing of the blood vessels

vasodilation—dilation of the blood vessels

vasospasm—contraction of the muscular coats of the blood vessels

vein—blood vessel that returns the blood supply to the heart

venipuncture—puncture of a vein to withdraw blood or inject fluid

ventricle—refers to the normal cavities of the heart

ventricular fibrillation—fine, rapid movements of the ventricular muscle that replace the normal contraction

venules—formed from convergence of the capillaries to begin return of the blood supply

CHAPTER 6

The Digestive (Gastrointestinal) System and Its Disorders

The overall function of the digestive system is the breakdown of foods into molecules that can be absorbed by the bloodstream for transport to cells of the body. The digestive, or **alimentary, canal** extends from the opening of the mouth down to the opening of the **rectum** or **anus.** (Figure 6.1). Those organs comprising this system are the mouth (with teeth, tongue, and **salivary glands), pharynx, esophagus, stomach,** and **intestines,** along with the **liver, pancreas,** and **gallbladder.**

Anatomy and Physiology

Digestion begins in the mouth. Both mechanical (chewing) and chemical (enzymatic) actions occur in the mouth, also sometimes referred to as the **buccal cavity** or **oral cavity.** The tongue serves to move the food into position for chewing, or mastication, by the teeth. Although this prepares the food for swallowing, it is not an integral part of the actual digestive process that begins with secretion of **saliva** by the **salivary glands.** The three largest pairs of salivary glands are the **parotids** (lying below the ears), the **submandibular** (on the medial side of the mandible), and the **sublingual** (on the floor of the mouth beneath the tongue). Saliva, which is composed of 99 percent water and 1 percent electrolytes and proteins, has several functions. It not only facilitates swallowing, but it begins the breakdown of carbohydrates with the enzyme **ptyalin** or **amylase.**

The **palate,** which is the roof of the mouth, is actually composed of two sections: the hard palate, which assists in mastication by providing a surface against which food can be manipulated, and the soft palate, which can move back and forth over the **nasopharynx** (nasal opening) to prevent food from entering the nasal cavity and to allow air to pass through.

Once the food is chewed into a soft mass ready for swallowing, it is called a **bolus.** The voluntary act of swallowing moves the **bolus** into the **pharynx,** where the muscular action becomes involuntary. At the pharynx, the digestive system branches from the pulmonary system since the pharynx opens into both the **esophagus** for the passage of food and the larynx for air. Food is prevented from entering the larynx by reflex closure of the **epiglottis.**

The esophagus in the adult is about ten inches in length. The bolus is propelled along this tube by alternating waves of contraction and relaxation, called **peristalsis.** The lower 4 cm of the esophagus consist of a band of smooth muscle, the **cardiac sphincter,** which

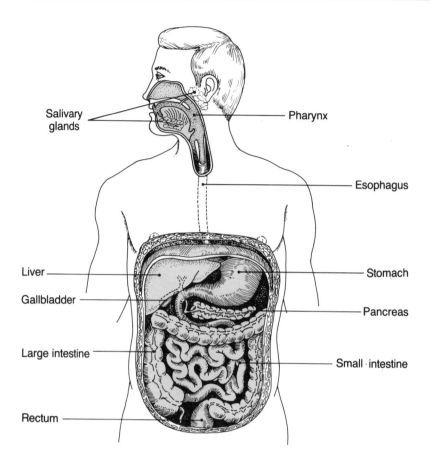

Figure 6.1—The Digestive System.
Anterior internal view, showing associated organs.

relaxes to permit food and liquids to enter the stomach. In its contracted state, the cardiac sphincter prevents the stomach contents, both food and hydrochloric acid, from being forced back up into the esophagus.

The stomach (see Figure 6.2) in an adult is usually up to ten inches long and six inches wide with a capacity of approximately 1.5 liters, although this varies greatly. The stomach is a single distinct cavity, but anatomists divide it into four primary areas on the basis of function and physiology. The **cardiac region** is nearest the esophagus and forms the entry into the stomach; the **fundus** is the body or large central portion; the **antrum,** which may be viewed as the upper part of the pylorus, is the portion where narrowing begins; and the **pylorus** leads out of the stomach.

Glands in the fundus primarily secrete **hydrochloric acid** and **pepsin,** while those in the cardia and pylorus primarily secrete **mucous.** Hydrochloric acid serves to release the digestive enzyme pepsin, which breaks down protein into amino acids. The mucus serves as a coating to protect the stomach lining from damage by the acid and enzymes. **Hypersecretion** refers to excessive amounts of these digestive enzymes.

By the time food leaves the stomach, it has been converted to the semiliquid, homogenous mixture called **chyme,** When this process has been completed, the **pyloric sphinc-**

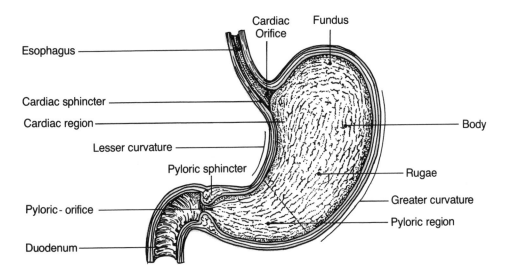

Figure 6.2—The Stomach.

ter opens to permit passage into the first portion of the small intestine, called the **duodenum.** An adult duodenum is approximately ten inches long and is the site where chyme is mixed with the secretions from the small intestine. These secretions provide the fluid necessary for action by enzymes from the pancreas and bile secreted in the liver, both of which enter the small intestine through the **common bile duct.**

The **pancreas,** located behind the stomach, contains digestive exocrine cells in addition to its endocrine function. Pancreatic enzymes are capable of digesting fats, carbohydrates, and proteins, and they are carried by an alkaline bicarbonate solution that neutralizes stomach acid. These juices act to convert the chemical environment from acidic to alkaline, which is more amenable to the intestines. Although the **liver** lies outside the digestive tract, it is considered a part of this system because of its many functions relating to digestion. It modifies all types of food substances, including fats, to enable utilization by body tissues. The **gallbladder,** a small, pear-shaped, sac-like organ located under the right lobe of the liver, serves as a storage area for excess bile before it passes into the duodenum.

Peristaltic contractions propel chyme from the duodenum, through the **jejunum** and **ileum,** sections of the small intestine approximately nine and thirteen feet in length respectively. During this process, all products of carbohydrate, fat, and protein digestion, along with most of the electrolytes, vitamins, and water, are absorbed. Bile salts and vitamin $B_{1}2$ are normally not absorbed until they reach the ileum.

After one to six hours in the small intestine, the chyme passes through the **ileocecal valve** into the **cecum,** the first part of the large intestine. Here the process of water and salt removal begins, converting liquid waste into feces. The large intestine, which frames the longer, but more compact, small intestine, consists of cecum, **ascending colon, transverse colon, descending colon,** and **sigmoid colon.** The **appendix** extends from two to six inches out from the side of the cecum, but it serves no known active role in the digestive process in humans. The terminal portions of the large intestines are the rectum, anal canal, and anus.

Normally, the waste products remain in the large intestine from twelve to thirty-six hours. Feces are usually stored in the sigmoid colon. The impulse to defecate, a response to the **gastrocolic reflex,** occurs when the rectum becomes distended with feces. Defecation is controlled by the **anal sphincter muscles.**

Anatomical Terminology

In discussing the digestive system and its associated diseases, members of the medical community use terms derived from basic system anatomy. For example, the alimentary canal is most frequently called the **gastrointestinal tract** (or GI tract), so called because it includes the stomach *(gastro-)* and the intestines. Indeed, the medical specialty dealing with the GI tract is called **gastroenterology.**

Nomenclature relating to the GI tract often follows the structures involved and position relative to those structures. For example, the submandibular salivary glands are medial to or ''under'' *(sub-)* the mandible, and the sublingual glands are under the tongue *(-lingual* = tongue). Lower in the GI tract, pain in the region of the stomach is epigastric pain *(epi-=* near; *gastric* = related to the stomach). Other terms simply combine roots to describe position, as in **nasopharyngeal, ileocecal** (between the ileum and the cecum), and **anorectal.**

Other structures are also named for their position. A sphincter is a band of muscle that constricts around an opening; the cardiac sphincter closes entry into the cardia of the stomach at the bottom of the esophagus, while the pyloric sphincter restricts emptying of the pylorus into the duodenum, and the anal sphincter controls evacuation of the rectum at the anus. Similarly, the portions of the large intestine are named for position. The ascending colon rises along the right side, the transverse colon lies across the body, and the descending colon leads down the left side. The sigmoid colon approximates an ''S'' shape, deriving its name from the Greek letter sigma (Σ), a variation on a positional name. With an understanding of basic GI anatomy, therefore, the pharmacist can decipher the meaning of most of the terms relating to structure, function, disease, or even treatment of the digestive system. Specialists who practice in the area of **gastroenterology,** treating disorders of the digestive system, are known as **gastroenterologists.**

Therapeutics

Diseases

Diseases affecting the digestive system can attack any portion of the gastrointestinal tract or its associated organs (see Table 6.1). Many of the diseases affecting the mouth only indirectly alter digestion by decreasing the effectiveness of chewing and are not usually considered digestive diseases (see Dental section). Other oral disorders, such as **stomatitis** (inflammation of the mouth), **glossitis** (inflammation of the tongue), and oral infections are often secondary to systemic diseases or are local disorders that do not affect digestion. Disorders of the remainder of the GI tract, however, are generally classified as digestive.

Clinical symptoms of esophageal disease include **dysphagia** (*dys-=* discomfort or difficulty; *-phagia* = swallowing), **pyrosis** (heartburn), and **odynophagia** (pain or burning on swallowing). **Gastroesophageal reflux disease** (GERD) is most commonly mani-

Table 6.1—Common Disorders of the Digestive System

Oral mucosa:	periodontitis
	gingivitis
	plaque
	dental caries
	alveolalgia
	alveolitis
	stomatitis
	lesions: pachyderma oris
	        leukoplakia
	        lichen planus
	        moniliasis
		Stomach:	ulcers
			gastritis
			Zollinger-Ellison syn-
			  drome
			gastrocele

Salivary glands:	parotitis sialadenitis sialolithiasis xerostomia	Pancreas:	acute pancreatitis chronic pancreatitis cystic fibrosis
Esophagus/ Pharynx	esophagitis GERD Barrett's syndrome pharyngocele pharyngitis	Gallbladder:	cholecystitis cholelithiasis choledocholithiasis acute cholangitis
Intestines:	enteritis enterocolitis enterocele diverticulosis diverticulitis appendicitis pyloric stenosis portal vein thrombosis hiatal hernia inguinal hernia polyposis dysentery ileus intussusception irritable bowel syn- drome ulcerative colitis	Rectum:	hemorrhoids anal fissures anal fistulas proctitis

Liver:	fatty liver	Other:	hyperphagia
	Reye's syndrome		dumping syndrome
	pyogenic liver abscess		polyphagia
	hepatorenal syndrome		peritonitis
	hepatic encephalopathy		neoplasms
	hepatic vein thrombosis		infectious diseases
	cirrhosis		
	hepatitis		

fested by mild to severe heartburn, which is often associated with regurgitation of acidic contents from the stomach and duodenum. GERD may be caused by a decrease or absence of lower esophageal sphincter tone, allowing reflux of gastric contents; dysfunction in the relaxation reflex of the esophageal sphincter, preventing normal esophageal emptying into the stomach; and decreased acid clearance due to impaired secondary peristalsis. Motor disorders of the esophagus include **achalasia** (or **cardiospasm,** a spasm of the cardiac sphincter), **scleroderma** (hardening [*sclero-*] of connective tissue [*-derma*]), and **diffuse esophageal spasm.** The general or lay term indigestion may be diagnosed as **dyspepsia,** gastric irritation, functional upper abdominal syndrome, non-ulcer dyspepsia (NUD) or gastric hyperacidity.

Ulceration occurs along the gastrointestinal tract, being a sore or lesion on the mucous membrane. These are described by various terms, sometimes denoting the location, such as peptic, esophageal, or duodenal. **Peptic ulcer disease** (PUD) of the stomach and duodenum results from a breakdown in the relevant mucosal defense mechanisms from *Helicobacter pylori* infection or other causes. The primary manifestation is burning or gnawing **epigastric** pain that is relieved by the ingestion of food or antacids. Complications include bleeding, perforation, obstruction of the gastric outlet, and intractable pain. **Zollinger-Ellison** syndrome is a peptic ulceration involving gastric hypersecretion and formation of a tumor (**gastrinoma**) also involving the pancreatic cells.

Nausea and **vomiting** generally occur together and can reflect the presence of acute

Table 6.2—Diagnostic Symptoms

Achalasia	Gastroesophageal reflux
Achlorhydria	Halitosis
Anorexia	Hyperemesis
Ascites	Jaundice
Bulimia	Leukoplakia
Constipation	Melena
Diarrhea	Nausea
Dysphagia	Steatorrhea
Emesis	Tenesmus
Eructation	Volvulus
Flatus	

abdominal emergencies, chronic indigestion, and acute systemic infections, as well as many diseases involving other body systems. They are often associated with abdominal pain. The medical term for vomiting is **emesis. Colic** can refer to spasmodic pains in the abdomen, to the paroxysms of pain seen in young infants, or to a variety of pain or cramping episodes due to a number of causes. **Anorexia** (loss of desire to eat) is a primary symptom in a number of disorders of the gastrointestinal tract and liver. **Diverticula** or pouches can occur along the intestinal wall. **Meckel's diverticulum** refers to such an area on the ileum that can produce ulceration and bleeding. **Diverticulosis** denotes the presence of multiple sites; **diverticulitis** specifically describes inflammation.

A number of disorders can cause **malabsorption** syndromes. These are generally classified as inadequate digestion, inadequate absorption, lymphatic obstruction, drug-induced malabsorption, hyperabsorptive malabsorption, or multiple mechanisms. Clinical features include edema; weight loss; oily, bulky, or watery stools; paresthesias; tetany; anemia; glossitis; abdominal distention; and flatulence.

Bleeding from the GI tract is another common clinical disorder. This may present as **hematemesis** (vomiting of blood), **melena** (black, tarry feces containing partly digested blood), or **hematochezia.** The vast majority of upper GI bleeding is due to peptic ulcers, gastritis, or esophagogastric varices. Lesions of the colon or anorectum are the most common causes of lower GI bleeding.

Diarrhea has been defined as an increase in stool liquidity and weight that may be associated with increased stool frequency, urgency, perianal discomfort, and/or fecal incontinence. It is associated with a number of diseases affecting various body systems, as well as bacterial and viral infections, use of antibiotics, parasitic infection, sexually transmitted diseases, and food poisoning.

The **irritable bowel syndrome** (IBS) is a common complex of symptoms including abdominal pain with alternating constipation and diarrhea for which no organic cause has been found. It is often linked to emotional stress.

Inflammatory bowel disease (IBD) is a term that encompasses both **idiopathic ulcerative colitis** and **Crohn's disease** or **regional enteritis.** Inflammation of the colon is present with classic symptoms of diarrhea, rectal bleeding, fever, weight loss, and abdominal pain. A number of extra-intestinal manifestations can also occur.

Gastrointestinal infections are caused by a number of pathogens and often associated with predominance of aerobic organisms in the large intestine. These include *Salmonella, Shigella, Campylobacter, Clostridium difficile, E. coli,* and *Staphylococcus.* Disease results from alteration in the intestinal microflora rather than introduction of a pathogen into a sterile site as in other infections.

Agents capable of causing acute **hepatitis** include several viruses, alcohol, toxins, and drugs. Viral hepatitis is primarily caused by hepatitis A virus (HAV), hepatitis B virus (HBV), or the non-A, non-B agents. Hepatitis B is a common cause of chronic hepatitis. Acute and chronic hepatitis are manifested clinically by fatigue, anorexia, weight loss, malaise, fever, and right upper quadrant abdominal pain. The additional symptoms of **spider telangiectases** (*tela-*= web-like; *angi-*= artery; *-ectasia* = dilation of a vessel), **palmar erythema,** gynecomastia, testicular atrophy, and diminished **libido** suggest **cirrhosis.** Severe viral hepatitis and cirrhosis are the most commonly observed causes of jaundice.

Cirrhosis of the liver occurs when hepatic cells are destroyed and replaced by fibrous connective tissue, causing **intrahepatic fibrosis.** Alcohol is the most frequent cause in the western world; hepatitis B can also result in cirrhosis. Fulminant hepatic failure can result from severe widespread hepatic necrosis. In severe liver disease, fluid frequently accumulates in the abdominal cavity; resulting in **ascites,** which is believed to result from low serum albumin concentration and/or increased portal venous pressure.

Diagnosis

A number of **radiographic** and **endoscopic** procedures have been developed to detect disorders or disease of the digestive system. Plain **radiographs** identify differences in tissue density, so plain X rays of the abdomen in the **supine** (lying on the back) and upright or **lateral decubitus** (lying on the side) positions are useful for detecting bowel obstruction, perforation of a hollow organ, infections with gas-forming organisms, and calcifications in the gallbladder or pancreas. **Contrast studies** incorporate a radiopaque medium into a body space to provide contrast on X ray. Contrast studies using barium sulfate can be used to detect mass (but usually not small or mucosal) lesions. Double contrast studies administering barium followed by a radiolucent substance are more effective in identifying all types of lesions. A **barium swallow** can be utilized to evaluate dysplasia, indicating whether the cause is mechanical obstruction or esophageal motor abnormality. If either of these is identified, an **esophagoscopy** with biopsy is performed to identify any lesion in the esophagus. Use of **fluoroscopy** during a barium swallow permits viewing of the movement of a swallowed radiopaque substance. These contrast examinations of the upper gastrointestinal tract, often referred to as an **upper GI series,** are widely used to detect mass lesions of the stomach and ulcers of the stomach and duodenum. An **endoscope** is the term for an instrument used to examine the interior of a canal or hollow organ. Specifically, a **gastroscope** would be utilized for inspecting the inner surface of the stomach.

The standard small bowel or **lower GI series** can detect mass lesions, obstructions, and fistulas. Either a lower GI series or **enteroclysis** (small bowel enema; literally, cleaning *[-clysis]* of the intestine *[entero-]*) is generally utilized to evaluate malabsorption, inflammatory bowel disease, or obstruction. Lesions of the colon are usually identified by **contrast radiographs.** Use of double-contrast or **pneumocolon** (air in the colon, which serves as a contrast medium) also detects polyps and early inflammatory bowel disease. The term **colonoscopy,** which is examination of the colon with a fiber-optic **colonoscope,** may be used in relation to this procedure.

Ultrasound (US) and **computed tomography** (CT) can provide visualization of the pancreas as well as complement barium studies. They are most useful in examination of the solid organs. The **liver-spleen scan** demonstrates mass lesions; the **99mTc-HIDA liver scan** reveals cystic duct obstruction, and the **99mTc-RBC scan** shows the approximate location of intermittently bleeding lesions. **Magnetic resonance imaging** (MRI), **oral cholecystography** (OCG), **percutaneous transhepatic cholangiogram** (PTC), **endoscopic retrograde cholangiopancreatography** (ERCP), **esophagogastroduodenoscopy, sigmoidoscopy, colonoscopy,** and **laparoscopy** are additional radiographic and endoscopic procedures employed in the diagnosis of disorders of the digestive system. The names of most of these procedures are self-explanatory to the pharmacist who knows the basic roots; esophagogastroduodenoscopy, for example, merely combines roots for the esophagus, stomach, and duodenum with-*oscopy,* visualization with a fiber-optic scope.

Angiography can demonstrate acutely bleeding lesions and define vascularity of mass lesions. Because it is an invasive procedure, however, its use is usually reserved for necessary follow-up of endoscopic examinations. Nasogastric (NG) intubation involves passage of a tube through the nose into the stomach and sometimes upper part of the small intestine to obtain contents for analysis.

Laboratory tests utilized to evaluate gastric secretion include the basal acid output, maximal histamine test, and the maximal Histalog test. A gastric analysis test will determine food/substance ingestion. Measurements of stool weight and stool fat, the D-xylose test, and lactase assay provide information on digestion. Microorganisms are detected by stool culture. The stool guaiac analysis reveals the presence of blood in the feces. This is often termed occult blood, meaning hidden, or amounts too small to be seen. Pancreatic secretion is evaluated by secretin stimulation testing. Laboratory tests of liver function are useful primarily to either test hepatic function or capacity, or as screening tests that suggest the presence and/or type of liver disorder. These include the serum albumin, serum bile acids, serum bilirubin, serum alkaline phosphatase (ALK), aspartate aminotransferase (AST; SGOT), alanine aminotransferase (ALT; SGPT), and prothrombin time. **Biopsy of the liver** is utilized in the differential diagnosis of cirrhosis, hepatitis, hemochromatosis, hepatomegaly, and neoplasms.

Treatment

Traditional management of diseases of the digestive system involves use of a number of pharmacologic agents, including antacids, antibiotics, H2 antagonists, corticosteroids, immunosuppressants, cathartics, and other specific agents to neutralize gastric acid or inhibit pepsin activity. Treatment of neoplasms is discussed in Chapter 18. Diet, botanical/nutritional therapies, colonic therapy, and stress management are utilized for some disorders such as irritable bowel syndrome. Ulcers have been treated with acupuncture, vitamin and mineral therapies, and stress reduction. **Phytotherapy,** use of plant-based preparations, has been utilized for upper abdominal complaints and infectious diseases of the gastrointestinal tract.

Surgical removal of organs are denoted by the suffix -*ectomy* along with the combining form denoting the site. Examples are **colectomy** (colon), **pancreatectomy** (pancreas), and **gastrectomy** (stomach). **Anastamosis** involves joining areas of the gastrointestinal tract after excision or ostomy procedures, which create an artificial opening between organs or from an organ, usually to the abdominal wall. These also are described by location: **sigmoidostomy, esophagojejunostomy, gastrostomy.** Incision into an organ (enterotomy—intestine; duodenotomy—duodenum) may be performed for exploration, biopsy, or foreign body removal. Suture *(-orrhaphy)* may be done for a perforated ulcer, diverticulum, wound injury, or rupture. Repair of the pyloric canal, known as **pyloroplasty,** is indicated in peptic ulcer disease. Likewise, a **palatoplasty** would correct deformities of the palate; **cheiloplasty** of the lips; and **pharyngoplasty** of the pharynx.

Surgical intervention most commonly would involve **colectomy** and **ileostomy** for inflammatory bowel disease, **vagotomy** or **antrectomy** for peptic ulcer disease, **cholecystectomy** for inflammation of the gallbladder, **appendectomy** for inflammation of the appendix, and repair of inguinal hernias by **herniorrhaphy. Paracentesis** or abdominocentesis (centesis = puncture) is a procedure done to remove fluid from the abdomen or peritoneal cavity.

Dental Terminology

Although chewing is not a major component of digestion, the teeth and associated structures are clearly part of the digestive tract. Dentistry, however, is a separate profession from other health care fields, and the terminology of dentition is often examined separately from the rest of the digestive system. Although incorporated here with digestion, dental terminology is also considered as an independent section.

The teeth are classified as either **deciduous** (from the Latin meaning "falling off"), commonly referred to as milk teeth or baby teeth, or **permanent.** Both sets are normally present in the gums at birth; the permanent teeth lying below the deciduous. Each jaw holds sixteen teeth: four **incisors,** two **canines** (eye teeth), four **premolars,** and six **molars** (millstone teeth). The teeth are held in their sockets by bundles of connective tissue called periodontal ligaments extending from the alveolar bone to the cement of the tooth.

The **periodontium** consists of the tissues that surround and support the teeth, which are the gingiva, periodontal ligament, cementum, and alveolar bone. The **gingiva** is the part of the oral mucosa that covers the alveolar process of the jaw and surrounds the neck of the tooth. **Periodontal ligaments** serve to attach teeth to the bone; to maintain gingival tissues in the proper relationship to teeth, as shock absorbers; and to provide a casing to protect the vessels and nerves. **Cementum** is the calcified or hardened tissue that forms the outer covering of the anatomic root. The process of its formation is variable, but continuous. The **alveolar bone** or tooth socket is the socket in the maxilla (upper jawbone) or mandible (lower jawbone) into which each tooth fits.

Each tooth consists of a root embedded in a socket of the jaw bone, a neck that is surrounded by the gum or gingiva, and a crown that projects upward from the gum. Teeth are composed of enamel, dentin, pulp, and cement (Figure 6.3).

Diseases

The most commonly encountered disease of the teeth is **plaque,** an accumulation of oral microorganisms and their products that adhere to the teeth and is not readily removed. Tooth decay, or **dental caries,** is a destructive process of loss of calcium of the tooth enamel resulting in continued destruction of enamel and dentin with cavitation of the tooth. **Malocclusion** refers to irregular alignment of the teeth that can cause periodontal disease. Diseases of the periodontal structures include **gingivitis,** inflammation of the gingivae or gums; **alveolitis,** inflammation of a tooth socket; and **alveolalgia** or dry socket, a painful secondary infection of the socket following tooth extraction. **Periodontitis** is a term for a slowly progressive inflammation extending from the gingiva and resulting in destruction of alveolar bone and periodontal membrane.

Diagnosis

Diagnostic methods employed in dental care include visual examination, dental **radiographs,** and **periodontal probe,** the clinical assessment of connective tissue destruction. An **odontoscope** is an optical device used to project the oral cavity onto a screen for multiple viewing. Iodine-125 (^{125}I) **absorptiometry** involves analysis of periodontal bone mass changes using a low-energy gamma beam originating from a radioactive source of iodine. **Photodensitometric analysis** technique is based on absorption of a beam of light

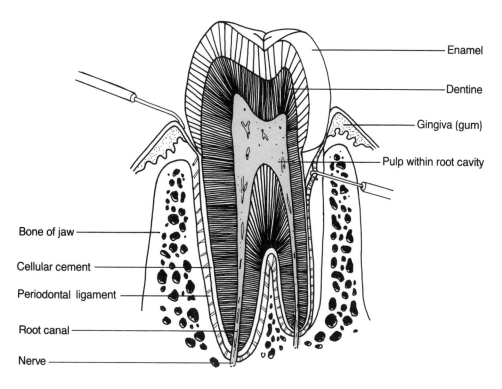

Enamel

Dentine

Gingiva (gum)

Pulp within root cavity

Bone of jaw

Cellular cement

Periodontal ligament

Root canal

Nerve

Figure 6.3—The Tooth.
Vertical section of tooth and gingiva.

by radiographic film. Computer-assisted subtraction radiography utilizes subsequent radiographs to show differences in relative densities. Nuclear medicine techniques are utilized to predict subsequent bone changes and provide a measure of disease activity. **Exfoliative cytology, darkfield** contrast **microscopy,** and **immunofluorescence microscopy** are microbiologic assays utilized in diagnosis of periodontal disease. **Latex agglutination** is an immunologic assay based on the binding of protein to latex used to detect periodontal pathogens.

Treatment

Dentistry (from the Latin *dens* meaning tooth) or **odontology** (from the Greek *odous*) refers to the specialty dealing with the prevention, diagnosis, and treatment of deformities or disorders of the teeth, oral cavity, and associated structures. **Orthodontics** is the branch of dentistry that specializes in the prevention and correction of dental and facial irregularities, often termed malocclusion. **Periodontics** is the branch of dentistry concerned with the study and treatment of abnormal conditions of the tissues surrounding the teeth. **Endodontics** is the branch of dentistry concerned with the study and treatment of the dental pulp and periapical (around the tip) tissues. **Pedodontics** is the branch of dentistry concerned with the teeth and dental care of children. Terms for the specialists in these areas are **dentist, odontologist, orthodontist, periodontist, endodontist**, and **pedodontist.**

Table 6.3—Eponyms Associated with Digestive Disorders

Andersen's disease	McArdle's disease
Barrett's esophagus/syndrome	Meyer's disease
Costen syndrome	Pompe's disease
Crohn's disease	Reye's syndrome
Dubin-Johnson syndrome	Rotikansky disease
Forbes' disease	Saunders' disease
Gierke's disease	Vincent's disease
Hirschsprung's disease	Von Gierke's syndrome
Mallory-Weiss syndrome	Zollinger-Ellison syndrome

The terms most often encountered relative to treatment of dental disorders include **amalgam restorations,** commonly referred to as "fillings," which are metal alloys applied to the surface of the tooth after removal of the caries. A **crown** refers to restoration of a major part of the crown of the tooth using gold, stainless steel, porcelain, or a composite. **Extraction** or removal of a tooth is performed either as a simple office procedure with a local anesthetic, or as part of a surgical procedure involving adjacent structures. A **root canal** involves approach from the top of the tooth (endodontic therapy), while a **root resection,** which usually follows, is an endodontic surgical procedure involving cutting and removal of the root. Replacement of missing natural teeth and adjacent tissues is generally termed artificial dentition. This may take the form of a bridge or partial **denture** or a complete dental **prosthesis,** commonly referred to as "false teeth." **Gingivectomy, alveoloplasty,** and **pulpectomy** are other surgical procedures involving the periodontal structures.

A number of eponyms reflect disorders of the digestive system; these are listed in Table 6.3. Abbreviations often encountered in reference to the digestive system, its disorders, and treatment are listed in Table 6.4.

Table 6.4—Abbreviations Associated with the Digestive System

AAC	agent-assisted colitis	**CAH**	chronic active/aggressive hepatitis
AAPC	antibiotic assisted pseudomembranous colitis	**CALD**	chronic active liver disease
ACBE	air contrast barium enema	**CBD**	common bile duct
ALD	alcoholic liver disease	**CD**	Crohn's disease
ALFT	abnormal liver function tests	**CDAI**	Crohn's Disease Activity Index
AMY	amylase		
ANP	atrial natriuretic peptide	**CDE**	common duct exploration
ARLD	alcohol-related liver disease	**CG**	cholecystogram
AVH	acute viral hepatitis	**CGB**	chronic gastrointestinal bleeding
BA	bile acid		
BaE	barium enema	**CIBD**	chronic inflammatory bowel disease
BHN	bridging hepatic necrosis		
BI	bowel impaction	**CLH**	chronic lobular hepatitis
BM	bowel movement	**CLLE**	columnar-lined lower esophagus
BO	bowel obstruction		
BOT	base of tongue	**CPH**	chronic persistent hepatitis
BS	bowel sounds	**CUC**	chronic ulcerative colitis

D & D	diarrhea and dehydration		**JI**	jejunoileal
DES	diffuse esophageal spasm		**JIB**	jejunoileal bypass
DU	duodenal ulcer		**LB**	large bowel
ECBD	exploration of common bile duct		**LBM**	loose bowel movement
			LBO	large bowel obstruction
EGTA	esophageal gastric tube airway		**LD**	liver disease
			LEHPZ	lower esophageal high pressure zone
FHF	fulminant hepatic failure		**LFS**	liver function studies
FME	full mouth extraction		**LFT**	liver function tests
FMX	full mouth extraction		**LSS**	liver-spleen scan
FNCJ	fine needle catheter jejunostomy		**NABS**	normoactive bowel sounds
			NANB	non-A, non-B hepatitis
FOBT	fecal occult blood test		**NBM**	no/normal bowel movement
FPD	fixed partial denture		**NBS**	normal bowel sound
FS	flexible sigmoidoscopy		**NEMD**	nonspecific esophageal motility disorder
GA	gastric analysis			
GB	gallbladder		**NGT**	nasogastric tube
GBP	gastric bypass		**N & V**	nausea and vomiting
GBS	gallbladder series		**NVD**	nausea, vomiting, diarrhea
GE	gastroenteritis		**OG**	orogastric (feeding)
GEP	gastroenteropancreatic		**PBC**	primary biliary cirrhosis
GER	gastroesophageal reflux		**PBD**	percutaneous biliary drainage
GIB	gastroileal bypass		**PEG**	percutaneous endoscopic gastrostomy
GIP	gastro-inhibitory peptide			
GIS	gastrointestinal series		**PMC**	pseudomembranous colitis
GIT	gastrointestinal tract		**PP**	postprandial
GJ	gastrojejunostomy		**PSP**	pancreatic spasmolytic peptide
GRD	gastroesophageal reflux disease			
			PU	peptic ulcer
GT	gastrotomy tube		**P & V**	pyloroplasty and vagotomy
HA	hepatitis, type A		**RDH**	Registered Dental Hygienist
HAA	hepatitis associated antigen		**RE**	regional enteritis
HB	hepatitis, type B		**SB**	small bowel
HBIG	hepatitis B immune globulin		**SBFT**	small bowel follow through
HbsAg	hepatitis B surface antigen		**SBO**	small bowel obstruction
HBV	hepatitis B vaccine		**S & D**	stomach and duodenum
HSM	hepato-splenomegaly		**SH**	serum hepatitis
H & V	hemigastrectomy and vagotomy		**TEN**	total enteral nutrition
			THC	transhepatic cholangiogram
IC	irritable colon		**TMC**	transmural colitis
IH	infectious hepatitis		**UC**	ulcerative colitis
IHO	intrahepatic duct		**UES**	upper esophageal sphincter
IJ	ileojejunal		**VH**	viral hepatitis
IOC	inoperative cholangiogram		**V & P**	vagotomy and pyloroplasty
IP	intraperitoneal		**ZES**	Zollinger-Ellison syndrome
IVC	intravenous cholangiogram			

Pronouncing Glossary of Roots

Root	Meaning	Example	Pronunciation
amylo-	starch	amylorrhea	am I lo RE ah
bili-	bile	biliuria	bill ee YOUR ee ah
chol-		cholelithiasis	kole lith EYE ah sis
bucco-	cheek	buccogingival	buk o JIN jee val
ceco-	cecum	cecocele	SEE ko seel
cheil-	lip	cheilosis	ki LOW sis
labio-		labiocervical	LAY bee oh sir veh kall
choledocho-	common bile duct	choledocholith	ko LED oko lith
col-	colon	colangitis	KOHL anj eye tes
dent-	tooth	dentalgia	dent AHL ja
odont-		odontoclasis	oh DONT oh klay ses
entero-	intestine	enterolith	enter oh LITH
gastro-	stomach	gastroscopy	gas TROS koh pee
gingivo-	gum	gingivitis	jin jee VI tis
gloss-	tongue	glossorrhaphy	glos OR ah fee
linguo-		linguiform	LING wee form
gluco-	sugar	glucogenesis	glu ko JEN eh sis
glyco-		glycemia	gli ko SEE me ah
hepato-	liver	hepatolysis	heh pat oh LIE sis
ileo	ileum	ileostomy	ih lee OSS toe me
jejuno-	jejunum	jejunostomy	je jun OST o me
lipo-	fat	lipolysis	li POL i sis
steato-		steatonecrosis	STE a to neh kro sis
litho-	stone	cholelithiasis	KO le li THI a sis
oro-	mouth	oronasal	oro NAZ el
stoma-		stomatitis	stohm ah TIE tis
palato-	palate	palatograph	PAL at o graf
pancreat-	pancreas	pancreatin	PAN kre ah tin
phago-	eating	phagocytic	FAG o sit ik
pharyngo-	pharynx	pharyngospasm	far EN go spahsm
procto-	rectum	proctoscopy	proc TOSS ko pee
recto-		rectocele	REK to seel

Root	Meaning	Example	Pronunciation
ptyl-	saliva	ptyalin	TI ah lin
pyloro-	pylorus, gatekeeper	pyloroplasty	pie LORO plastee
sial-		sialadenitis	sEYE ALL addn eye tes
sigmoido-	sigmoid colon	sigmoidoscopy	SIG moy dos ko pee
typhlo-	cecum	typhlomegaly	TIF lo MEG ah lee

Glossary

achalasia—obstruction that develops in the lower esophagus due to loss of motor innervation

achlorhydria—absence of hydrochloric acid from the gastric juice

alimentary—relating to nourishment or nutrition

alveoloplasty—surgical preparation of the alveolar ridges for the reception of dentures

alveolus—cavity in the jaw containing the root of the tooth

anal fissure—a painful linear ulcer in the mucous membrane of the anus

anal fistula—an opening at or near the anus, usually near the rectum

anorexia—an aversion to food; loss of appetite

antrectomy—surgical removal of the antrum (distal half) of the stomach

appendectomy—surgical removal of the appendix

appendicitis—inflammation of the appendix

ascites—an accumulation of serous fluid in the peritoneal cavity

Barrett esophagus—chronic peptic ulcer of the lower esophagus

bulimia—a mental disorder characterized by binge eating

cement—the layer of modified bone covering the root and neck of the tooth

cheilitis—inflammation of the lips

cholangiogram—roentgenographic examination of the bile ducts

cholangitis—inflammation of a bile duct

cholecystectomy—surgical excision of the gallbladder

cholecystitis—inflammation of the gallbladder

cholecystography—visualization of the gallbladder by X ray after administration of a radiopaque substance

choledocholithiasis—presence of a gallstone in the common bile duct

cholelithiasis—presence of a stone in the gallbladder

cirrhosis—progressive disease of the liver with fibrosis and degeneration

colectomy—surgical excision of all or part of the colon

colitis—inflammation of the colon

colonoscopy—visual examination of the inner surface of the colon

Crohn's disease—regional enteritis

cystic fibrosis—a congenital metabolic disorder of the pancreas

dentin—the sensitive bulk of the tooth surrounding the pulp cavity

diverticulitis—inflammation of a diverticulum, especially of the small pockets in the wall of the colon

diverticulosis—presence of a number of diverticula in the intestine

diverticulum—a pouch or sac-like opening from a tubular organ

dumping syndrome—a series of symptoms that occur after eating in patients who have had surgical removal of part of the stomach

dysentery—frequent watery stools containing blood and mucus, characterized by pain, fever, tenesmus, and dehydration

dyspepsia—gastric indigestion

dysphagia—difficulty in swallowing

electrolyte—an ionizable substance in solution

enamel—hard substance covering the exposed part of the tooth

endoscopy—examination of the interior of a canal or hollow organ by means of a special instrument

enteritis—inflammation of the intestine

enterocele—an intestinal hernia

enterocolitis—inflammation of the mucous membrane of both small and large intestines

enteroclysis—high enema

enterohepatic—referring to the intestine and liver

epigastric—referring to the region of the abdomen located between the margins of the ribs and the subcostal plane below

eructation—belching

esophagitis—inflammation of the esophagus

esophagogastroduodenoscopy—examination of the interior of the esophagus, stomach, and duodenum by means of an endoscope

esophagoscopy—inspection of the interior of the esophagus

feces—the matter discharged from the bowel during defecation

flatus—gas or air in the gastrointestinal tract

fluoroscopy—examination of the tissues and deep structures of the body by X ray

gastrin—hormone secreted in the mucosa of the stomach

gastritis—inflammation of the stomach

gastrocele—hernia of a portion of the stomach

gastrocolic—relating to the stomach and the colon

gastroenteritis—inflammation of the stomach and intestine

gastroesophageal—relating to the stomach and esophagus

gastroileal—relating to the stomach and ileum

gastrointestinal—referring to the stomach and intestines

gingiva—the gum; the mucous membrane that covers the border of the jaw

gingivectomy—surgical resection of the gingival (gum) tissue

gingivitis—inflammation of the gums

glossitis—inflammation of the tongue

guaiac—a resin from the wood of trees used as a reagent

halitosis—offensive odor of the breath

hematemesis—vomiting of blood

hematochezia—passage of bloody stools

hemochromatosis—a disorder of iron metabolism

hemorrhoids—a varicose condition of the external hemorrhoidal veins

hepatitis—inflammation of the liver
hepatomegaly—enlargement of the liver
hepatorenal—referring to the liver and kidneys
hernia—protrusion of a part or structure through the tissues normally containing it
herniorrhaphy—a suture operation for hernia
hiatal hernia—hernia of part of the stomach through the esophageal opening of the
　　diaphragm
hyperphagia—overeating; gluttony
hypogastric—relating to the lower belly area
icterus—jaundice
ileostomy—establishment of an opening from the ileum to the outside of the body
ileus—obstruction of the bowel with severe colicky pain, vomiting, fever, and
　　dehydration
inguinal hernia—hernia in the groin area
intussusception—unfolding of one segment of the intestine within another
jaundice—yellowish staining of the skin and deeper tissues
jejunostomy—operative establishment of an opening from the abdominal wall into the
　　jejunum
laparoscopy—examination of the contents of the peritoneum with a scope passed
　　through the abdominal wall
leukoplakia—presence of patches or plaques on the mucous membrane
malabsorption—a disorder of gastrointestinal absorption of nutrients
melena—passage of dark-colored, tarry stools
moniliasis—Candidiasis; a type of fungus infection
mucous—referring to mucus, the clear secretion of the mucous membranes
odynophagia—dysphagia; difficulty swallowing
pancreatitis—inflammation of the pancreas
parotid—located near the ear
parotitis—inflammation of the parotid gland
pepsin—the principal digestive enzyme of the gastric juice
perianal—located near or around the anus
periodontitis—an inflammatory disease involving alveolar bone, gingiva, and
　　periodontal membrane
peritonitis—inflammation of the membrane covering the abdominal cavity
pharyngitis—inflammation of the mucous membrane and underlying parts of the
　　pharynx
pharyngocele—a herniation of the pharynx
pneumocolon—gas in the colon
polyphagia—excessive eating
polyposis—presence of several polyps
portal vein—large vein located near the liver
proctitis—inflammation of the mucous membrane of the rectum
pulp—the soft connective tissue in the tooth containing blood vessels, nerves, and
　　lymphatics
pulpectomy—excision of the entire pulp structure of the tooth
pyloric stenosis—narrowing of the gastric pylorus
pyogenic—relating to pus formation
pyrosis—heartburn; substernal pain or burning sensation

radiography—examination of any part of the body by X ray

regurgitation—the return of gas or small amounts of food from the stomach

sialadenitis—inflammation of a salivary gland

sialolithiasis—formation or presence of a salivary calculus

sigmoidoscopy—establishment of an artificial anus by opening into the sigmoid colon

steatonecrosis—the death of adipose (fat) tissue

steatorrhea—fat indigestion characterized by passage of large amounts of feces

sublingual—below or beneath the tongue

submaxillary—beneath the mandible or lower jaw; submandibular

tenesmus—urgent desire to evacuate the bowel, accompanied by painful spasm of the anal sphincter

vagotomy—division of the vagus nerve

varices—dilated veins in the lower segment of the esophagus that are subject to ulceration and bleeding

volvulus—a twisting of the intestine causing obstruction

xerostomia—a dryness of the mouth caused by lack of sufficient salivary secretion

CHAPTER 7

The Musculoskeletal System and Its Disorders

The musculoskeletal system serves as the basic framework and motor system of the body and consists of the muscles, tendons, ligaments, joints, and bones of the skeleton. All of these components are interconnected and work together to support the body and to allow movement.

System Anatomy

Muscles are the contracting tissues that provide the force needed for both locomotion and stability. Likewise, the skeletal **bones** form the structural component. From these two basic components comes the name of the system—musculoskeletal. The working relationship between muscles and bones involves several other components. Muscles are attached to the bones by **tendons,** and bones are bound together by tough bands of tissue known as **ligaments. Cartilage** is the flexible tissue that forms the connecting structures of the skeleton, acting as a shock absorber. To provide both fine and coarse movements, bones come together at **joints** called **articulations;** within these joints is a cavity containing synovial fluid to provide the lubrication necessary between the bones. The bursae (singular: **bursa**) are sacs or sac-like cavities found in areas subject to friction, as over an exposed part or where a tendon passes over a bone (Figure 7.1).

Of the 206 bones in the body, three are located in each ear and transmit the vibrations of sound rather than function as a support mechanism; the remainder are divided between the **axial** skeleton—the skeleton of the central axis—and the **appendicular** skeleton of the appendages such as the arms (Figure 7.2). In addition, small **sesamoid** bones develop within the tendons. These are named for their general size and shape (literally, ''in the form of a sesame seed'') and act to reduce friction and sometimes function as pulleys to influence the direction of muscle pull.

The **skull** consists of the eight bones of the **cranium,** which form the cranial vault to house the brain, and the fourteen bones that form the face. Except for the jawbone or **mandible,** these bones are immovable and joined together by serrated joints called **sutures.**

The spine or **vertebral** column in most adults consists of thirty-three separate bones called **vertebrae.** The vertebral column is divided into five regions. Just below the skull is the cervical (*cervix* = neck) region. Below the cervical region, in the chest area, is the thoracic (*thorax* = chest) region, which is followed in turn by the lumbar (*lumbar* = loin) region. Below the lumbar region is the spade-shaped bone called the **sacrum.**

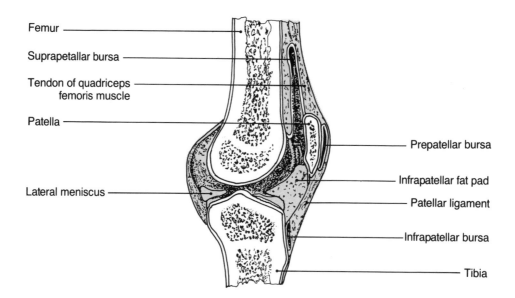

Femur

Suprapetallar bursa

Tendon of quadriceps femoris muscle

Patella

Lateral meniscus

Prepatellar bursa

Infrapatellar fat pad

Patellar ligament

Infrapatellar bursa

Tibia

Figure 7.1—The Bursa.
Lateral sectional view.

Finally, the **coccyx** is formed from additional fused vertebrae. These last two regions are sometimes referred to as false vertebrae because, unlike the bones in the upper three regions, they are not separate and movable.

The thoracic vertebrae articulate with the **ribs** to form the thorax or chest cavity. The upper seven ribs also join in the front of the body with the breast bone or **sternum**. The eighth, ninth, and tenth ribs are known as vertebrochondral ribs because they join the cartilage of the seventh rib (*chondro-* denotes cartilage). The lowest two ribs are referred to as floating ribs because they are not connected in front. The pelvic girdle includes the sacrum and coccyx and joins with the vertebral column above and the thigh bones or femurs below.

The large bone located above the knee in the leg is the **femur**. The **tibia** is the largest bone below the knee, located in front of the **fibula**. The ankle bones or **tarsals**, the foot bones or **metatarsals** (literally, "after the tarsals"), and the toe bones or **phalanges** (singular: **phalanx**) complete the lower extremity. The upper extremity is composed of the collar bone or **clavicle**, which articulates with the wingbone or **scapula**, the long bone of the upper arm known as the **humerus**, the **radius** and **ulna** below the elbow and joining the wrist bone or **carpals**, the bones of the hand or **metacarpals**, and the **phalanges** of the fingers.

Names of the specific muscles are not encountered as frequently as are those of the bones; however, several listed in Figures 7.3 and 7.4 may be familiar. Derivation of the muscle names varies, with some reflecting proximity to specific areas or body parts: **occiput**—back of the head; **frontalis**—in front; **pectoralis** major—from pectus, breast bone; **rectus abdominis**—abdominal area; **gluteus**, from the Greek *gloutos*, buttock; or **peroneus**—fibula. Others have more unique associations, such as **sartorius** (Latin *sartor*, "tailor"), named for its use in crossing the legs in the tailor's position, or **deltoid**, named after the Greek letter shaped like a triangle.

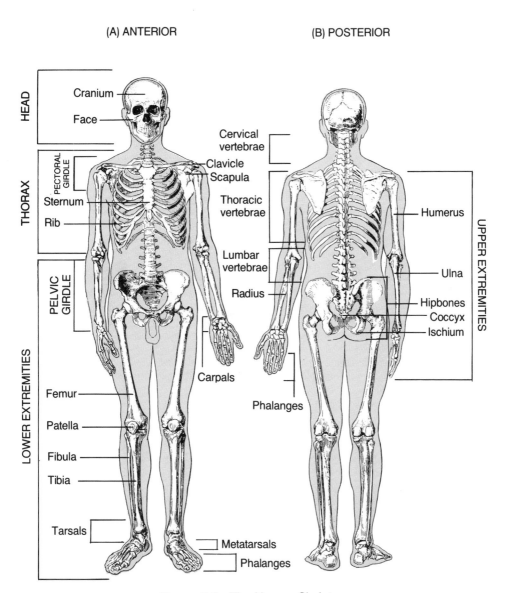

Figure 7.2—The Human Skeleton.
(A) Anterior internal view. (B) Posterior internal view.

Anatomical Terms

Bones may be classified according to shape, structure, or embryonic development. Terms used to denote shape could include simple descriptors as long, short, irregular, flat, etc. A bone's structural classification is determined by examination under a microscope. **Compact bone** is hard and dense; on the other hand, **spongy bone,** also referred to as **cancellous** bone (from the Latin for "lattice"), contains many small cavities filled with marrow. All bones contain both types of tissue, but classification is made by the

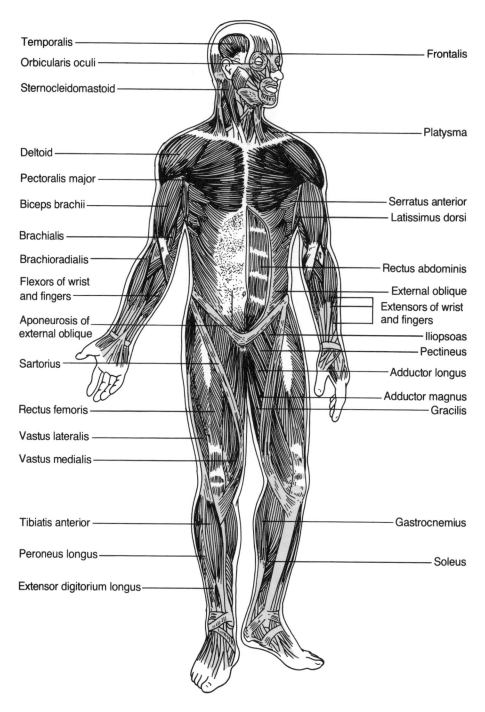

Temporalis

Orbicularis oculi

Sternocleidomastoid

Deltoid

Pectoralis major

Biceps brachii

Brachialis

Brachioradialis

Flexors of wrist
and fingers

Aponeurosis of
external oblique

Sartorius

Rectus femoris

Vastus lateralis

Vastus medialis

Tibiatis anterior

Peroneus longus

Extensor digitorium longus

Frontalis

Platysma

Serratus anterior

Latissimus dorsi

Rectus abdominis

External oblique

Extensors of wrist
and fingers

Iliopsoas

Pectineus

Adductor longus

Adductor magnus

Gracilis

Gastrocnemius

Soleus

Figure 7.3—The Muscular System.
Anterior internal view.

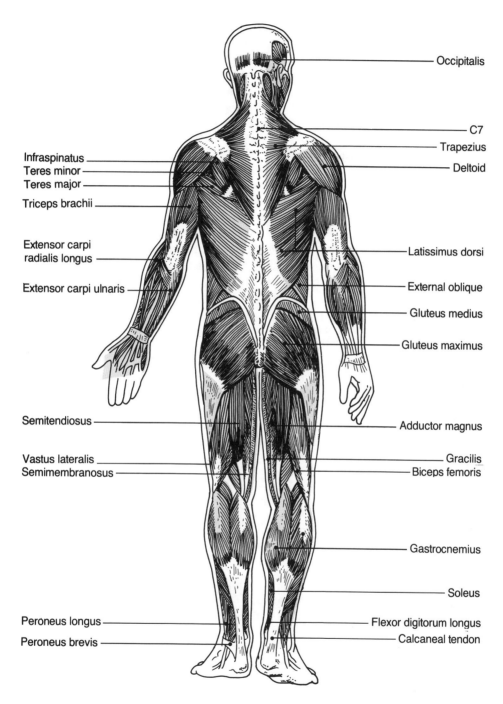

Figure 7.4—The Muscular System.
Posterior internal view.

Occipitalis

C7

Trapezius

Deltoid

Infraspinatus

Teres minor

Teres major

Triceps brachii

Extensor carpi
radialis longus

Latissimus dorsi

Extensor carpi ulnaris

External oblique

Gluteus medius

Gluteus maximus

Semitendiosus

Adductor magnus

Vastus lateralis

Semimembranosus

Gracilis

Biceps femoris

Gastrocnemius

Soleus

Peroneus longus

Flexor digitorum longus

Peroneus brevis

Calcaneal tendon

predominating type. The third method of classification, by embryonic development, groups bones into those that arise in the embryo from cartilage (**cartilaginous**) or those arising from membrane (**membranous**).

The inner cavity of the bone is referred to as the **medullary cavity** or **marrow cavity** because it contains the bone marrow (medulla osseum). The cavity is lined by connective tissue called the **endosteum** (*endo-*= inner; *osteum* or *osteo-* = bone). The outer sheath of tissue surrounding the bone is known as the **periosteum,** which covers all of the bone except the articular end, the part forming a joint with another bone. Bone tissues are traversed by a system of canals through which blood vessels, lymph vessels, and nerves enter the bone via the periosteum.

A long bone consists of two parts, the **diaphysis,** which is the shaft or main body of the bone, and the **epiphysis,** the end of the bone. Yellow bone marrow, consisting primarily of fat cells, is found in the marrow cavity in the center of long bones, while the epiphysis is filled with red marrow that produces blood cells. Vertebrae consist of a rounded body at the front and a spring arch at the back. Through the center is the **vertebral foramen,** the opening that houses the spinal cord. Spiny projections called **processes** project from the vertebrae to allow attachment of muscles and ligaments. Discs of cartilage between the vertebrae act as shock absorbers.

Muscles are sheathed in a dense fibrous tissue called **deep fascia**. Named for the Latin word for "band," these deep fasciae are bands of tissue that enclose blood and lymphatic vessels and separate the individual muscles they enclose. **Superficial fascia** is the term for the tissue lying just beneath the skin (subcutaneous).

Body movement results from the action of a group of muscles rather than a single muscle. Both **flexion** and **extension** require a prime mover or **agonist** pulling in one direction and an **antagonist** that contracts with an opposite action. **Fixation** muscles are groups that hold body parts steady to facilitate muscle action. **Synergists** function by preventing unnecessary muscle action. Functions of some specific muscles are summarized in Table 7.1.

Therapeutics

Diseases

Treatment of musculoskeletal disorders most frequently comes under the specialty of **orthopedics** focused on bones, **rheumatology** focused on the joints, **osteopathy** focused on adjustment, or **chiropractic** focused primarily on the relationship between the spinal column and the nervous system. The practitioners are termed orthopedist (or more commonly, orthopedic surgeon), rheumatologist, osteopath, and chiropractor, respectively. The most commonly encountered disorders of the bones include fractures, herniated disk, spina bifida, spinal curvatures, tumors, and infections (see Table 7.2).

A **fracture** is a break in bone tissue and can vary from a minor hairline crack to the complete separation of bone segments. A fracture may be referred to as simple (closed), with no open wound in the skin, or compound (open), with an open wound. Other terms denoting types of fractures include impacted, compression, comminuted, greenstick, and Colles'. Fractures of the vertebral column may be either compression or extension fractures, depending on whether the spine is pressed together or stretched apart. Spinal cord

Table 7.1—Muscle Functions

biceps brachii	flexion, supination of the arm
brachialis	flexion of the forearm
brachioradialis	flexion of the forearm
deltoid	flexion, extension, rotation of the arm
frontalis	move the scalp
gastrocnemius	flexion of the foot
gluteus maximus	extend the thigh
gluteus medius	abduct, rotate the thigh
latissimus dorsi	extend, adduct, rotate the arm
pectoralis major	adduct, rotate the arm
peroneus	movement of the foot
rectus abdominis	straight muscle of the abdomen
rectus femoris	straight muscle of the thigh
sartorius	flexion, rotation of the thigh and leg
sternocleidomastoid	flexion of the neck; extension of the head
temporalis	close the jaw
tibialis anterior	movement of the foot
trapezius	rotate the shoulder
vastus	extension of the leg

injury can result from extension fractures and **dislocations,** which usually affect the posterior portions of the vertebral column.

A **herniated disk** (also called a ruptured or slipped disk) results when the soft center or nucleus pulposus protrudes through the outer ring of an intervertebral disk.

Spina bifida or cleft spine is a developmental disorder in which the neural arches of the vertebra do not close completely, making the spinal nerves subject to injury or infection. Three abnormal spinal curvatures occurring in adolescents or adults are **kyphosis** (*kypho* = hunchback), **lordosis** (*lordo* = bent backward), and **scoliosis** (*scoli* = crooked).

Osteoporosis, sometimes referred to as **osteomalacia,** denotes increased porosity with softening of bones. This decrease in density results in brittleness and deformity accompanied by rheumatic pain. A **bunion** is a deviation of the big toe toward the second toe, with formation of a bursa and callus at the bony prominence of the first metatarsal bone.

An inflammation of bone is called **osteitis.** Inflammation of the bone marrow and adjoining bone is **osteomyelitis** (*osteo* = bone, plus *myel* = marrow). It can be caused by direct infection of the bone by an outside source or can result from spread of an infection from nearby tissue, as is sometimes seen after surgical reduction of a fracture. **Osteochondritis** (*chon* = cartilage) denotes inflammation of a bone and its cartilage.

Tumors of the bone can be benign such as an **exostosis** (*ex-* meaning out,-*osis* meaning condition), **osteoma, osteochondroma,** or **bunion.** Malignant bone tumors include **osteosarcoma,** also known as osteogenic sarcoma and **Ewing's sarcoma.** The most common joint disorders are arthritis, fibrositis, gout, immune disorders, trauma, tumors, and infections.

The general term for inflammation of a joint is **arthritis** (*arthro* = joint, *itis* = inflammation). It occurs most commonly in joints of the hands, knees, hips, low back, and

Table 7.2—Common Disorders of the Musculoskeletal System

Bones	fractures
	herniated disk
	hydrocephalus
	kyphosis, lordosis, scoliosis
	spina bifida
Joints and Surrounding Areas	fibrositis
	bone lesions
	bursitis
	soft tissue inflammation
	tendonitis
Joints, Cartilage, and Ligaments	acromegaly and other metabolic disorders
	degenerative joint disease (osteoarthritis)
	trauma
Joints and Synovium	ankylosing spondylitis
	gout
	rheumatoid arthritis
	psoriasis
	Reiter's syndrome
	scleroderma
	septic infections
	serum sickness
	synovial trauma
	synovitis
	systemic lupus erythematosus
Muscles	alcoholic myopathy
	amyotrophic lateral sclerosis
	botulism and other poisonings
	dermatomyositis
	hereditary adynamia
	metabolic myopathy
	myositis and other infections
	myasthenia gravis
	myotonia
	neural muscular atrophy (Charcot-Marie-Tooth disease)
	polymyositis
	progressive bulbar palsy
	progressive muscular dystrophy
	pyogenic abscess
	tetanus, tetany
	trauma: rupture, hemorrhage
	tumors

shoulders. The most common type of arthritis is **osteoarthritis (OA)** or degenerative joint disease **(DJD)**, which is a chronic, progressive, degenerative disease usually affecting the weight-bearing joints. A term likely to be associated with this disease is **Heberden's nodes,** pea-size enlargements of the fingers as the tubercles (small rounded protuberance on the bone) enlarge.

Rheumatoid arthritis (RA) is the most debilitating form of chronic or long-term arthritis. It is an inflammatory disease, most often affecting the fingers, wrists, and knees. Associated terms include **ankylosis,** which is a stiffening or fixation of a joint with fibrous or bony union across the joint, and **pannus** (from the Latin, "cloth") which is a membrane of granulation tissue covering the articular cartilages.

Spondylitis (*spondyl-* meaning "vertebra") is the term for inflammation of one or more vertebrae. **Ankylosing spondylitis,** also called Marie-Strumpell disease, denotes arthritis of the spine. It eventually leads to ossification (change into bone) of ligaments and bony bridging between the bodies or main parts of the vertebrae with irreversible skeletal immobility. Herniation of an intervertebral disk occurs when the cartilage pad protrudes into the spinal nerve or nerve canal. This condition is often referred to as a slipped disk.

Psoriatic arthritis is also an inflammatory arthritis occurring in association with psoriasis, lesions on the skin. **Reiter's syndrome** involves arthritis of the spine, along with inflammation of the urethra and iridocyclitis (iris and ciliary body of the eye). **Septic arthritis** or **infectious arthritis** is usually acquired from the blood but may also result from the spread of osteomyelitis to the joint. Lyme disease or arthritis is an inflammatory disorder with multiple symptoms involved; transfer is by a tick.

The term **gout** refers to a group of disorders displaying elevated uric acid blood levels (hyperuricemia), crystalline deposits in tissues (tophi), and recurrent episodes of acute (gouty) arthritis. **Chondrocalcinosis** results from deposits of calcium pyrophosphate dihydrate (CPPD) crystals in cartilage. **Pseudogout** is an acute inflammatory arthritis also involving CPPD crystals.

A **dislocation,** also known as a **luxation** (or when incomplete, a subluxation) occurs when two articulating surfaces become separated as a result of injury, associated disease, or a congenital disorder. It occurs most often in the shoulder joint and occasionally in the jaw. A **sprain** is the tearing of ligaments associated with sudden wrenching of a joint. This occurs most often in the ankle and is associated with loss of mobility and discoloration of the skin caused by hemorrhaging into the surrounding tissue. **Carpal tunnel syndrome (CTS)** occurs when the wrist ligament compresses the median nerve where it passes (tunnels) between the ligament and bones and tendons of the wrist (carpus).

Inflammation of the bursa, or **bursitis,** results from infection or physical stress related to activity or injury. It occurs most frequently near the shoulder, knee, and elbow.

Disorders of the tendons include **tendonitis,** which is an inflammation of the tendon and tendon sheath, usually from a sports injury or strain. It occurs most often in the shoulder area, hamstring, or calcaneal tendon. **Tennis elbow** is a term that refers to epicondylitis or inflammation of the tendon fibers or ligaments of the elbow joint.

Nonarticular rheumatism designates a group of disorders that affect the fascia, tendons, ligaments, bursae, and intervertebral disks. The **fibromyalgia syndrome** is the most common of these, causing generalized muscle aching, joint pain and stiffness, fatigue, paresthesias, and irritable bowel syndrome.

Systemic lupus erythematosus (SLE) is a chronic inflammatory disorder that involves the joints as well as connective tissue—tendons, ligaments, bones, and cartilage. Another rheumatic disease is **scleroderma** (*sclerosis,* meaning "hard," plus *derma,* "skin"), causing sclerosis of the skin and some organs.

Diseases of the muscles include infections, muscular dystrophy, myasthenia gravis, tetanus, and hernias (see Table 7.2).

Myositis (containing the root *myo-,* meaning "muscle") denotes inflammation of a muscle. **Polymyositis** and **dermatomyositis** are specific inflammatory muscle disorders (myopathies) of unknown cause. Polymyositis causes proximal muscle weakness; this is accompanied by a skin rash in dermatomyositis.

Muscular dystrophy is a general term for degeneration of muscles as the result of a group of inherited diseases. This disorder, usually beginning in childhood, is characterized by degeneration and reduction in size of muscle fibers with an increase in connective tissue and fat deposits. The most common form is called **Duchenne's dystrophy,** where muscles enlarge as fat replaces those that have degenerated or atrophied.

Myasthenia gravis is a disease related to improper transmission of nerve impulses at the neuromuscular junction. As a result, any muscular exertion causes extreme fatigue. It is fatal when respiratory muscles fail (see Chapter 12 for further discussion).

Although **tetanus** or lockjaw is a disease affecting the nervous system, it may also be classified as musculoskeletal because it produces spasms and painful convulsions of the skeletal muscles. Tetanus is caused by infection by *Clostridium tetani* bacteria, which may be introduced into a puncture wound, cut, or burn by contamination with infected soil.

A **hernia** or rupture is the protrusion of any organ or body part through the muscular wall that should contain it. The most common are **inguinal** hernias, so named because they occur in the inguinal region (the area of the groin), and they usually occur in males. **Hiatal** hernias develop from a defect in the diaphragm that allows part of the stomach to pass through an opening for the esophagus into the thoracic cavity. **Femoral** hernias just below the groin involve a portion of the bladder and peritoneum, most frequently in females. **Umbilical** hernias protruding at the naval are most common in newborns, obese females, and females following multiple pregnancies. An **incisional** hernia forms around an improperly healing surgical wound.

Myalgia denotes pain in a muscle. Injury can involve **myorrhexis,** a tear in the muscle, or **myostasis,** stretching. Muscular spasms may cause **myotonus** or myospasm.

Myoma is a benign tumor of muscular tissue. Malignant muscle tumors include **myosarcoma, leiomyosarcoma,** and **rhabdomyosarcoma.**

Diagnosis and Therapy

Orthopedics (*ortho-* from the Greek *orthos,* meaning correct or straight) is the term for the medical specialty that corrects deformities caused by disease or damage to the bones and joints. Similarly, **orthodontics** (Greek *odous,* tooth) refers to the branch of dentistry concerned with the correction and prevention of irregularities and malocclusion of the teeth. An **orthopedist** or **orthopedic surgeon** and **orthodontist** are the specialists in these fields.

A fracture in the bone undergoes several stages of healing after the fragments of the broken bone are manipulated or **reduced** back to their original position. The bone is usually then **immobilized** by a splint, cast, or traction. Follow-up **surgery** and/or **physical therapy** are sometimes necessary. Procedural terms relating to treatment of bones include manipulation, skeletal traction, percutaneous skeletal fixation, bone grafts, amputation, and **osteoplasty.** Photon **absorptiometry** and bone scans are diagnostic procedures.

The primary treatment for vertebral column injuries is **immobilization** to allow the bone to heal and prevent damage to the spinal cord. **Surgery** is performed when needed to repair severe damage to the vertebrae or tissues or to relieve pressure.

Treatment of a herniated disk usually consists of **bedrest, heat** applications, an **exercise** program, and sometimes **traction** with **muscle relaxant** or **analgesic** medications. If these therapies are not effective, a **laminectomy** may be performed to remove the protruding nucleus pulposus.

In addition to the symptoms of fever, swelling, erythema, and bone tenderness in the affected area, osteomyelitis is usually diagnosed based on a significant increase in the number of **leukocytes** (white blood cells) along with an elevated **erythrocyte sedimentation rate** (ESR). The infecting organism is usually present in the blood and identified by a **blood culture.** Such a culture is generally tested with a variety of agents to indicate to which **antibiotics** the organism is sensitive or resistant. Besides the appropriate spectrum, of course, the selected antibiotic must have the ability to penetrate into the bone to effectively treat osteomyelitis.

Diagnostic procedures involving the joints include **arthroscopy,** visual examination of the inside of a joint, also used for repairs; **arthrography,** injection of contrast material into a joint with X-ray visualization; and **arthrocentesis,** puncture of a joint space for removal of synovial fluid.

Joint dislocation is treated with **reduction** or relocation to prevent muscle spasm, swelling, and further damage to surrounding tissues. **Immobilization** may also be required. Treatment of joint damage has traditionally been by immobilization; however, a technique called **continuous passive motion** (CPM) is now being utilized following surgical procedures to stimulate the flow of synovial fluid and prevent adhesion of cartilage to the synovial membrane.

Several laboratory tests are used in the diagnosis of rheumatoid arthritis. The first is usually the ESR, which indicates the presence of an inflammatory response. Another test associated with a systemic inflammatory response is the **C-reactive protein** (CRP). **Serum immunoglobulin levels** can also be measured to detect acute or chronic inflammation. Antibodies called rheumatoid factors are increased during the chronic infections that can lead to rheumatoid arthritis; therefore, the immunoglobulins **IgG** and **IgM** are often measured. Autoantibodies directed against nuclear and/or cytoplasmic (*cyt* = cell) antigens are often found in serum when rheumatic diseases are present; therefore, the **antinuclear antibody** (ANA) test will often be ordered. The earliest **X-ray** evidence of rheumatoid arthritis is soft tissue swelling, followed by osteoporosis around the affected joint. Large cystic erosions can be seen in advanced disease.

Basic treatment of rheumatoid arthritis involves rest **(splinting),** passive exercise and heat, and emotional support. **Anti-inflammatory** and **analgesic** agents are used for pain and management of inflammation. If this is not sufficient, **gold salts, methotrexate, antimalarial** drugs, **penicillamine, azathioprine,** or **corticosteroids** may be effective. Surgical procedures include **joint replacement** and **synovectomy.**

Osteoarthritis is diagnosed by symptoms in the affected joints. **Crepitation** (meaning ''crackling'') can be heard on joint motion. Osteoarthritis has no specific laboratory features allowing identification. It is characterized by normal values for ESR, serum complement levels, synovial fluid analysis, and blood count. Management of osteoarthritis requires several approaches including exercise, orthoses and adaptive devices, analgesics and anti-inflammatory agents, and, in some patients, reconstructive joint surgery.

Gout is diagnosed by its painful arthritis, most frequently in the first toe joint (the metatarsophalangeal joint between the metatarsal and phalanx), along with an elevated **serum urate** level (**hyperuricemia**) and eventually **tophi** deposits and kidney stones (**nephrolithiasis**). If the uric acid level is not elevated, analysis of **synovial fluid** will still show urate crystals in the white blood cells. Acute gout is treated with **colchicine, nonsteroidal anti-inflammatory agents,** or **corticosteroids.** For recurrent episodes, **uricosuric** agents such as probenecid and sulfinpyrazone are utilized to prevent increased serum urate levels. **Allopurinol** is used to decrease uric acid production. Additional terms associated with this disorder include **monosodium urate, purines,** and **podagra.**

No laboratory tests are specific for ankylosing spondylitis. The **sedimentation rate, alkaline phosphatase,** and the genotype **HLA-B27** are used for a possible association. Treatment is with a vigorous exercise program and cautious use of **nonsteroidal antiinflammatory agents** (NSAIDs).

Systemic lupus erythematosus is diagnosed by presentation of a number of clinical symptoms, most commonly arthralgia (*arth* = joint, *algia* = pain) and arthritis. Laboratory tests show abnormal ANA titer, positive LE cell test. Several different drugs are utilized in the treatment of systemic lupus erythematosus. **Aspirin** and the **NSAIDs** are used to manage arthralgias or synovitis (inflammation of the synovium), pleurisy, headache, and low-grade fever. The antimalarial agent **hydroxychloroquine** is effective in treating arthralgias, arthritis, and skin disease. **Corticosteroids** are used to control the inflammatory response. Connective tissue disorders are treated by rest and exercise, physical and occupational therapy, heat, supportive or rehabilitative devices, education, nutrition, and orthopedic surgery.

Polymyositis and dermatomyositis are diagnosed by measuring the **creatinine phosphokinase** (CPK); **ANA** and **rheumatoid factor** (RF) are present in some cases.

Electromyogram (EMG) findings are abnormal. A **muscle biopsy** can confirm diagnosis by showing degeneration of muscle fibers. Treatment of these diseases includes **physical therapy, corticosteroids,** and **immunosuppressive agents** if necessary.

Scleroderma is often diagnosed by what is called the **CREST** syndrome, the presence of calcinosis, Raynaud's phenomenon, esophageal dysfunction, sclerodactyly, and telangiectasia. Since there is no specific treatment, general supportive therapy is indicated.

Treatment of muscular dystrophy generally includes **exercises, physical therapy, braces,** and sometimes **surgery;** however, progressive deterioration cannot be permanently stopped.

Treatment for tetanus consists primarily of prevention with the combined vaccine for diphtheria, pertussis, and tetanus (DPT), which is given to children as a permanent **immunization** against the disease.

Traditionally less utilized treatment approaches for musculoskeletal disorders of all types include relaxation therapy, thermotherapy, kerotherapy, massotherapy, naprapathy, electrotherapy, fangotherapy, fomentation, diathermy, and crenotherapy.

Surgical procedures involving the musculoskeletal system are summarized in Table 7.3.

Physical Medicine and Rehabilitation

The medical specialty of physical medicine and rehabilitation (**PM & R**), although not limited entirely to the musculoskeletal system, can be considered within this context

Table 7.3—Common Surgical Procedures of the Musculoskeletal System

Bones	autogenous bone graft
	osteotomy
	diaphysectomy
	osteoplasty
	scapulopexy
	sequestrectomy
	skeletal fixation
	skeletal traction
Joints and Surrounding Areas	arthrectomy
	arthrocentesis
	arthrodesis
	arthroplasty
	arthrotomy
	condylectomy
	meniscectomy
	synovectomy
Muscles	myectomy
	myotomy
Tendons	tenolysis
	enotomy
General	amputation
	cheiroplasty

Table 7.4—Terms Associated with Physical Medicine and Rehabilitation

apraxia	goniometer
asthenia	hydrotherapy
ataxia	hypokinesia
atonic	isometric
balneotherapy	isotonic
crenotherapy	kerotherapy
diathermy	kinesalgia
dynamometer	massotherapy
dyskinesia	orthosis
dyslalia	prosthesis
dyslogia	psychrotherapy
ergometry	relaxation therapy
fangotherapy	thermotherapy
fluidotherapy	
fomentation	

because of the extent of involvement with the bones, joints, and other supporting structures of the body.

Physiatrics is that branch of medicine concerned with diagnosis and treatment of disease of the neuromuscular system with physical elements (heat, cold, water, electricity, etc.) to bring about maximal restoration of physical, physiological, social, and vocational function. A **physiatrist** is a physician who specializes in physiatry. Other health care practitioners in this field include physical therapists (PTs), occupational therapists (OTs), speech pathologists, and vocational counselors.

Conditions commonly treated that should be familiar to the pharmacist are, first, those associated with recovery from cerebrovascular accidents: **hemiplegia,** or **hemiparesis, aphasia,** and **dysphasia;** second, conditions of paralysis from trauma such as **paraplegia** and **quadriplegia;** and third, post**amputations** of the extremities.

Treatment modalities include the employment of **orthotic** and **prosthetic** (from the Greek, ''placed instead'') devices, as well as a number of therapies. Terms often encountered within this realm are listed in Table 7.4 and defined in the glossary.

Abbreviations relating to the musculoskeletal system in general are listed in Table 7.5.

Table 7.5—Abbreviations Associated with the Musculoskeletal System

AAROM	active assistive range of motion	**BJ**	bone and joint
ADL	activities of daily living	**BJM**	bone, joint, muscles
ADR	acute dystonic reaction	**BK**	below-knee
AE	above elbow (amputation)	**BKA**	below-knee amputation
AFO	ankle–foot orthosis	**BMT**	bone marrow transplant
AGA	acute gonococcal arthritis	**CaBI**	calcium bone index
AGE	angle of greatest extension	**CCF**	compound comminuted fracture
AGF	angle of greatest flexion	**CDH**	congenital dysplasia of the hip
AIMS	arthritis impact measure scale	**CDLE**	chronic discoid lupus erythematosus
AINS	anti-inflammatory nonsteroidal	**CLC**	cork, leather, and elastic (orthotic)
AK	above-knee	**CMJ**	carpometacarpal joint
AKA	above-knee amputation	**CORF**	comprehensive outpatient rehabilitation facility
ALS	amyotrophic lateral sclerosis	**CP**	chondromalacia patella
AMG	acoustic myography	**CPA**	costophrenic angle
AMP	amputation	**CPM**	continuous passive motion
A-Mpr	Austin-Moore prosthesis	**CPPB**	continuous positive pressure breathing
APL	abductor pollicis longus	**CPPV**	continuous positive pressure ventilation
AROM	active range of motion	**CREST**	calcinosis, Raynaud's phenomenon, esophageal dysmotility, sclerodactyly, and telangiectasia
AS	ankylosing spondylitis		
ATL	Achilles tendon lengthening		
ATNR	asymmetrical tonic neck reflux		
ATR	Achilles tendon reflex	**CRST**	calcinosis, Raynaud's phenomenon, scleroderma, and telangiectasia
BC	bone conduction		
BDAE	Boston Diagnostic Aphasia Examination		
BE	below elbow		
BFO	balanced forearm orthosis		
BIH	bilateral inguinal hernia		

CRUMBS	continuous remote, unobtrusive monitoring of biobehavioral systems
CTR	carpal tunnel release
CVA	costovertebral angle
CVAT	costovertebral tenderness
D1,D2	dorsal vertebra #1, #2
DDD	degenerative disk disease
DEXA	dual energy X-ray absorptiometry
DILE	drug-induced lupus erythematosus
DIP	distal interphalangeal
DISH	diffuse idiopathic skeletal hyperostosis
DJD	degenerative joint disease
DLE	discoid lupus erythematosus
DM	dermatomyositis
DMARD	disease-modifying antirheumatic drug
DMD	Duchenne's muscular dystrophy
DMX	diathermy, massage, and exercise
DTR	deep tendon reflexes
EAST	external rotation, abduction stress test
ECEMG	evoked compound electromyography
ECRL	extensor carpi radialis longus
ECU	extensor carpi ulnaris
EDF	extension, derotation, flexion
EMF	electromotive force
EMG	electromyelogram
EORA	early onset rheumatoid arthritis
EPB	extensor pollicis brevis
EPL	extensor pollicis longus
EPS	electrophysiologic study
ESR	erythrocyte sedimentation rate; electric skin resistance
FCC	fracture compound and comminuted
FCMD	Fukiyama's congenital muscular dystrophy
FCR	flexor carpi radialis brevis
FCU	flexor carpi ulnaris
FDP	flexor digitorum profundus
FDS	flexor digitorum superficialis
FES	functional electrical stimulation
FIM	functional independent measure
FMH	fibromuscular hyperplasia
FPB	flexor pollicis brevis
FPL	flexor pollicis longus
FRJM	full range of joint motion
FROM	full range of movement
FSHMD	facioscapulohumeral muscular dystrophy
FWB	full weight bearing
FWW	front wheel walker
Fx	fracture
FXR	fracture
HD	hip disarticulation
HH	hiatal hernia
HIVD	herniated intervertebral disc
HKAFO	hip-knee-ankle-foot orthosis
HKO	hip-knee orthosis
HLD	herniated lumbar disc
HMX	heat massage exercise
HNP	herniated nucleus pulposus
HP	hemiplegia
HS	heel spur
HV	hallux valgus
ICM	intracostal margin
ICS	intercostal space
ICT	inflammation of connective tissue
IH	inguinal hernia
IM	intramuscular, intrametatarsal
IMF	intermaxillary fixation
IPJ	interphalangeal joint
ISMA	infantile spinal muscular atrophy
JAMA	juvenile autoimmune myasthenia gravis
JDMS	juvenile dermatomyositis
JF	joint fluid
KAFO	knee-ankle-foot orthosis
KAO	knee-ankle orthosis
KBM	a below-knee prosthesis
KD	knee disarticulation
L1,L2	lumbar vertebra #1, #2
LAC	long arm cast
LAPMS	long arm posterior molded splint
LBT	lupus band test
LE	lupus erythematosus
LED	lupus erythematosus disseminatus
LFA	low friction arthroplasty
LHP	left hemiparesis
LIH	left inguinal hernia
LLB	long leg brace
LLC	long leg cast
LLSB	left lower sternal border
LOM	limitation of motion
LORS	Level of Rehabilitation Scale
LOT	left occiput transverse
LRND	left radical neck dissection
L-S	lumbosacral
LSA	left sacrum anterior

LSB	left sternal border	RCM	right costal margin
LSP	left sacrum posterior	RES	rehabilitation evaluation system
LST	left sacrum transverse	RICE	rest and immobilization, ice, compression, elevation
LT	lumbar traction		
LVL	left vastus lateralis		
MAS	mobile arm support	RICS	right intercostal space
MCH	muscle contraction headache	RIH	right inguinal hernia
MCP	metacarpophalangeal joint	RLR	right lateral rectus
MCTD	mixed connective tissue disease	RM	repetitions maximum
		RMI	repetitive motion injuries
MD	muscular dystrophy	RMR	right medial rectus
MG	myasthenia gravis	RND	radical neck dissection
MLF	median longitudinal fasiculus	ROA	right occiput anterior
MMT	manual muscle test	ROM	range of motion
MP	metacarpal phalangeal joint	ROP	right occiput posterior
MPJ	metacarpophalangeal joint	ROT	right occipital transverse
MS	musculoskeletal; muscle strength	RPO	right posterior oblique
		RRND	right radical neck dissection
MSR	muscle stretch reflexes	RS	Reiter/Reye's syndrome
MSS	muscular subaortic stenosis	SAARD	slow-acting antirheumatic drugs
MTP	metatarsal phalangeal		
NMD	normal muscle development	SAC	short arm cast
NSAID	nonsteroidal anti-inflammatory drug	SACH	solid ankle cushion heel
		SAFE	stationary attachment and flexible endoskeletal (prosthesis)
OA	osteoarthritis		
OMT	osteopathic manipulative treatment	SB	spina bifida
		SCLE	subcutaneous lupus erythematosus
ORIF	open reduction internal fixation		
		SC/SP	supracondylar/suprapatellar prosthesis
OT	occupational therapy/therapist		
OTR	occupational therapist, registered	SIG	sacroiliac joint
		SKA	supracondylar knee-ankle orthosis
PACO	pivot ambulating crutchless orthosis		
		SLB	short leg brace
PID	prolapsed intervertebral disc	SLC	short leg cast
PIP	proximal interphalangeal joint	SLE	systemic lupus erythematosus
PIVD	protruded intervertebral disc		
PLS	primary lateral sclerosis	SLRT	straight leg raising cast
PMF	progressive massive fibrosis	SLWC	short leg walking cast
PMR	physical medicine and rehabilitation	SMA	spinal muscular atrophy
		SMR	skeletal muscle relaxant
POS	parosteal osteosarcoma	SPMA	spinal progressive muscle atrophy
POSM	patient-operated selector mechanism		
		STJ	subtalar joint
PP	proximal phalynx	T1,T2	thoracic vertebra #1, #2
PPD	posterior polymorphous dystrophy	TAA	total ankle arthroplasty
		TAL	tendon Achilles lengthening
PRE	progressive/passive resistive exercise	TARA	total articular replacement arthroplasty
PROM	passive range of motion		
PsA	psoriatic arthritis	TEA	total elbow arthroplasty
PSF	posterior spinal fusion	THA	total hip arthroplasty
PT	physical therapy/therapist	THR	total hip replacement
PTA	physical therapy assistant	TKA	total knee arthroplasty
PTB	patellar tendon bearing	TKR	total knee replacement
RA	rheumatoid arthritis	TMJ	temporomandibular joint

TORP	total ossicular replacement prosthesis	USB	upper sternal border
		UTO	upper tibial osteotomy
TSA	total shoulder arthroplasty	YORA	younger-onset rheumatoid arthritis
TSR	total shoulder replacement		
TTA	total toe arthroplasty		

Pronouncing Glossary

Root	Meaning	Example	Pronunciation
acro-	extremity	acromion	ah KRO me an
ankylo-	bent, crooked	ankylosis	ANK ki LO sis
arth-	joint	arthrodesis	ar thro DEE sis
brachi-	arm	brachialgia	brak ee AL ja
calcaneo-	heel	calcaneodynia	kal KA ne o DIN ee a
caudo-	tail	caudal	KAW dull
cheiro-	hand	cheiroplasty	KI ro plas ti
chiro-		chiropractic	ki ro PRAK tic
chondr-	cartilage	chondromalacia	kon dro mah LAY-shee ah
cleido-	clavicle	cleidocranial	kli do KRAN ee al
costa-	rib	costophrenic	kost oh FREN ik
coxa-	hip	coxalgia	kox AL ja
crani-	skull	craniotomy	kran ee OT oh mee
dactylo-	finger, toe	dactylitis	dak tee LI tis
desmo-	ligament	desmodynia	des mo DIN ee ah
fibro-	fiber	fibroblast	FI bro blast
gnath-	jaw	gnathoplasty	NATH oh plas tee
ilio-	ilium	iliofemoral	il ee oh fem OR al
leio-	smooth	leiomyoma	LI oh my O ma
myel-	marrow	myelitis	MI ehl eye tis
myo-	muscle	myocardium	my oh KARD ee um
omo-	shoulder	omodynia	ohm oh DINN ee ah
orth-	straight, correct	orthopedic	or tho PEED ik

Root	Meaning	Example	Pronunciation
oss-	bone	osseous	OSS ee us
osteo-		osteoporosis	ost ee oh pur O sis
pelvi-	pelvis	pelvioplasty	PEL vee o plas tee
pero-	deformed	peroneal	per o NE al
pubo-	pubic	pubofemoral	PU bo FEM or al
rachi-	spine	rachicentesis	rak ee sin TEE sis
radio-	radius	radiocarpal	RA dee o CAR pal
rheum-	watery discharge	rheumatoid	ROO mah toy d
sacro-	sacrum	sacroiliac	say kro ILL ee ak
scapulo-	scapula	scapulopexy	SKAP u lo PEX ee
spondyl-	vertebra	spondylitis	spon dee LI tis
sterno-	breastbone	sternocostal	STER no KOS tal
tendo-	tendon	tendonitis	ten do NI tes
tibio-	tibia	tibiofemoral	TIB e oh fem OR al

Glossary

absorptiometry—procedure for determining the amount of gas absorbed by a given quantity

adynamia—weakness, loss of normal vitality

amputation—the surgical removal of a limb or other projecting part

ankylosing spondylitis—rheumatoid arthritis of the spine

ankylosis—stiffening or fixation of a joint

antihyperuricemic—indicating a drug or mode of treatment that reduces uric acid in the blood

aphasia—impaired or absent communication by speech, writing, or signs, caused by dysfunction of brain centers

appendicular—referring to the appendix or dependent part attached to a main structure

apraxia—a disorder of voluntary movement with inability to execute purposeful movements

arthralgia—severe pain in a joint

arthritis—inflammation of a joint

arthrocentesis—aspiration into a joint; withdrawal of fluid through a puncture needle

asthenia—weakness or debility

ataxia—inability to coordinate the muscles in execution of voluntary movement

atonic—relaxed, without normal tone or tension

atrophy—wasting of tissues or organs

axial—relating to or situated in the central part of the body

balneotherapy—treatment by baths

bone—a hard tissue consisting of cells in a matrix of ground substance and collagen fibers

bone scan—use of an ultrasonic beam to mark or trace structure of a bone

bunion—a localized swelling of the first metatarsophalangeal joint resulting in displacement of the toe

bursitis—inflammation of the bursa

carpal—relating to the wrist

cartilage—specialized connective tissue characterized by its nonvascularity and firm consistency

chondrocalcinosis—calcification of cartilage

chrysotherapy—treatment of disease by the administration of gold salts

clavicle—collarbone; a doubly curved long bone that forms part of the shoulder girdle

coccyx—tail bone

cranium—skull

C-reactive protein—a beta-globulin found in the serum of individuals with inflammatory, degenerative, and neoplastic diseases

crenotherapy—treatment by mineral water

dermatomyositis—a condition characterized by muscular weakness and necrosis with a nonspecific eczematous inflammation of the skin

diaphysis—the shaft of a long bone

diathermy—therapeutic healing of a body part by conversion of high-frequency electrical current

dynamometer—ergometer; an instrument for measuring the degree of muscular power

dyskinesia—difficulty in performing voluntary movements

dyslalia—disorder of articulation

dyslogia—impairment in the power of speech

dysphasia—lack of coordination in speech and failure to communicate understandably

dystrophy—defective nutrition

Ewing's sarcoma—a connective tissue neoplasm; a malignancy of the bones of the extremities

electromyogram—a graphic recording of the somatic electric currents associated with muscular action

electrotherapy—includes diathermy, ultrasound, infrared and ultraviolet radiation, and so on

endosteum—a thin membrane lining the inner surface of bone in the central medullary cavity

epicondylitis—infection or inflammation of an epicondyle, a projection from a long bone near the articular extremity above or upon the condyle

epiphysis—the end of a long bone distinct from the shaft or separated from it by a layer of cartilage

ergometry—measurement of the amount of work done by muscular contractions

erythema—inflammatory redness of the skin

ESR—erythrocyte sedimentation rate; the rate at which red blood cells settle out of suspension in blood plasma measured under standardized conditions

exostosis—a cartilage-shaped bony projection

fangotherapy—therapeutic application of mud of volcanic origin as packs or baths

fascia—a sheet of fibrous tissue that envelops the body beneath the skin and encloses the muscles and various body organs

femur—thigh bone

fibromyalgia—muscular pain stemming from fibrous tissue

fibrosis—the formation of fibrous tissue

fibrositis—inflammation of fibrous tissue

fibula—calf bone

fixation, percutaneous skeletal—placement of pins across the fracture site, usually under X-ray imaging

fluidotherapy—type of dry heat treatment for a hand or foot

fomentation—external application of a hot, moist substance or object

foramen—an opening into or through a bone or a membranous structure

fracture, Colles—break in the lower end of the radius with displacement

fracture, comminuted—fracture in which the bone is broken into pieces

fracture, green-stick—bending of a bone with incomplete fraction

fracture, impacted—fracture in which one of the fragments is driven into the tissue of the other fragment

goniometer—calibrated device designed to measure the arc or range of motion of a joint

gout—an arthritis caused by an inherited metabolic disorder characterized frequently by an elevated blood uric acid level

graft, bone—bone transplanted from a donor site to a recipient site

Heberden's nodes—hard nodules about the size of a pea found on the terminal phalanges of the fingers in osteoarthritis

hemarthrosis—blood in a joint

hemiparesis—slight paralysis affecting one side of the body only

hemiplegia—paralysis of one side of the body

hernia—the protrusion of an organ or part of an organ or other structure through the wall of the cavity normally containing it

humerus—the bone of the arm, articulating with the scapula above and the radius and ulna below

hydrotherapy—use of water by external application for pressure effect or as a means of applying physical energy to the tissues

hyperkinesia—excessive motility or muscular action

hyperuricemia—high levels of uric acid in the blood

hypokinesia—diminished or slow movement

hypotonia—a condition in which there is a diminution or loss of muscular activity

iliococcygeal—relating to the ilium and coccyx

interphalangeal—located between two phalanges, bones between joints of the fingers and toes

isometric—of equal measure; refers to activity of a muscle during which its length does not change

isotonic—of equal tone; refers to the activity of a muscle during which its tension (tone) remains constant while length changes

kerotherapy—treatment by external use of liquid paraffin

kinesalgia—pain occurring during muscle movement

kyphosis—an abnormal curvature of the spine, with convexity backward

ligament—a sheet of fibrous tissue connecting two or more bones, cartilage, or other structures or serving as support for muscles

lordosis—hollow or saddle back; anteroposterior curvature of the spine

luxation—dislocation

mandible—jaw bone

manipulation—attempted reduction or restoration of a fracture or joint dislocation to its normal anatomic alignment by the application of manual force

marrow—the soft, fatty substance filling the medullary cavities of the long bones

massotherapy—treatment by manipulation of soft tissues; massage

metacarpophalangeal—relating to the metacarpus, one of five bones of the hand between the carpus and the phalanges

metatarsophalangeal—relating to the metatarsal bones and the phalanges of the foot

monosodium urate—salt of a uric acid

muscle—tissue that consists microscopically predominantly of contractile cells

muscular dystrophy—abnormality of muscle associated with dysfunction and ultimately with deterioration

myasthenia gravis—a chronic progressive disorder of neuromuscular function

myopathy—any abnormal condition or disease of the muscular tissues

myositis—inflammation of a muscle

myotonia—delayed relaxation of a muscle after an initial contraction

nucleus pulposus—the soft fibrocartilage central portion of the intervertebral disk

orthosis—general term for a device applied to a part for a supportive, assistive, adaptive, preventive or corrective purpose

osteoarthritis—degenerative joint disease

osteochondroma—a benign cartilaginous neoplasm

osteoma—a benign neoplasm consisting of osteoblastic connective tissue

osteomyelitis—inflammation of the bone marrow and adjacent bone and epiphysial cartilage

osteopenia—abnormally reduced bone mass due to inadequate osteoid synthesis

osteoplasty—bone grafting; repair or plastic surgery of the bones

osteoporosis—atrophy of skeletal tissue

osteosarcoma—osteogenic sarcoma; most common and malignant of bone tumors, arising from bone-forming cells and affecting ends of long bones

paraplegia—paralysis of both lower extremities, usually including the trunk

periosteum—the thick fibrous membrane covering the entire surface of a bone except its articular cartilage

phalanges—bone between two joints of the fingers and toes

podagra—gout, especially of the big toe

polyarthritis—simultaneous inflammation of several joints

prosthesis—artificial part of the body

pseudogout—articular chondrocalcinosis; a disease characterized by calcified deposits in synovial fluid

psoriasis—a chronic hereditary skin condition characterized by the eruption of reddish, silvery-scaled maculopapules

psychrotherapy—treatment by the application of cold

quadriplegia—tetraplegia; paralysis of all four limbs

Reiter's syndrome—a seronegative spondyloarthritis characterized by arthritis along with inflammation of the urethra and conjunctiva

relaxation therapy—conscious education of the muscular tonus, aimed at achieving relaxation of the body, hence of the mind

rheumatism—an indefinite term applied to various conditions with pain or other symptoms of the musculoskeletal system

rheumatoid factor—globulins in the serum of patients with rheumatoid arthritis that enhance agglutination of suspended particles

sacrum—the segment of the vertebral column forming part of the pelvis

scapula—the shoulder blade

sclerodactyly—acrosclerosis; stiffness and tightness of the skin of the fingers with atrophy of the soft tissue and osteoporosis of the distal phalanges

scoliosis—lateral curvature of the spine

serositis—inflammation of a serous membrane

spina bifida—limited defect in the spinal column, with absence of the vertebral arches, through which the spinal membranes may protrude

spondyloarthritis—arthritis of the vertebrae

spondylodynia—pain in the spine

sternocostal—relating to the sternum and the ribs

sternum—the breastbone

subluxation—a dislocation where contact between joint surfaces remains

synovial fluid—a fluid that functions as a lubricant in a joint

synovectomy—excision of a portion or all of the synovial membrane of a joint

tarsal—relating to the instep of the foot

tendon—a fibrous cord or band that connects a muscle to a bone

tendonitis—inflammation of a tendon

tetanus—a disease marked by painful tonic muscular contractions, caused by the toxin of *Clostridium tetani*

thermotherapy—treatment by heat of any kind: hot air, hot water, hot pack, infrared radiation, diathermy

tibia—shin bone, shank bone

tophi—pleural of tophus, a deposit of uric acid and urates in fibrous tissue, cartilage of the external ear or kidney found in gout

traction, skeletal—use of pulling force on a bone fracture by use of a pin, screw, clamp, or wire inserted into the bone

vertebra—one of the segments of the spinal column

vertebrochondral—denoting the three false ribs that are connected with the vertebrae

The Integumentary (Dermatologic) System and Its Disorders

The integumentary system consists of the skin, glands, nails, and hair. The origin of the name of this system is the Latin word *integumentum,* which means "cover." In addition to covering and protecting the underlying tissues, the integumentary system also functions to regulate body temperature, excrete waste materials, serve as a sense organ, and convert and store nutrients.

Anatomy and Physiology

The skin, which covers the body's entire surface, is its largest organ. It is composed primarily of two layers. The outer layer is the **epidermis,** named for the prefix *epi-,* meaning "upon" (as in *epigastric,* the area "upon" the stomach, and *epidural,* on or over the dura mater) and the root *derm.* The second layer is the **dermis** or **corium,** the thicker layer of connective tissue beneath the epidermis and named for the Greek word for skin (see Figure 8.1).

The epidermis is composed of up to five layers called **strata.** There are no blood vessels in these epithelial tissues, and the epidermis contains the **melanocytes** that produce the pigment **melanin** and dead cells containing the fibrous protein **keratin.** Skin pigmentation results from the presence of melanin (*mela* = black), the yellow pigment **carotene** (the yellow pigment in carrots), and the color of blood reflected through the epidermis. The main function of melanin is to screen out excessive ultraviolet radiation. The thickness and number of these layers of the epidermis varies throughout the body.

The dermis or "true skin" is a strong, flexible meshwork of fibrous connective tissue. The upper or **papillary** layer derives its name from the Greek word for pimple, the same root denoting the bumps in a "maculopapular rash"; the papillary layer contains numerous small projections that join it to the epidermis. The lower reticular layer contains blood and lymph vessels, nerves, fat (or **adipose** cells), oil glands, and hair roots (see Figure 8.1).

The **hypodermis** or subcutaneous layer of loose, fibrous connective tissue lies below the dermis. It contains lymph and blood vessels, nerves, sweat gland ducts, and hair follicle bases, as well as the adipose cells.

The **sudoriferous** or **sweat glands** are found over almost the entire surface of the skin, particularly on the palms of the hands and soles of the feet. These glands function to regulate body temperature. There are two types of sweat glands; the eccrine glands are embedded in the hypodermis, and the apocrine glands are found in the armpits, dark

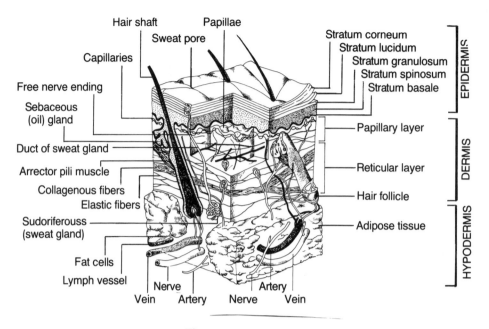

Figure 8.1—The Skin.
A "textbook" drawing of skin structure, showing components in an ideal arrangement.

region around the nipples, and the anal and genital regions. Apocrine glands are larger and more deeply located than the eccrine glands and respond to stress rather than heat. The female breasts are apocrine glands that have adapted to the secretion of milk rather than sweat. For this reason, study of the breasts is sometimes included in the integumentary system.

Hair grows out of the hair **follicles** in the epidermis. It is composed of threads of cells that function in protection from temperature and injury. The **sebaceous** (oil) glands are located between a hair follicle and a strip of smooth muscle and are found throughout the body, except on the palms and soles. These secrete the fatty substance **sebum** to lubricate the skin and help protect it from the elements. Activity of these glands is low until puberty.

The nails arise from the epidermis. They are composed mostly of a semitransparent **keratin** plate surrounded proximally and laterally by folds of skin.

The sensory information provided by the skin is caused by the abundant supply of sensory nerve fibers, along with autonomic fibers that innervate secreting glands, smooth muscle, and blood vessels. The primary sensations are pain, pressure, touch and temperature. Itching is also associated with the pain receptors.

Blood supply in the skin provides nourishment and also functions in regulation of body temperature and blood pressure.

Words describing the integumentary system often include the roots *cutis* or *derm,* both of which mean skin. The term **dermatology** is used to denote the study or diagnosis and treatment of the integumentary system (the suffix *-ology* means "study of"). A **dermatologist** is a physician specializing in the diagnosis and treatment of skin disorders. Similarly, **dermatitis** is the general term referring to any inflammation of the skin. Words containing the root *onycho* refer to a condition involving the nails, such as **onychosis,** which is any disease or deformity of the nails. Most terms relating to hair include the word parts *pilo*-such as **pilosis** (excessive development of hair) and pilosebaceous (relating to the hair follicles and their associated sebaceous glands) or *tricho*-as in trichomycosis (any hair disease caused by a fungal infection) or **trichosis** (any disease of the hair).

Therapeutics

Diseases

Alterations in the skin are collectively termed **lesions.** There are several types of lesions that can be classified in two primary ways—by the level of elevation or depression in relation to the normal skin or by the component of the skin that is primarily involved. Terms that should be recognized as types of skin lesions include **macule** (freckle), **papule** (pimple), **plaque, vesicle** (blister), **bulla, pustule** (abscess), **nodule, cyst, ulcer, wheal** (hive), **scale,** and **crust.** A number of terms will be found in the medical literature to further describe shape, surface features, color, etiology, or other condition of these lesions. These terms include **symmetrical, scaling, erythematous** (red), **macerated** (softened by soaking), **pyogenic** (pus producing), **exudative** (leaking fluid and cellular debris), **atopic** (caused by a hereditary predisposition to an allergic reaction), **allergic, exfoliative** (falling off in layers or scales), **circumscribed** (surrounded with a distinct edge), **ulcerated, purulent** (containing pus), indolent (slow growing, causing little pain), **necrotic** (containing dead tissue), **ecchymoses** (small, nonelevated hemorrhagic spots) and **purpura** (purplish or brownish red hemorrhagic spots). Diseases associated with the various types of skin lesions are numerous and are included in Table 8.1 to provide an indication of their relation to dermatology. A few are discussed in greater detail because the terms appear so commonly in the medical literature or are related to other terms with which pharmacists should be familiar.

Psoriasis is a chronic skin disease characterized by recurring exacerbations and remissions of thick, scaly lesions. The cause is unknown. **Desquamation** (*squama* meaning scale) is the term for scaling of the skin or cuticle. Another term for shedding of the skin is **keratolysis** (*kerat* = horny, plus *lysis* = loosening). **Xerosis,** a condition of "dry skin," is derived from the root *xero*-meaning dry and the suffix-*osis* denoting state of or disease. **Hidrosis,** the formation and excretion of perspiration (*hidros* = sweat), more commonly refers to excessive sweating. Conversely, **anhidrosis** is an abnormal deficiency of perspiration.

A number of skin infections occur in various locations throughout the integumentary system. An organism may infect only the outer layers of the skin, causing a superficial infection. For example, **folliculitis** is a superficial inflammation of hair follicles. Similarly, **erysipelas** is an infection of the superficial layers of the skin caused by group A *Streptococcus*. It is usually seen on the face as a bright raised lesion with sharply demarcated edges. **Impetigo** is another superficial infection of the skin, also usually caused by group A *Streptococcus*, although it may be staphylococcal. Impetigo starts as a red patch and develops into small pustules, which may join and form yellow, crusty sores. Other skin infections are deeper. **Furuncles** (commonly called boils) and **carbuncles** (groups of furuncles with common drainage channels) are subcutaneous abscesses caused by an infection with *Staphylococcus aureus*. **Cellulitis** is an infection of the deeper layers

Table 8.1—Common Disorders of the Integumentary System

allergic responses:	eczematous dermatitis	
	poison ivy	
	poison oak	
	poison sumac	
	psoriasis	
skin infections:	bacterial:	acne vulgaris
		carbuncle
		cellulitis
		dermatitis
		dermatophytosis
		ecthyma gangrenosum
		folliculitis
		furuncle
		impetigo
		pyoderma gangrenosum
	fungal:	candidiasis
		tinea (ringworm)
	parasite:	pediculosis (lice)
		scabies (mites)
	virus:	Herpes simplex
		Rickettsial pox
		Varicella-zoster
skin lesions:	pemphigus	
	pityriasis rosea	
	scleroderma	
skin growths:	nevus	
	keratosis	
	lipoma	
	sebaceous cyst	
	steatoma	
	verrucae	
	basal cell epithelioma/carcinoma	
	malignant melanoma	
	squamous cell carcinoma	
pressure sores:	decubitus ulcer	
	stasis ulceration	
	diabetic ulceration	
skin trauma:	burns	
	bruises	
	solar elastosis	

of the skin, usually seen in the lower extremities after injury to the skin. **Ecthyma gangrenosum** manifests as a vesicle or papule with an erythematous halo that develops into a necrotic ulcer. It indicates the presence of a gram-negative rod infection. The most common fungal infection is **tinea pedis,** also known as **athlete's foot.** Mild infection may cause slight erythema and scaling along with mild pruritus and peeling. More severe forms may be macerated, edematous, vesicular, and more pruritic and painful.

Acne vulgaris is the primary disease of the sebaceous glands in humans. It is characterized by a variety of inflammatory and noninflammatory lesions including **comedones** ("blackheads" or "whiteheads"), nodules, papules, pustules, and cysts. This condition is believed to develop from primary inflammation in the follicle wall that ruptures, spreading the inflammatory process.

Ulcers occur when the epidermis and papillary layer of the dermis are destroyed. These are found most frequently on the legs and feet, usually from disturbances in circulation. **Pressure sores** (also called **bedsores** or **decubitus ulcers**) occur at weight-bearing sites when movement is severely limited. Patients who remain in a lying position will rapidly develop skin necrosis at the sacrum, spine, and heels, causing bedsores. Those on their sides will ulcerate in the hip area. **Stasis ulcers** occur with swelling in the lower extremities, the ulcer being formed as a result of stasis of the blood.

Pruritus is the medical term for itching. This can occur in response to a localized lesion, as a symptom of systemic disease, or in reaction to stress.

Disorders of melanin pigmentation are classified as **hypomelanosis** (*hypo* = low, *osis* = condition; thus, relative lack of melanin) or **hypermelanosis** (presence of increased melanin). **Albinism** is an extreme example of hypomelanosis; others include **phenylketonuria** and **vitiligo.** Both freckles (**ephelides**) and moles (**nevi**) are types of hypermelanosis.

A number of skin changes and disorders are caused by exposure to ultraviolet radiation from the sun. The **sunburn** reaction is a complex inflammatory process, including swelling and capillary leakage. Skin cancer is also known to be caused by solar radiation, as are degenerative changes of the skin such as wrinkling, **keratoses, telangiectasia,** and **atrophy.** Cutaneous **photosensitivity** is a general term for any abnormal reaction of the skin to the stimulus of light. A large number of chemicals, including many drugs, also can produce this reaction.

Hypersensitivity to food, drugs, or physical agents; infections; or stress may produce a transient condition called **urticaria,** commonly referred to as "hives." This is a reaction of the blood vessels with the appearance of slightly elevated red or pale patches or wheals accompanied by severe itching. Allergic **contact dermatitis** is most often caused by poison ivy. Poison oak and sumac contain the same sensitizing oleoresin and produce the same inflammation. Typically, the rash is erythematous, vesicular, and sometimes oozing and ulcerated. Other agents that frequently cause allergic contact dermatitis include soaps, detergents, and fragrances. The term *contact dermatitis* is also frequently used generically for any skin inflammation, even without a hypersensitivity reaction; for example, a reaction to a caustic may sometimes be described as a contact dermatitis, although the term technically should be reserved for allergic reactions.

Many adverse drug reactions are most commonly recognized by eruptions on the skin. These are most often seen as **morbilliform** (measles-like) or **scarlatiniform** (scarlet fever-like) eruptions.

Diagnosis

Diagnosis of skin lesions involves physical examination to determine the lesion's type, color, response to touch, shape, arrangement (for multiple lesions), extent of involvement, and pattern and location of distribution. The patient is questioned to determine the length of time the lesions have been present and if they itch.

Visual aids to diagnosis of a lesion include viewing under magnification, **translumination** or sidelighting, **diascopy** (examination of superficial skin lesions) and illumination with long-wave ultraviolet light or **Wood's lamp.** Patch testing is used primarily to detect contact sensitivity.

Laboratory procedures include examination for bacteria in crusts and biopsy specimens, examination for **mycelia** (the growth threads of fungi), and the **Tzanck test** (a microscopic examination of cells from the base of vesicles to detect the presence of herpes simplex/zoster and varicella). **Dark-field examination** of serum from ulcers and erosions on the genitalia is used to detect *Treponema pallidum.* Biopsies of skin tissue are frequently utilized in diagnosis since these are easy to obtain.

Therapeutics

Topical administration (direct application) of a drug involves passage of the drug through the epidermis and penetration directly into the dermis. Drug molecules may then be absorbed into the general circulation through the capillary network, allowing a systemic effect. Sweat glands and pilosebaceous units (hair follicles and associated sebaceous glands) admit only a small amount of topically applied drugs.

Numerous topical dosage forms are available. Wet dressings provide evaporative cooling, which causes constriction or narrowing of the blood vessels. Wet dressings are utilized to soothe and cool inflammation, dry oozing lesions, soften crusts, and aid in cleaning and draining of wounds. They are most useful for acute inflammatory lesions, erosions, and ulcerations. Agents used include normal saline and solutions of aluminum acetate, potassium permanganate, silver nitrate, and acetic acid. Other forms of topical administration are baths, powders, emulsions, gels, creams, ointments, and aerosols. Ointment bases are most useful for chronic scaling lesions that are **lichenified** (having thickened layers that appear in patches; named for lichen, a moss-like plant that grows in patches on rocks and other surfaces). Ointments are used for their occlusive properties. Gels are colloidal suspensions that have set to form a jelly-like substance and are used similarly to ointments. Powders are used primarily to decrease friction and irritation in **intertriginous** areas (literally, "between triangles"; areas where two skin surfaces touch, such as between fingers and under the arms). Powders, therefore, are often used to treat athlete's foot, **jock itch,** and **diaper rash.** They are also utilized for prevention of decubitus ulcers or bedsores. Lotions are used to treat superficial skin disorders or if significant inflammation and tenderness are present, such as in acute contact dermatitis. Liquid oil-in-water or water-in-oil emulsions are useful in conditions where dry skin predominates. They are utilized as vehicles for insoluble medications. Creams, which are semisolid, oil-in-water emulsions, are the vehicles used most often in dermatology. They are useful for application on nonirritable chronic skin conditions. Aerosols are useful if direct contact with the skin causes pain.

Several drugs are commonly used in topical or systemic preparations for dermatological conditions. Topical corticosteroids are used in the treatment of **atopic eczema,** all inflammatory and pruritic eruptions, and **hyperplastic** and **infiltrative** disorders. Brief courses of systemic corticosteroids are indicated for severe contact dermatitis.

Topical antibiotics are used for bacterial infection of the skin, especially if the infection is severe, deep, and associated with fever or other systemic manifestations. Those with a suitable spectrum of activity include bacitracin, gentamicin, gramicidin, neomycin, and polymyxin B. Benzoyl peroxide is widely used for mild to moderately severe acne. Effective systemic antibiotics for dermatological use include tetracycline, erythromycin, clindamycin, trimethoprim/sulfamethoxazole, doxycycline, and minocycline.

Topical use of the vitamin A preparation tretinoin is an effective adjunctive to treatment of acne if initial irritation is tolerated. This product is also widely used by the lay public as an "anti-aging" remedy.

Coal tar preparations are available in gels or oils for use in treating psoriasis. Subsequent ultraviolet radiation and/or topical corticosteroids can increase the clinical response. **Photochemotherapy,** used in the treatment of psoriasis, includes administration of a drug (psoralens) and subsequent exposure of the skin to a predetermined amount of ultraviolet radiation. This therapy is sometimes denoted by the abbreviation **PUVA.**

Sunscreens are categorized as chemical agents that absorb ultraviolet radiation (e.g., PABA) and physical agents that reflect and scatter the rays (e.g., zinc oxide).

For the topical administration of systemically active drugs, other dosage forms are available. Skin patch delivery systems, generally known as **transdermal patches,** have been designed to deliver drugs directly into the bloodstream through the skin. Examples of drugs administered by this route are estrogen and nitroglycerin. Certain solvents can also be used to enhance dermal absorption of drugs, and some could provide direct administration of many drugs through the skin.

Abbreviations likely to be encountered in reference to the dermatological system are included in Table 8.2.

Table 8.2—Abbreviations Associated with the Integumentary System

BCC	basal cell carcinoma	**PPD**	purified protein derivative
BSA	body surface area	**PUVA**	psoralen-ultraviolet light
BSB	body surface burned	**SA**	surface area
BSPM	body surface potential	**SC**	subcutaneous
	mapping	**SCC**	squamous cell carcinoma
CIU	chronic idiopathic urticaria	**SD**	scleroderma
CMM	cutaneous malignant	**SPF**	sun protective factor
	melanoma	**SSM**	superficial spreading
DCH	delayed cutaneous		melanoma
	hypersensitivity	**ST**	split thickness
DCR	delayed cutaneous reaction	**STD**	skin test dose
DPV	delayed pressure urticaria	**STSG**	split thickness skin graft
HNT	hereditary hemorrhagic	**TBSA**	total burn surface area
	telangiectasis	**UV**	ultraviolet
ID	intradermal	**UVA**	ultraviolet A light
IPK	intractable plantar keratosis	**UVB**	ultraviolet B light
LCR	late cutaneous reaction	**UVL**	ultraviolet light
LMM	lentigo maligna melanoma	**UVR**	ultraviolet rays
NHD	normal hair distribution	**VZ**	varicella zoster

Pronouncing Glossary

Root	Meaning	Example	Pronunciation
cutis-	skin	subcutaneous	sub q TA nee us
derm-	epidermis	ep eh DER mus	
omphalo-	navel	omphaloncus	ahm ful ONK us
onych-	nail	onychomycosis	ah nee ko my KO sis
pilo-	hair	pilomotor	PI lo mo ter
sarco-	flesh	sarcoadenoma	sar ko ad en OH ma
seb, sebi-	sebum, sebaceous	seborrhea	seb o REE ah
sudor	sweat, perspiration	sudoresis	soo oh REE sis
tricho-	hair	trichoglossia	tri ko GLOSS ee ah

Glossary

abscess—a localized collection of pus surrounded by damaged and inflamed tissues

acne—general term for any of the varieties of inflammatory eruptions involving the sebaceous glands

athlete's foot—tinea pedis; a fungal infection, usually found between the toes and on the soles of the feet

bulla—a large blister containing serous fluid

candidiasis—infection caused by a yeastlike fungus of the genus *Candida,* usually the species *Candida albicans*

carbuncle—infection of several hair follicles with formation of pus and connected sinuses

carotene—a yellow/red pigment found in plants and animals that includes precursors of the A vitamins

cellulitis—inflammation of the connective tissue between adjacent tissues and organs

cerumen—earwax; the waxy material secreted by the sebaceous glands of the ear

ceruminous—relating to cerumen

chemexfoliation—chemabrasion; a chemosurgical technique involving superficial destruction of the outer layers of skin to remove scars or treat chronic skin lesions

comedo (comedone)—a plug formed of fatty material (sebum and keratin) in the outlet of a sebaceous gland in the skin

cutaneous cyst—an abnormal sac or closed cavity in the skin filled with liquid or semisolid matter

dermatitis—inflammation of the skin

dermatophytosis—any fungus infection of the skin

dermis—the true skin; the thick layer of living tissue that lies beneath the epidermis

diascopy—examination of superficial lesions by means of pressure on a flat glass plate

ecthyma—a pus forming skin infection containing crusts and ulceration

eczema—a superficial inflammation of the skin causing itching and rash with small blisters that weep and become crusted

epidermis—the outer layer of the skin

epilation—the act or result of removing hair

epithelial—pertaining to the tissue that covers the external surface of the body and lines the hollow structures

eponychium—the thin skin attached to the nail surface

exfoliative—marked by desquamation or profuse scaling

folliculitis—inflammation of the hair follicles

furuncle—inflammation of a hair follicle with pus formation; a boil

herpes simplex—infections caused by the herpes simplex virus, such as cold sores, fever blisters, etc.

herpes zoster—shingles; a herpes virus infection characterized by groups of vesicles following the course of a nerve

hyponychium—the thickened layer of the epidermis beneath the free border of the nail

impetigo—a contagious infection of the skin with vesicles that rupture and crust

keloid—hard, irregular elevated scar tissue that progressively increases in size due to collagen formation

keratin—a fibrous protein that primarily forms the body's horny tissues, such as nails, hair, epidermis, and tooth enamel

keratolytic—relating to keratolysis, loosening or separation of the horny layer of the epidermis

keratosis—any circumscribed overgrowths of the horny layer of the epidermis

lesion—an area of tissue with impaired function as a result of damage from disease or trauma

lipoma—a benign neoplasm of adipose tissue

macule—a spot, discoloration, or thickening of the skin that forms a distinct area from the surrounding normal surface

mammary—relating to the breast

melanin—a dark pigment occurring in the hair, skin, iris, and some tumors

melanosis—a disorder in the body's production of the pigment melanin

nevus—a birthmark or benign growth of melanin-forming cells

nodule—a small swelling or aggregation of cells detectable by touch

oleaginous—oily; greasy

papule—a small, circumscribed, solid elevation on the skin

pemphigus—refers to any of the blistering skin diseases

photosensitivity—abnormal and severe reaction of the skin to sunlight

pilosebaceous—pertaining to the hair follicles and their associated sebaceous glands

pityriasis rosea—a skin disorder with self-limited eruption of macules or papules, usually involving the trunk and extremities

plantar—relating to the sole of the foot

pruritus—itching

psoriasis—a chronic hereditary skin disease in which itchy red scaly patches form on various parts of the body, especially the scalp and extremities

purpura—disorders involving a skin discoloration resulting from bleeding into the skin from capillaries

pustule—a small pus-containing lesion on the skin

pyoderma—any pus-forming infection of the skin

scleroderma—a thickening of the skin caused by thickening of the underlying fibrous tissue

sebaceous—relating to or secreting sebum; oily, fatty

sebum—secretions of the sebaceous glands composed of fat and epithelial debris

solar elastosis—degeneration of the yellow fibers in connective tissues and skin, caused by exposure to sunlight

steatoma—tumor of a sebaceous gland

stratum—a layer of tissue or cells, such as those of the epidermis of the skin

subcutaneous—beneath the skin

telangiectasis—localized collection of dilated capillary blood vessels

trichiasis—condition where the eyelashes grow inward and contact the eyeball

trichomycosis—any hair disease caused by a fungal infection

ulcer—a skin or mucous membrane lesion, usually caused by inflammation and caused by loss of tissue

urticaria—hives; elevated wheals on the skin, accompanied by itching

vesicle—a small blister of the epidermis

vitiligo—a progressive condition in which areas of skin lose their pigmentation

wheal—a pale red swollen area of the skin seen in urticaria

CHAPTER 9

The Respiratory System and Its Disorders

The respiratory system is composed of all the organs involved in the exchange of gasses between the body and its environment, the process commonly known as **respiration**. This process, which is essential for the body to carry on life functions, involves the intake of oxygen through **inspiration** (or **inhalation**) and the elimination of carbon dioxide and other volatile waste products by **expiration** (or **exhalation**). In a broader sense, respiration also includes the exchange of gasses at the cellular level, providing the cells with oxygen for metabolic processes and transporting the carbon dioxide to the lungs for elimination. In addition to the exchange of oxygen and carbon dioxide, the respiratory system also functions as the source of sound for vocalization.

Anatomy and Physiology

Breathing or **ventilation** can be done through the mouth; however, it most often occurs through the **nares** or **nostrils**. As air is inhaled through the nostrils, it is cleaned and filtered by the lining of short, stout hairs found in the dilated part of the nostrils just inside the opening called the **vestibule**. Above the vestibule, the nostrils are lined with a layer of mucous membrane from which grow **cilia**. These microscopic hair-like projections serve to filter the air as it passes through. Smaller particles of matter pass into the upper nostril and are entrapped in **mucus** secreted by the mucous membrane lining. Some of these particles then move out of the vestibule; others pass along a channel leading to the mouth where they can be **expectorated** (spit out) or swallowed. During this part of the respiratory process, the air is also warmed and moistened by the mucous membrane in the nostrils.

The two nostrils are separated by a wall of cartilage and bone called the **septum**. In the bone surrounding the nasal cavity are eight small air pockets called the **paranasal sinuses: maxillary, ethmoid, sphenoidal**, and **frontal**. The primary function of these four paired sinuses is to warm and humidify inhaled air, remove airborne debris, increase sensitivity to smell, and impart resonance to the voice. The secretions of these sinuses drain into the **nasal cavity** that fills the space between the base of the skull and roof of the mouth.

Air from the nostrils passes into the **pharynx**. The pharynx may be subdivided into three areas: the **nasopharynx** (the part above the soft palate and nearest the nose), the **oropharynx** (at the back of the mouth), and the **laryngopharynx** (the lower part nearest the larynx). In the oropharynx are the **tonsils**, lymphoid structures that are functionally part of both the pharynx and the immune system. From the pharynx, air travels to a tube in front of the esophagus called the **larynx** or voice box. In the front part of the larynx is the thyroid cartilage or "Adam's apple."

At the opening of the larynx where it bifurcates from the esophagus is a disc of cartilage and mucous membrane called the **epiglottis**. When food is swallowed, an automatic nerve–muscle action closes the epiglottis and prevents the food from entering the larynx. Continuing below the larynx is another tubular structure called the **trachea**, commonly referred to as the "windpipe." These two tubes are connected by the **cricoid cartilage**. At the base of the larynx just above the cricoid cartilage are the paired strips of stratified squamous epithelium known as the **vocal cords**.

In the chest, the trachea divides into a left and right **bronchus** (plural: **bronchi**) leading to the left and right lungs. The ridge where the bronchi begin is known as the **carina**. Irritation of the carina triggers the cough reflex.

Within the lungs, the left and right bronchi branch into smaller and smaller passageways. As these tubes become small enough to remain barely visible without a microscope, they still contain the cartilage rings found in the trachea and left and right bronchi, so they are still referred to as bronchi. As the size continues to decrease, however, only muscle tissue remains. These smallest branches are called **bronchioles**, meaning "little bronchi." Bronchioles terminate in small air sacs called **alveoli** from which oxygen passes into the bloodstream for transport throughout the body (Figure 9.1).

The alveoli are located in the **lungs**, considered to be the primary organs of respiration. The lungs are located in the **thoracic cavity**, also called the **pleural** cavity because of the serous membrane (**pleura**) which covers the lungs. The thoracic cavity is divided into two parts by the **mediastinum**, which contains all the major organs of the thoracic cavity except the lungs, which lie on either side.

Deep fissures in the lungs divide them into **lobes**. The right lung contains three lobes, which are called the superior, middle, and inferior lobes. In the left lung are the superior and inferior lobes and the **cardiac notch** where the heart projects into the thoracic cavity.

The lungs rest on a large muscle called the **diaphragm**. During inspiration, the diaphragm contracts and moves downward, increasing the size of the thoracic cavity. It relaxes and moves upward to decrease the cavity size during expiration.

Respiration also results from pressure changes. The pressure within the thorax, called **intrathoracic pressure**, is usually less than atmospheric pressure. This creates a slight vacuum within the thorax that exerts suction on the elastic lungs so that they never fully collapse. During inspiration, intrathoracic volume increases and the lungs expand, causing intrathoracic pressure to decrease. Because of the lower pressure, air rushes in to fill the lungs and the pressure accordingly increases. During expiration, intrathoracic volume decreases and intrathoracic pressure increases, forcing the air out of the lungs. The amount of air inhaled and exhaled during normal unstrained (quiet) respiration is called **tidal volume** and averages about 500 ml for the adult male. During one respiratory cycle, only about 350 ml of this air actually reaches the alveoli; the remainder, called **dead space air**, remains in the respiratory passages. The total amount of air that can be forcibly expelled from the lungs after a maximal inspiration is called the **vital capacity (VC)**, a measure of maximum respiratory volume. This is about 4000 ml in the adult male.

The process by which oxygen passes from the alveoli into the bloodstream and carbon dioxide passes from the bloodstream into the alveoli is **diffusion**. Once the carbon dioxide from the blood reaches the alveoli, it is forced up and out through the respiratory passages

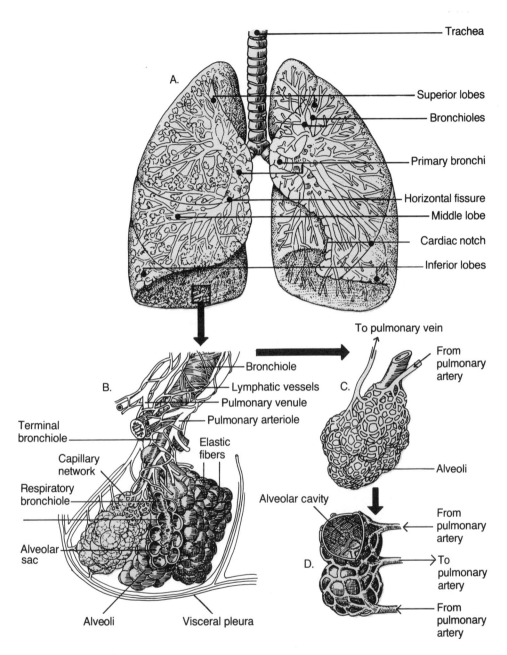

Figure 9.1—The Respiratory System.
(A) Lower portion of the respiratory tract. (B) Lung lobe, showing alveolar sacs.
(C) Detail of alveolar sac. (D) Cluster of alveoli are surrounded by a capillary network,
where exchange of oxygen and carbon dioxide takes place.

during expiration (Figure 9.2). The oxygen that has entered the bloodstream is carried to cells throughout the body by the protein molecule called **hemoglobin**. The term **oxyhemoglobin** refers to the molecule of hemoglobin when it is combined with oxygen.

Regulation of the respiratory cycle is controlled by respiratory centers in the brain. These centers respond primarily to the carbon dioxide content in the blood. An increase in carbon dioxide content increases the rate of respiration, while a decrease in the CO_2 content results in a decreased respiratory rate.

Therapeutics

Diseases

Dyspnea (difficulty breathing) is a primary symptom experienced by many patients with respiratory disorders. The term is derived from the prefix *dys-*, indicating difficulty or pain, and the root *-pnea* from the Greek word for breath *(pnoia)*, which appears in many terms referring to specific breathing disorders. The term for abnormal slowness of respiration is **bradypnea** *(brady* = slow); conversely **tachypnea** *(tachy* = rapid) denotes rapid breathing. Dyspneic patients may also present with **chest pain (thoracodynia, thoracalgia,** both literally "pain in the thorax"). Chest pain in a patient with a respiratory disorder is often pleuritic in origin and may be caused by inflammation of the pleura from a pneumonia, pulmonary thromboembolism, tuberculosis, or malignancy, among other possible sources. Pleuritic pain is related to movements of the thorax and to respiration and is usually localized on one side of the chest.

Cough and **expectoration** (discharge of sputum from the mouth) are also classic signs of pulmonary disease. Paroxysmal or episodic cough may be present in bronchial asthma. The **sputum** may be described as pink, frothy, watery, mucoid, mucopurulent, rusty, thick, gelatinous, or blood-streaked, depending on the disorder. When sputum is bloody, the term applied is **hemoptysis,** the coughing up of blood. Other terms frequently encountered to describe respiratory symptoms include **rales, rhonchi, wheeze,** pleural friction rub, and adventitious breath sounds.

The group of diseases that interfere with ventilation, primarily by limiting expiratory flow rates, are known as the **chronic obstructive lung diseases (COLD), chronic obstructive pulmonary diseases (COPD),** or **chronic obstructive airway diseases (COAD).** These include asthma, chronic bronchitis, and emphysema. Patients with these diseases have symptoms of cough, sputum, wheezing, or dyspnea.

Asthma is a general term sometimes used to describe difficulty in breathing. Asthma results from the constriction of smooth muscles in the walls of the bronchi and bronchioles accompanied by excess mucus secretion and insufficient contraction of the alveoli. It is characterized by relatively symptom-free periods between attacks of dyspnea and labored breathing, reversibility of airway obstruction, and increased **bronchomotor** response to a variety of inhaled substances. **Aeroallergens,** airborne substances that induce allergic reactions, include such substances as pollen, mold, household dust, or animal dander; all of these aeroallergens can precipitate an asthma attack. Between attacks, asthma patients may have episodes of **bronchospasm,** a narrowing of the bronchi by muscular contraction.

Chronic **bronchitis** (inflammation of the bronchi) is a condition of chronic or excessive

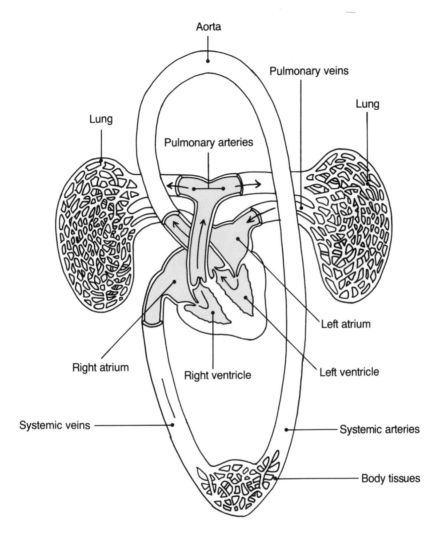

Figure 9.2—Respiratory Circulation.
Schematic diagram of pulmonary and systemic circulation.

mucous secretion in the bronchial tree resulting in coughing and may evolve from several causes.

Emphysema is a condition in which the alveoli do not contract properly and do not expel enough air. Manifestations include a lowered diffusing capacity and a loss of elastic recoil in the lung. Diagnosis is made by pathological (laboratory) results rather than by symptoms.

Disturbances of ventilation include the abnormally slow breathing of **hypoventilation,** which results in an increase in the level of carbon dioxide and a decrease in partial pressure of oxygen in alveolar gas and arterial blood. These results of hypoventilation are referred to as **hypoxemia** (deficiency of oxygen in the blood) and **hypercapnia** or **hypercarbia** (increased CO_2 content in the blood). Another result of hypoventilation can be **hypoxia,** deficiency of oxygen at the tissues, a condition that often occurs with, but technically is different from, hypoxemia. Conversely, **hyperventilation** is abnormally rapid breathing and causes the level of carbon dioxide (pCO_2) to fall below normal. Terms associated with this condition include **Kussmaul breathing** (also called **Kussmaul-Kien respiration** or **Kussmaul's respiration**), a paroxysmal air hunger causing gasping; **hypoxia** because it may induce hyperventilation; and **Cheyne-Stokes respiration,** which is a form of periodic breathing characterized by alternating periods of **apnea** (lack of breathing) and **hyperpnea** (carbon dioxide retention). **Asphyxia** or asphyxiation occurs from impaired or absent exchange of oxygen and carbon dioxide during ventilation.

The inability of the lungs to eliminate carbon dioxide results in a condition called **respiratory acidosis,** a decrease in serum pH from the excess carbonic acid of dissolved CO_2. **Alkalosis** is a condition that results when the lungs eliminate too much carbon dioxide, increasing serum pH. Diseases that impair the ability of the lungs to transfer oxygen to the blood may produce **hypoxia,** in which oxygen in the blood is insufficient for the tissues, or **anoxia,** in which no oxygen enters the blood.

Hypersensitivity disease of the lung includes a number of related disorders that involve both inflammation and an immunologic cause. Some of the more frequently encountered of these terms include hypersensitivity pneumonitis, allergic alveolitis, farmer's lung, and allergic bronchopulmonary aspergillosis.

Environmental lung disease results when substances other than oxygen are inhaled. Such substances include allergens, viruses, smoke, bacteria, toxic gas, and dust. Disease terms related to occupational exposure are byssinosis, baritosis, pneumoconiosis, and silicosis, among others; other terms frequently encountered include specific agents to which an individual may be exposed, such as asbestos.

Rhinitis (from the Greek *rhin-,* meaning ''nose'') is inflammation of the nasal mucous membrane and is characterized by nasal discharge, sneezing, and congestion. A general term applied to any nasal inflammation, rhinitis is often modified to indicate the other structures affected. Infectious rhinitis includes viral infections that can result in symptoms such as **coryza** or the common cold. **Rhinosinusitis,** affecting both the nose and sinuses, is caused by a bacterial infection. **Allergic rhinitis,** also called ''hayfever,'' and nonallergic perennial rhinitis show similar symptoms of nasal stuffiness and itching, rhinorrhea, sneezing, and conjunctivitis (inflammation of the eye covering), although one is caused by an allergic reaction and is cyclic, while the other is chronic and not allergic in origin.

Bronchiectasis is the condition of a permanent abnormal dilatation, or stretching, of one or more bronchi. All forms of bronchiectasis are associated with bacterial infection. **Broncholithiasis** refers to the presence of bronchial calcifications or stones.

Tuberculosis, caused by the microorganism *Mycobacterium tuberculosis,* can occur in many parts of the body but is generally considered a respiratory disorder because the lungs are most often the site of infection. Associated terms include Mantoux skin test, purified protein derivative (PPD), tuberculin, bacillus Calmette-Guerin (BCG) vaccine, necrosis, liquefaction, and atelectasis.

Infections of the respiratory tract include numerous other disorders, the most common of which are listed in Table 9.1, along with terms that may be used to describe symptoms, diagnosis, or treatment of each. Many of the related terms are associated with several of the respiratory disorders and are not repeated for each (e.g., erythema is a redness that may appear in the nose, pharynx, larynx, or practically any other structure in relation to a host of disorders).

Table 9.1—Common Infections of the Respiratory Tract

Area Infected	Term	Related Terms
Nose	rhinitis	rhinorrhea, nasal congestion, erythema, auscultation, rhonchi
Pharynx	pharyngitis	hoarseness, lymphadenopathy, pharyngeal/tonsillar exudate
Larynx	laryngitis	hoarseness, dysphagia, aphonia
Larynx, trachea, bronchi	bronchitis; laryngo-tracheo-bronchitis; laryngotracheitis; spasmodic croup; diphtheria; pertussis	cough, dyspnea, hypoxemia, rales, rhonchi, wheezing, airway obstruction
Trachea	tracheitis	stridor, purulent sputum, exudate, sub-glottic structures
Epiglottis	supraglottitis; epiglottitis	aryepiglottic folds, dysphagia, respiratory distress, drooling, erythema
Sinuses	sinusitis	purulent nasal discharge, intranasal
Bronchi	bronchitis	sputum, rales, rhonchi, rhinovirus, coronavirus, adenovirus, postural drainage
Lungs	pneumonias*; pneumonomycosis	aspiration, rales, rhonchi, cavitation, pleural effusions, pathogens, rigor, pleuritic pain

*Pneumococcal pneumonia, *Hemophilus influenzae* pneumonia, *Legionella* pneumophila (Legionnaire's disease), *Mycoplasma* pneumonia, staphylococcal pneumonia, aerobic gram-negative bacilli (AGNB) pneumonia, aspiration pneumonitis, *Pneumocystis carinii* pneumonia.

Cystic fibrosis (CF) is primarily a disorder of increased production of exocrine gland (e.g., paranasal sinuses) secretions, which produce chronic lung infections, along with several other manifestations. Complications for the respiratory system include development of pneumonia, bronchiectasis, atelectasis, abscesses, empyema, pneumothorax, and hemoptysis.

Pneumothorax is a collection of gas in the pleural space that results in collapse of the lung. **Hemothorax,** or the presence of blood in the thoracic cavity, can occur following trauma to the chest and may require drainage or thoracotomy. **Empyema** or **pyothorax** refers to the presence of infected liquid or pus in the pleural space. **Pleurisy** is an inflammation of the pleura caused by microorganisms and exhibits stages of fibrinous dry pleurisy, serofibrinous pleurisy, and purulent pleurisy or empyema.

Pulmonary edema results from an increase in pulmonary venous pressure with engorgement of the pulmonary vessels and tachypnea (rapid breathing). **Adult respiratory distress syndrome (ARDS),** also known as shock lung, wet lung, or primary/noncardiogenic edema, results from injury to the vascular system in the lungs, allowing accumulation of tissue edema fluid.

Orthopnea is the term that describes dyspnea (difficulty in breathing) in the lying-down position (the prefix *ortho-* means "straight" or "flat," as in *orthostatic hypertension*). Orthopnea is often seen in cardiovascular disorders involving elevation of the pulmonary venous and capillary pressures.

Sleep apnea (*a*-meaning "without") occurs when breathing periodically stops during sleep as a result of upper airway obstruction. **Sudden infant death syndrome (SIDS** or crib death) is considered a respiratory disorder even though the cause is unknown. Either spasmodic closure of the air passages or dysfunction of the respiratory centers may produce respiratory failure, causing SIDS.

Bronchopulmonary dysplasia (BPD) is a chronic lung disorder of infants. **Hyaline membrane disease,** also known as "glassy-lung" disease because the lungs assume a glassy or hyaline appearance, is a failure at birth to produce sufficient surfactant to allow the alveoli to fill with air properly.

Traumas to the respiratory system include **drowning** and **choking. Cyanosis** (from the Greek *cyano-,* meaning dark blue) occurs whenever breathing is stopped and the pulse is weak or absent. The skin develops a bluish color, resulting from the buildup of deoxygenated hemoglobin.

Lung cancer is an oncologic disorder of the respiratory organs (see discussion in Chapter 18).

Drug-induced pulmonary disorders include asthma, pulmonary edema, pulmonary fibrosis, and Löffler's syndrome.

Disorders of the respiratory tract are summarized in Table 9.2.

Diagnosis

Physical assessment is significant in diagnosing disorders of the respiratory tract. Terms often encountered include auscultation, percussion, rhonchi (wheezes), rales (crackles), stridor, pleural rub, and sputum. Laboratory diagnostic tests used to evaluate the respiratory system include measurement of the **arterial blood gases** (ABGs), PO_2 (partial pressure of oxygen, oxygen tension), $PaCO_2$ (arterial carbon dioxide tension), and serum pH. **Oximetry** measures the oxygen saturation of hemoglobin in a sample of blood.

Pulmonary function tests determine the presence, type, and extent of dysfunction in the airways, alveoli, and pulmonary vascular bed caused by obstruction or restriction or both. These tests are of three general types: (1) airway flow rates measure flow to assess airway patency and resistance; (2) lung volume and capacity measure compartments of the lung to assess air-trapping and differentiate impairments; and (3) gas exchange (diffusion capacity) measures rate of gas transfer across the alveolar-capillary membranes. The **spirometer** is a device used to measure lung volume; the procedure is called **spirometry.** The peak expiratory flow rate (**PEFR,** maximal flow that can be produced during forced expiration), pulmonary venous congestion (**PVC),** forced expiratory vol-

---

Table 9.2—Common Disorders of the Respiratory System

Adult respiratory distress syndrome	Hypersensitivity disease
Asthma	Hyaline membrane disease
Atelectasis	Infections (see Table 9.1)
Bronchiectasis	Neoplasms
Bronchopulmonary dysplasia	Pneumonias
Chronic bronchitis	Pleurisy
Chronic obstructive lung/pulmonary/airway disease	Pneumothorax
Cystic fibrosis	Pulmonary edema
Drug-induced disorders	Respiratory acidosis/alkalosis
Emphysema	Rhinitis
Empyema/pyothorax	Rhinosinusitis
Environmental lung disease	Sudden infant death syndrome
Hemothorax	Tuberculosis

---

ume **(FEV),** and the mean forced expiratory flow **(FEF)** during the middle of the forced vital capacity **(FVC)** can be measured by flow meters.

Exercise stress testing is done to evaluate fitness, functional capacity, and other limiting factors in obstructive and restrictive disorders. This assesses ventilation, gas exchange, and cardiovascular function during increased demands. It can also provide nonspecific responses to assist in diagnosing many conditions.

Body **plethysmography,** using a **pneumotachometer,** is another diagnostic technique used to measure airway mechanics, although this procedure is primarily used only in research laboratories. The specific airway conductance (SGAW) can be determined by this method.

Roentgenographic examination (radiographs) of the chest, sometimes referred to as simply chest X ray, provides assistance in diagnosis of pulmonary disease. Magnetic resonance imaging **(MRI), laminagraphy,** computerized **tomography,** and pulmonary **photoscanning** are also useful procedures.

The fiberoptic **bronchoscope** is an instrument utilized for visual examination of the bronchi through the procedure of **bronchoscopy** and may be used to obtain bronchial brushings and biopsies. **Mediastinoscopy** is the examination of the mediastinum and its lymph nodes, particularly in suspected malignancy. Use of an endoscope to inspect the larynx is **laryngoscopy. Thoracoscopy** denotes examination of the pleural cavity. **Fluoroscopy** is a type of radiographic technique that allows visualization of the thoracic contents in a dynamic manner and provides a range of views.

Pulmonary **scintiphotography** is a technique that provides a visual image of the distribution of blood flow and ventilation in the lungs. Pulmonary **angiography** permits visualization of the pulmonary vessels and is frequently used to detect emboli or lesions.

Cultures of sputum, pleural fluid, and bronchial washings identify organisms causing infections. Material for cultures of the lung can be obtained by **transtracheal** (meaning "through the trachea") catheter and percutaneous needle aspiration (suction) or by direct percutaneous aspiration. Lung **biopsy** can be performed with the bronchoscope, by aspiration, or after a **thoracotomy** or **pleurotomy,** which indicates incision into the chest

---

Table 9.3—Surgical Procedures of the Respiratory Tract

Location	Procedure
Nose	rhinoplasty
Sinuses	antrostomy, ethmoidectomy, turbinectomy, antrotomy, sinusotomy, Caldwell-Luc (radical sinusotomy)
Pharynx	pharyngectomy, pharyngoplasty, pharyngotomy
Tonsils	tonsillectomy
Trachea	tracheostomy, tracheotomy, tracheoplasty
Larynx	laryngectomy, laryngoplasty, laryngostomy, laryngotomy
Bronchi	bronchoplasty, bronchorrhaphy, bronchotomy
Lungs	lobectomy, pneumonectomy, wedge resection, thoracentesis
Thoracic cavity	thoracentesis, thoracostomy, thoracoplasty, thoracotomy, pleuracentesis, pleurotomy

---

wall. **Thoracentesis,** puncture of the thoracic cavity, is performed to obtain pleural fluid and pleural biopsy specimens.

Treatment

Infections of the respiratory tract are treated with a variety of bactericidal and bacteriostatic **antibiotics,** depending on the organisms cultured. Other pharmacologic agents employed in treatment of upper respiratory infections include **antitussives, bronchodilators, expectorants,** and **mucolytics.**

Treatment of asthma involves the use of sympathomimetic and anticholinergic **bronchodilators, methylxanthines** (particularly theophylline), **anti-allergic agents,** and **corticosteroids.**

Immunotherapy or **desensitization** is a means of treatment employed for allergic rhinitis.

Mechanical devices used in treatment of upper respiratory infections and asthma include the **turboinhaler, metered dose inhaler, nebulizer,** and **nebulized bronchodilators.**

Terms used to describe the delivery of medication and respiratory support include **ventilator, respirator, percussinator, endotracheal** (ET) tube, and positive end-expiratory pressure (**PEEP**).

Surgical procedures involving various structures of the respiratory tract are listed in Table 9.3 and are defined in the glossary. Abbreviations commonly encountered in association with the respiratory system are included in Table 9.4.

Table 9.4—Abbreviations Associated with the Respiratory System

AAVV	accumulated alveolar ventilatory volume	**CPR**	cardiopulmonary resuscitation
ABC	airway, breathing, circulation	**CSR**	Cheyne-Stokes respiration
AFB	acid-fast bacillus (causes tuberculosis)	**CT & DB**	cough, turn, and deep breathe
AGNB	aerobic gram-negative bacilli	**CTA**	clear to auscultation
AMV	assisted mechanical ventilation	**CV**	closing volume
AND	anterior nasal discharge	**CXR**	chest X ray
A & P	auscultation and percussion	**DB & C**	deep breathing and coughing
ARD	adult/acute respiratory distress	**DBE**	deep breathing exercises
ARDS	adult/acute respiratory distress syndrome	**DBS**	diminished breath sounds
ARF	acute respiratory failure	**DILD**	diffuse infiltrative lung disease
BAE	bronchial artery embolization	**DL**	direct laryngoscopy
BAL	bronchoalveolar lavage	**DNS**	deviated nasal septum
BBS	bilateral breath sounds	**DOE**	dyspnea on exertion
BCG	bacillus Calmette-Guérin (vaccine)	**DPT**	diphtheria, pertussis, toxoid
		DTT	diphtheria, tetanus toxoid
BD	bronchial discharge	**E-A**	say EEE, comes out as A,A,A upon auscultation of lung
BPD	bronchopulmonary dysplasia		
BPM	breaths per minute	**ECMO**	extracorporeal membrane oxygenation
BPS	bronchopulmonary segmental drainage	**Endo**	endotracheal
BS	breath sounds	**EOA**	esophageal obturator airway
CAL	chronic airflow limitation	**ERV**	expiratory reserve volume
CAO	chronic airway obstruction	**ET**	endotracheal
CB	chronic bronchitis	**FEC**	forced expiratory capacity
CBA	chronic bronchitis and asthma	**FICO$_2$**	fraction of inspired carbon dioxide
CDB	cough, deep breathe	**FIO$_2$**	fraction of inspired oxygen
CF	cystic fibrosis	**FMF**	forced midexpiratory flow
CFP	cystic fibrosis protein	**FOB**	fiberoptic bronchoscope
CHFV	combined high frequency of ventilation	**FR**	flow rate
		FVL	flow volume loop
CLD	chronic lung disease	**HBO**	hyperbaric oxygen
CMV	controlled mechanical ventilation; cool mist vaporization	**HHN**	hand-held nebulizer
		IC	inspiratory capacity
		ICPP	intubated continuous positive pressure
CNP	continuous negative pressure	**IDV**	intermittent demand ventilation
COAD	chronic obstructive airway disease	**IMV**	intermittent mechanical ventilation
COLD	chronic obstructive lung disease	**INB**	intermittent nebulized beta-agonists
COPD	chronic obstructive pulmonary disease	**IPA**	invasive pulmonary aspergillosis
COPE	chronic obstructive pulmonary emphysema	**IPPB**	intermittent positive pressure breathing
CPAP	continuous positive airway pressure	**IPPV**	intermittent positive pressure ventilation
CPE	chronic pulmonary emphysema; cardiogenic pulmonary edema	**IRV**	inspiratory reserve volume
		IS	incentive spirometer; induced sputum

ISB	incentive spirometry breathing	**PND**	paroxysmal nocturnal dyspnea
IT	inhalation therapy		
LAR	late asthmatic response	**Pnx**	pneumothorax
LLL	left lower lobe (of lung)	**PORT**	postoperative respiratory therapy
LUL	left upper lobe (of lung)		
MBC	maximum breathing capacity	**P & PD**	percussion and postural drainage
MDI	metered dose inhaler		
MEF	maximum expired flow rate	**PS**	pulmonary stenosis
MEFV	maximum expiratory flow volume	**PTE**	pulmonary thromboembolism
		PVC	pulmonary venous congestion
MFEM	maximum forced expiratory maneuver	**PVOD**	pulmonary vascular obstructive disease
MMEFR	maximal midexpiratory flow rate	**PVS**	percussion, vibration, and suction
MMF	mean maximal flow	**PWP**	pulmonary wedge pressure
MMFR	maximal midexpiratory flow rate	**Px**	pneumothorax
		R	respiration
MVV	maximum voluntary ventilation	**R(AW)**	airway resistance
		RD	respiratory disease
NAEP	National Asthma Education Program	**RDS**	respiratory distress syndrome
		RHC	respiration has ceased
NET	naso-endotracheal tube	**RICU**	respiratory intensive care unit
NIF	negative inspiratory force	**RLL**	right lower lobe (of lung)
NSDA	non-steroid-dependent asthma	**RM**	respiratory movement
		RML	right middle lobe (of lung)
NT	nasotracheal	**RQ**	respiratory quotient
NTS	nasotracheal suction	**RR**	respiratory rate; regular respirations
NTT	nasotracheal tube		
OER	oxygen enhancement ratios	**RT**	respiratory therapist
OHP	oxygen under hyperbaric pressure	**RUL**	right upper lobe
		RURTI	recurrent upper respiratory tract infection
OSA	obstructive sleep apnea		
OTS	orotracheal suction	**RV/TLC**	residual volume to total lung capacity ratio
OTT	orotracheal tube		
P & A	percussion and auscultation	**SAS**	sleep apnea syndrome
PA/PS	pulmonary atresia/stenosis	**SDA**	steroid-dependent asthmatic
PAOP	pulmonary artery occlusion pressure	**SIDS**	sudden infant death syndrome
PAP	pulmonary artery pressure	**SIMV**	synchronized intermittent mandatory ventilation
PAS	pulmonary artery stenosis		
PAWP	pulmonary artery wedge pressure	**SMI**	sustained maximal inspiration
		SMR	submucous resection
PCP	pneumonocystitis carinii pneumonia; pulmonary capillary pressure	**SO$_2$**	oxygen saturation
		SOB	shortness of breath
		SPN	solitary pulmonary nodule
PCWP	pulmonary capillary wedge pressure	**T & A**	tonsillectomy and adenoidectomy
PDE	paroxysmal dyspnea on exertion	**TBB**	transbronchial biopsy
		Tbc	tuberculosis
PE	pulmonary embolism; pleural effusion	**T & C**	turn and cough
		TCDB	turn, cough, deep breathe
PECO$_2$	mixed expired CO2 tension	**TCH**	turn, cough, hyperventilate
PEG	pneumoencephalogram	**TD**	tidal volume; tetanus-diphtheria toxoid
PFR	peak flow rate		
PFT	pulmonary function test	**TLV**	total lung volume
PIE	pulmonary interstitial emphysema	**Trach**	tracheostomy

TSBB	transtracheal selective bronchial brushing	**USN**	ultrasonic nebulizer
T set	tracheotomy set	**V & P**	ventilation and perfusion
TV	tidal volume	**WC**	whooping cough
UAO	upper airway obstruction	**WLS**	wet lung syndrome
		ZEEP	zero end-expiratory pressure

Pronouncing Glossary

Root	Meaning	Example	Pronunciation
aero-	air, gas	aerotherapy	ar o THER ah pee
alveolo-	alveolus	alveolotomy	al ve o LOT o me
antro-	cavity, sinus	antroscopy	an TROS ko pee
broncho-	bronchus, windpipe	bronchorrhea	BRONG ka RE ah
laryngo-	larynx	laryngopathy	LAR ing GOP a thee
oxa-	oxygen	hypoxia	hi POX ee ah
naso-	nose	nasopharynx	nay so FAR nix
rhino-		rhinoplasty	RHIN o plas tee
pharyngo-	pharynx	pharyngospasm	fa RING go spazm
phreno-	diaphragm	phrenoplegia	FREN o play ja
pleuro-	pleura, side, rib	pleurodynia	plur o DINN ee ah
pneo-	breath, breathing	pneograph	NEW oh graff
pneum-	air, lung	pneumonia	NEW mon ee ah
pulmo-	lung	pulmonary	PULL mon ary
sino-	sinus	sinusitis	SIN u sit es
spiro-	coil, breathe	spirometer	spi ROM eh ter
thoraco-	chest	thoracentesis	thor ah sen TEE sis
tonsillo-	tonsil	tonsillitis	ton sil I tes;
tracheo-	trachea	tracheocele	TRAK ee oh seel

Glossary

acidosis—actual or relative decrease of alkali in bodily fluids in proportion to the content of acid

adenovirus—adenoidal-pharyngeal-conjunctival virus, the type associated with minor respiratory infections of children

aeroallergens—allergens in the air

alkalosis—abnormally high alkali reserve of the blood and other body fluids, tending to increase pH of the blood

angiography—radiography of vessels after injection of a radiopaque material

anoxia—absence of oxygen in arterial blood or tissues

antitussive—relieving cough

antrostomy—the formation of an opening into any antrum or nearly closed cavity

antrotomy—incision through the wall of any antrum

aphonia—loss of the voice caused by disease or injury of the organ of speech

apnea—the absence of breathing

aryepiglottic folds—a fold of mucous membrane stretching between the lateral margin of the epiglottis and the cartilage on either side

asphyxia—deficiency or lack of exchange of oxygen and carbon dioxide during ventilation

aspiration—entrance of fluid or foreign body such as vomitus during inspiration; use of suction to remove gas or fluid from a body cavity

asthma—a condition in which there is widespread narrowing of airways of the lungs

atelectasis—airlessness of the lungs due to failure of expansion or resorption of air from the alveoli

auscultation—listening to the sounds made by any of the internal parts of the body

bronchiectasis—chronic dilation of the bronchial tubes as the result of inflammatory disease or obstruction

bronchiole—one of the terminal subdivisions of the bronchial tubes

bronchitis—inflammation of the mucous membrane of the bronchial tubes

bronchodilator—an agent that causes an increase in the caliber of a bronchus or bronchiole

bronchomotor—an agent that can dilate or contract the bronchi or bronchial tubes

bronchoplasty—the surgical repair of any defect in the bronchi

bronchorrhaphy—suture of a wound of the bronchus

bronchoscope—an instrument for use in inspecting the interior of the tracheobronchial tree for diagnostic purposes or for the removal of foreign bodies

bronchoscopy—inspection of the interior of the tracheobronchial tree by means of a lighted endoscope

bronchospasm—spasmodic narrowing of the lumen of a bronchus due to muscle contraction

bronchotomy—incision of a bronchus

bronchus—one of the subdivisions of the trachea that functions to convey air to and from the lungs

carina—any of several anatomical structures forming a projecting central ridge, as where the bronchi begin

cavitation—the formation of a cavity, as occurs in the lung in tuberculosis or pneumonias

Cheyne-Stokes respiration—a pattern of breathing with gradual increase in depth and sometimes in rate to a maximum, followed by a decrease resulting in apnea

cilia—the motile extensions of a cell surface

coronavirus—a virus that causes respiratory infections in humans

coryza—acute rhinitis; cold in the head

cricoid cartilage—the lowest of the laryngeal cartilages

croup—inflammation of the larynx, trachea and bronchi in infants and young children, caused by a parainfluenza virus

cyanosis—a dark blue or purple discoloration of the skin and mucous membranes caused by deficient oxygenation of the blood

cystic fibrosis—fibrocystic disease of the pancreas also involving chronic lung infections and other manifestations

diaphragm—the muscular membranous partition between the abdominal and thoracic cavities

diffusion—the random movement of free molecules or ions or small particles under the influence of thermal motion toward a uniform distribution throughout a solution or suspension

dysphagia—difficulty in swallowing

dysplasia—abnormal tissue development

dyspnea—shortness of breath; subjective difficulty in breathing

edema—accumulation of an excessive amount of fluid in cells, tissues, or serous cavities

effusion—the escape of fluid from the blood vessels or lymphatics into the tissues

emphysema—increase in the size of air spaces near the bronchioles, either from dilation or from destruction of the walls

empyema—pus in the pleural cavity

epiglottis—a leaf-shaped plate of elastic cartilage covered with mucous membrane, at the root of the tongue, which folds back to cover the opening of the larynx during the act of swallowing

epiglottitis—inflammation of the epiglottis

erythema—inflammatory redness of the skin

ethmoid sinus—protrusion of the mucous membrane of the middle and superior meatus of the nasal cavity considered as one sinus on each side

ethmoidectomy—removal of the mucosal lining and bony partitions between the ethmoid sinuses

expectorant—an agent that increases bronchial secretion and facilitates its expulsion

expectoration—spitting; sputum expelled by coughing

expiration—breathing out; exhalation

exudate—fluid that has oozed out of tissue or capillaries

fluoroscopy—examination of the inner parts of the body by means of the fluoroscope

frontal sinus—a hollow formed on either side in the lower part of the frontal bone

hemoglobin—the red, respiratory protein of red blood cells that transports oxygen from the lungs to the tissues

hemoptysis—the spitting of blood from the lungs or bronchial tubes

hemothorax—an effusion of blood into the pleural cavity

hoarseness—an unnaturally deep and harsh quality to the voice; dysphonia

hypercapnia—the presence of an abnormally large amount of carbon dioxide in the circulating blood

hypercarbia—hypercapnia

hyperventilation—overventilation resulting in a decrease of alveolar carbon dioxide pressure

hypoventilation—underventilation, resulting in increased alveolar carbon dioxide pressure

hypoxemia—decreased levels of oxygen in arterial blood

hypoxia—decrease below normal levels of oxygen in air, blood, or tissue

immunotherapy—treatment directed at the reduction of allergic sensitivity or reactions to the specific allergen

inspiration—the act of breathing in; inhalation

intrathoracic—within the cavity of the chest

intubation—the insertion of a tube into the throat or nose for control of ventilation

Kussmaul breathing—deep, rapid respirations characteristic of diabetic acidosis or coma

laminagraphy—tomography; examination of any part of the body for diagnostic purposes by means of roentgen rays, the record of the findings being impressed upon a photographic plate

laryngectomy—excision of the larynx

laryngoplasty—reparative or plastic surgery of the larynx

laryngoscopy—inspection of the larynx by means of the laryngoscope

laryngostomy—establishment of a permanent opening from the neck into the larynx

laryngotomy—laryngofissure; operative opening into the larynx

larynx—the organ of voice production that lies between the pharynx and trachea

liquefaction—the change from solid to liquid

lobectomy—excision of a lobe of any organ or gland

lymphadenopathy—any disease process affecting a lymph node

Mantoux skin test—the intracutaneous tuberculin test

maxillary sinus—an air cavity in the body of the maxilla, communicating with the middle meatus of the nose

mediastinoscopy—exploration of the mediastinum through an incision above the sternum used for biopsy of paratracheal lymph nodes

mediastinum—the area containing the structures that lie between the lungs

mucolytic—capable of dissolving, digesting or liquefying mucous

Mycoplasma—a genus of bacteria containing Gram-negative cells

nares—nostrils

nasopharynx—the part of the pharynx that lies above the soft palate and opens anteriorly into the nasal cavity

nebulizer—an atomizer, an apparatus for projecting a liquid in the form of a fine spray or vapor

orthopnea—discomfort on breathing in any but the erect sitting or standing position

oximetry—measurement of the oxygen saturation of hemoglobin in a sample of blood

oxyhemoglobin—hemoglobin in combination with oxygen

paranasal—alongside the nose

pathogen—any virus, microorganism, or other substance causing disease

percussion—tapping over the lung area to distinguish between presence of air and fluid

perfusion—blood flow through pulmonary vessels

pertussis—whooping cough

pharyngectomy—excision of the pharynx

pharyngoplasty—reparative or plastic surgery of the pharynx

pharyngotomy—incision into the pharynx

pharynx—the throat or upper extended portion of the digestive tube between the mouth and esophagus

photoscanning—the photographic display of the distribution of an internally administered radiopharmaceutical

plethysmography—measurement and recording of changes in volume of an organ or other part of the body

pleura—the serous membrane surrounding the lungs and lining the walls of the pleural cavity

pleuracentesis—insertion of a hollow needle or a trocar and cannula into the pleural cavity; thoracentesis

pleural rub—grating sound heard when inflamed surfaces make contact

pleurectomy—excision of a pleura, the serous membrane lining the wall of the pleural cavity

pleurisy—inflammation of the pleura

pleurotomy—any cutting operation on the chest wall; thoracotomy

pneumococcal—pertaining to or containing the pneumococcus, a species of Gram-positive diplococci

pneumonectomy—removal of pulmonary lobes from a lung

pneumonia—inflammation of the lungs with exudation and consolidation

pneumonitis—inflammation of the lungs

pneumonomycosis—disease of the lung caused by the presence of fungi

pneumotrachometer—an instrument for measuring the instantaneous flow of respiratory gases

pneumothorax—the presence of air or gas in the pleural cavity

postural—relating to or affected by the position of the limbs or carriage of the body

purified protein derivative of tuberculin—purified tuberculin containing the active protein fraction

pyothorax—pus in the pleural cavity

radiography—the making of a record by means of X rays or by a radioactive body or substance

rale—a sound heard on auscultation of the chest in diseases of the lungs, indicative of the presence of fluid

respiration—ventilation; the act of breathing

rhinitis—inflammation of the nasal mucous membranes

rhinoplasty—reparative or plastic surgery of the nose

rhinorrhea—a discharge from the nasal mucous membrane

rhinosinusitis—inflammation of the mucous membrane of the nose and sinuses

rhinovirus—a virus responsible for the common cold

rhonchi—abnormal crackling sounds heard during inspiration denoting presence of fluid in the bronchi

rigor—rigidity or chill

septum—a thin wall dividing two cavities or masses of softer tissue, such as the nares

sinusitis—inflammation of the lining membrane of any sinus, especially of one of the paranasal sinuses

sinusotomy—incision into a sinus

sphenoidal sinus—one of a pair of cavities in the body of the sphenoid bone communicating with the nasal cavity

spirometer—an instrument for measuring the volume of respiratory gases

sputum—expectorated material

stridor—a high pitched, noisy respiration, indicative of respiratory obstruction
subglottic—below the glottic opening between the vocal cords
supraglottitis—inflammation of the area above the glottis
thoracalgia—pain in the chest
thoracodynia—pain in the chest
thoracostomy—the establishment of an opening into the cavity of the chest
thoracentesis—insertion of a hollow needle into the pleural cavity
thoracoplasty—reparative or plastic surgery of the thorax
thorax—the chest
tomography—sectional X rays taken by a tube with curvilinear motion
tonsillectomy—removal of the tonsils
tonsil—a collection of lymphoid nodules on the posterior wall of the nasopharynx
trachea—the windpipe
tracheitis—inflammation of the lining membrane of the trachea
tracheoplasty—reparative surgery of the trachea
tracheostomy—formation of an opening into the trachea
tracheotomy—the operation of opening into the trachea
tuberculin—a diagnostic test of a glycerin broth culture of *Mycobacterium tuberculosis*
tuberculosis—a disease caused by the presence of *Mycobacterium tuberculosis* usually affecting the lung
turbinectomy—surgical removal of the inferior turbinated one on the lateral wall of the nasal cavity
ventilation—movement of gases in and out of the lung; respiration
ventilator—an apparatus to assist respiration
vestibule—the anterior part of the nasal cavity enclosed by cartilage
vocal cords—the sharp edge of a fold of mucous membrane stretching along either wall of the larynx
wheeze—to breathe noisily and with difficulty

CHAPTER 10

The Reproductive System and Its Disorders

The function of the reproductive system is preservation of the species by the production of offspring. The male reproductive system consists of organs and ducts responsible for the production of male sex cells, their storage and transport, and their mixing with glandular secretions for ejaculation into the female vagina during coitus. The reproductive system in the female consists of organs that form the female sex cells and transport them to other organs where they are fertilized and the new individual develops.

In many anatomy texts, the reproductive system is described as a component of the genitourinary (GU) system; after all, some anatomic structures are involved both in the excretion of waste products through urination and in reproduction, and the organs of both systems are located in the pelvis and abdomen. Despite the anatomical overlap, the two systems serve different functions, and the terminology is in many instances quite distinct.

Anatomy and Physiology

Anatomical Terminology of the Male Reproductive System

In the male, reproduction begins with the formation of spermatozoa (sperm) in the male gonads, the two testicles (Figure 10.1). The testicles are suspended by the spermatic cord within the scrotum, a sac of skin that hangs downward from the junction of the abdomen and perineum. The interior of each testicle is divided into lobules filled with the convoluted seminiferous tubules, so named because they are literally "twisted seed-producing small tubes"; it is in these tubules where sperm production takes place. Each tubule straightens and joins others at efferent ductules ("small ducts"), which pass into the epididymis, the storehouse and location of maturation for sperm cells. A distinction exists between the terms *testicle* and *testis*, although both are derived from the same source. Technically, the testis is an organ made up primarily of convoluted seminiferous tubules and is responsible for spermatogenesis (sperm formation). The testicle, on the other hand, consists of the testis and its associated ducts such as the epididymis and vas deferens.

Numerous other structures and cells exist within the testicles; for example, Sertoli cells may nourish developing sperm cells, and Leydig cells (interstitial cells) produce the male hormone androgen. Yet much of the medical terminology related to testicular function, disease, and treatment is derived from a few basic sources. The Greek word for testis is

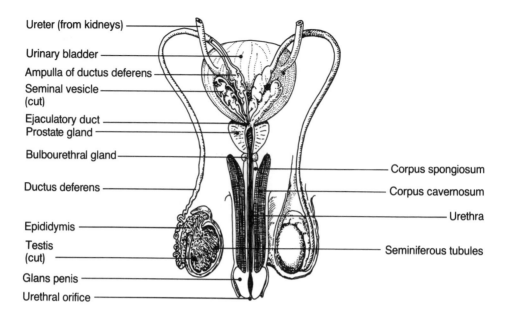

Ureter (from kidneys)
Urinary bladder
Ampulla of ductus deferens
Seminal vesicle (cut)
Ejaculatory duct
Prostate gland
Bulbourethral gland
Ductus deferens
Epididymis
Testis (cut)
Glans penis
Urethral orifice

Corpus spongiosum
Corpus cavernosum
Urethra
Seminiferous tubules

Figure 10.1—Male Reproductive Anatomy.
Anterior view of the male reproductive system. Sectional view of portions of the penis and right testis to show interior structures.

orchis, and the prefixes *orchi-*, *orchio-*, and *orchido-* refer to testes in such terms as **orchidotomy** (incision into the testis, usually for biopsy), **orchidectomy** (removal of the testis), **orchitis** (inflammation of the testis), **orchidalgia** (pain in the testicle), and **cryptorchidism** (failure of the testicle to descend into the scrotum; also called **cryptorchism**).

The sperm cells are excreted from the testicle through the **ductus deferens** (or **vas deferens**). In conjunction with a bundle of other fibrous and vascular structures, the ductus deferens is part of the spermatic cord suspending the testicles. After passing through the inguinal canal and over the iliac vessels, the duct turns downward toward the posterior surface of the bladder. The ductus deferens then becomes dilated into the **ampulla** (Latin for "bottle," the same source as the pharmaceutical term "ampul"), which is connected to the **seminal vesicle**. The seminal vesicle gets its name from the Latin for "seed bladder," which is at least partly appropriate. It does not store sperm cells (or "seed"); instead, this glandular outgrowth of the ductus deferens contributes a secretion to the seminal fluid in which the sperm cells are suspended. The seminal fluid from the testicles and the secretions of the seminal vesicle combine to form semen. Both the ampulla and the seminal vesicle narrow at the base of the bladder and join to form the **ejaculatory duct** and enter the **prostate gland**.

The prostate gland is located just below the bladder and surrounds the prostatic urethra. Consisting of three lobes, the prostate in older men is susceptible to **benign hypertrophy** (also called BPH, for benign prostatic hypertrophy or benign prostatic hyperplasia). BPH is a condition in which the prostate, particularly the median lobe, becomes enlarged and presses on the urethra and base of the bladder, interfering with the flow of urine. The gland is also a major site of cancer in men.

The **penis** is the external male genital organ and serves several functions. It conveys the penile urethra from the prostate gland to its opening at the external urethral meatus; in its flaccid state, the penis conveys urine to the surface of the body. The penis also may be stiffened in an erection by the congestion of blood within the three cylinders of erectile tissues that constitute the main mass of the penis. The two **corpora cavernosa** lie along the anterolateral (forward outside) surfaces, and the **corpus spongiosum** extends along the lower surface of the penis medially. The term *corpus cavernosum*, which is the singular form, means "cave-like body," named for its meshwork of cavernous spaces which become engorged with blood during sexual stimulation. Parasympathetic vasodilation of the penile arteries allows blood to enter the penis and cause swelling while the same stimulation prevents drainage of the blood into the veins; after ejaculation or cessation of sexual stimulation, sympathetic stimulation dilates the veins and returns the penis to its flaccid state. Similarly, **corpus spongiosum** means "spongy body" because of its meshwork structure; it becomes engorged in the same way as the corpora cavernosa.

Externally, the penis consists of the body or shaft, which terminates in the **glans penis**, a cap-like extension of the corpus spongiosum. The word *glans* is from the Latin for "acorn," so the term is often used for any rounded mass or gland-like structure (for example, **glans clitoridis** is the erectile tissue at the end of the clitoris). The glans penis is molded into an expanded rim called the **corona** (from the Greek for "crown," as in *coronary*). The **prepuce** or foreskin, a fold of skin between the corona and shaft of the penis, folds forward over the glans unless removed by the surgical procedure known as circumcision.

Anatomical Terminology of the Female Reproductive System

In the female, reproduction begins in the female gonads—the two **ovaries**—with the development of the **ova** (singular: **ovum**). The process through which ova are formed is called **oogenesis** ("formation of eggs"). Thus, the medical community uses two prefixes—both oo- (or *oophor-*) and *ovo-*, respectively, from the Greek and Latin words for "egg"—to refer to the ova or ovaries. For example, **oophoritis** is inflammation of the ovaries, **oophorectomy** is the surgical removal of an ovary, either an **oocyte** or an **ovocyte** is a developing ovum, and an **oviduct** is a tube that carries an ovum from an ovary to the uterus. Like the testicle, the ovary is a small ovoid (same root again!) body that produces both germinal cells and hormones. The ovaries are located within the pelvis on the lateral walls close to the ureters (Figure 10.2). They rest on the broad ligament of the uterus and are attached with a short mesentery, the mesovarium, which supplies blood vessels to the ovaries; they are also attached with two other ligaments. In spite of these attachments, the ovaries can normally rise with the uterus and be moved about during a pelvic examination.

At birth, the ovaries contain all the ova that will be formed during the individual's lifetime. Contained in minute cellular chambers called **primitive follicles** (or **primordial follicles**), most of the thousands of ova originally present never progress beyond this stage; instead, most atrophy, while others develop into **mature follicles**. Ordinarily, only one follicle and ovum reach maturity at a time, usually alternating between the two ovaries with each menstrual cycle. In response to hormonal stimulation, the mature follicle ruptures in the process called **ovulation**, releasing the ovum into the peritoneal cavity in a miniature gush of follicular fluid. The follicle then collapses and transforms into the **corpus luteum** as the ovum is transported to the uterus.

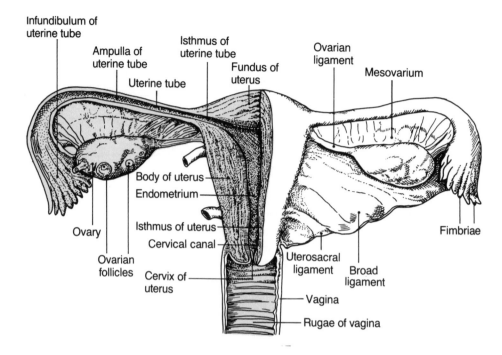

Figure 10.2—Female Reproductive Anatomy.
Anterior view of the female reproductive system. Sectional view of portions of the organs on the right side to show interior structures.

The **uterus** is a hollow organ suspended in the midline of the pelvis and opening into the vagina. It is connected to the abdominal cavity near the ovaries by the uterine tubes. It is through the uterine tubes (also called **fallopian tubes** or oviducts) that the ovum reaches the uterus. One end of the uterine tube is the **infundibulum**, a flared structure like a trumpet, which rests near the ovary. Projecting from the infundibulum are fringed processes called **fimbriae** (singular: **fimbria**), which clasp the surface of the ovary and guide the ovum into the uterine tube. The main body of the uterine tube, called the **ampulla** because of its shape (Latin for "bottle" or "jug"), is a thin-walled muscular tube that arches over the ovary. The ampulla then narrows into a short, thick-walled segment called the **isthmus** (narrowing, just as in the geographical term), which leads into the uterus. The entire length of the fallopian tube has a mucosal lining bearing hair-like **cilia**, which create a current flowing into the uterus and, in conjunction with the peristalsis of the tube, propelling the ovum along the oviduct.

Fertilization usually occurs during the passage of the ovum through the fallopian tube. Spermatozoa deposited in the vagina during **coitus** swim through the uterine cavity, into the tubal opening, and along the tube to reach and penetrate the ovum. The fertilized ovum continues its passage through the uterine tube and undergoes the first cellular divisions in the development of the new individual before reaching the uterus.

In rare instances, the fertilized ovum becomes attached to the wall of the ovarian tube resulting in a **tubal pregnancy**, which presents insufficient blood supply for the growing fetus and may cause the tube to rupture. Even more rarely, the ovum may escape the fimbriae entirely, be fertilized, and become implanted upon the wall of an abdominal organ in an **abdominal pregnancy**. Both of these situations are called **ectopic pregnancies** because they are ectopic or "outside the normal position."

In its nonpregnant condition, the uterus is a small muscular organ with thick walls encompassing the narrow triangular uterine cavity. Rising above the vagina and bent forward at an angle of 90 degrees, the uterus is normally in a position of **anteversion** (literally "turning before" or forward). All of the uterus except the cervix, however, is somewhat mobile and can become lifted back in **retroversion** or flexed and folded back in **retroflexion**; either abnormal position can decrease fertility. Above the level of the uterine tubes lies the widest part of the uterus, the **fundus**. The **body of the uterus** is the main portion that extends down and backward to the constricted area called the isthmus or neck of the uterus. Below the isthmus, the **cervix** is a more fixed tubular portion that extends into the upper portion of the vagina and forms the opening called the **ostium** of the uterus (or the **external os, cervical os,** or **cervical orifice**).

The uterine cavity is lined with the **endometrium** (*endo-*: within; *metra*: uterus), a mucosal layer that undergoes cyclic changes under the influence of the ovarian hormones estrogen and progesterone. These cyclic changes prepare the endometrium to support the implantation of the fertilized ovum. If a fertilized ovum is not implanted in the uterus, the endometrium is sloughed in a hemorrhagic process known as **menstruation** or **catamenia** in which blood and endometrial tissue, called **menses**, is discharged through the vagina. The endometrium then regenerates to complete the menstrual cycle. During the menstrual cycle, the endometrium goes through four phases. Regeneration after the previous cycle in response to estrogenic hormone from the maturing follicle is known as the **follicular** phase. With ovulation, usually between the tenth and sixteenth day, the endometrium enters the **progravid** (*pro-* = before; *gravid* = pregnant) phase and becomes thickened and engorged in preparation for pregnancy. If fertilization does not occur, the **ischemic** phase reduces the blood supply to the endometrium, which begins to shrink before being sloughed off during the **menstrual** phase.

Below the cervix of the uterus lies the **vagina**, a fibromuscular tube that receives the penis during coitus, serves as the outlet for menstrual flow, and forms the birth canal along with the cavity of the uterus. Normally collapsed, the walls of the vagina are capable of significant dilation, especially during childbirth, and are lined with mucous membrane. At the upper end of the vagina, the anterior, posterior, and lateral **fornices** (singular: fornix) of the vagina are recesses between the vaginal wall and the cervix of the uterus. The vagina opens externally at a vertical slit called the **vaginal orifice**.

The external genitalia in the female, often referred to collectively as either the **vulva** or the **pudendum**, consist of several structures in the urogenital triangle of the perineum. The vaginal orifice, along with the urethra above it, opens into the vestibule (an entry, as in architecture) of the vagina. The orifice is partly closed by a thin membrane called the **hymen**, which is reduced to tags of tissue as sexual relations are established and children are born. At each side of the orifice are the bulbs of the vestibule, which cover the greater vestibular glands. These glands, whose ducts open at the margin of the hymen, form a mucous secretion during sexual activity to lubricate the lower end of the vagina.

The vestibule is surrounded by two folds of skin, the **labia minora** (singular: **labium minor**, literally meaning "small lip"). The labia minora join superiorly to form a hood over the **clitoris**, the female homologue of the male penis. Composed of the **corpora cavernosa**, which are two small bodies of erectile tissue, the body of the clitoris ends in a small knobby projection called the **glans clitoridis**. Like the glans of the penis, the glans clitoridis is extremely sensitive to the touch and becomes engorged with blood during sexual excitation.

On either side of the labia minora are the **labia majora** (singular: **labium majus**), elevations of skin and fatty tela subcutanea, the loose connective tissue beneath the skin. When the legs are close together, the labia majora touch medially to form the pudendal cleft. The labia majora are homologous to the male scrotum and enclose and protect the other external genital organs. Superior to the pudendal cleft is the **mons pubis** (commonly called the pubic mound), a rounded elevation of tissue similar to the labia majora and covering the **symphysis pubis** (the joint of the pubic bones; symphysis = "growing together"). After puberty, the mons pubis and labia majora become covered with short coarse pubic hairs.

The primary function of the genital organs is reproduction, which is accomplished through **conception** and **pregnancy**. Pregnancy occurs if an ovum is fertilized by a sperm, the process of conception, and then becomes implanted into the endometrium where it develops into an embryo. At the embryonic stage, the **placenta** and **amniotic sac** also develop. Within the placenta, blood of the embryonic circulation is exposed to maternal blood. Although there is no direct mixing of these two blood supplies, the thin placental membrane permits absorption of nutritive materials, oxygen, and some harmful substances into the fetal blood and release of carbon dioxide and nitrogenous waste from it. Sometimes referred to as the "bag of waters," the amniotic sac envelops the embryo and is filled with **amniotic fluid**, which serves to protect the embryo and permit movement. The **umbilical cord** connects the embryo and the placenta to the mother and is the stalk containing the umbilical arteries and veins.

After the first two months of pregnancy until the time of birth, the unborn child is usually referred to as a **fetus** instead of an embryo. In a normal pregnancy, the fetus remains in the uterus for forty weeks after pregnancy begins. This time span is referred to as the **gestation** period (derived from the Latin *gesto-*, which translates as "to bear"). The time before birth is also referred to as the **antenatal** (*ante-*, before; *natus,* birth), **prenatal**, or **antepartum** (Latin *partus*, "to bring forth") period.

During this prenatal period, a woman is commonly referred to as pregnant, but medical records usually rely on another set of terms that are more specific. A woman who is pregnant is said to be **gravid**, from the Latin for "heavy" or "loaded." **Gravida**, the noun form, simply means a pregnant woman, and the sequence of the pregnancy in the woman's life is denoted numerically by a Latin prefix (e.g., *primi-, secundi-, terti-*, etc.) or by a Roman numeral for each occurrence. For example, a woman in her first pregnancy is indicated by the terms *primigravida* or *gravida I*. Likewise, **para** (like *partus*, meaning "to bring forth") is the term given to a woman who has given birth to a viable fetus, whether the child was living or not. The nulliparous woman has never given birth, while the multiparous one has undergone more than one delivery. The numerical sequence of the birth, like the sequence of a pregnancy, is denoted by either the Latin prefix (e.g., primipara) or the Roman numeral (para I). The number refers to the sequence of the birth, not the number of children; therefore, the birth of twins will count only as one birth. Thus, a woman who is pregnant for the third time, although she may not have carried either fetus to term, is tertigravida (or gravida III); after giving birth to twins, she will be primipara (para I), although she will have two children. As is evident from this example, such terminology conveys more information than the more common terms *pregnant* and *mother*.

The process of giving birth is called **parturition**. This includes **labor**, which is divided into four stages, and **delivery**, the passage of the fetus and placenta from the genital canal into the external world. Terms associated with the birth process refer to presentation of the fetus (**breech, vertex, transverse, face, cephalic,** depending on which fetal structure faces the cervix) or to procedures involved (**episiotomy, hysterotomy, Cesarean section**). Immediately after delivery of the fetus, the **secundines** or "afterbirth," which includes the placenta and attached umbilical cord, are expelled as the final stage of labor. **Lochia** refers to the discharge of mucus, blood, and tissue debris that continues for a period of time following childbirth.

The period immediately after birth and continuing through the first 28 days of life is described as the **neonatal** period when referring to the infant or neonate and the **postpartum** period when referring to the pregnancy. **Lactation,** the production of milk by the mammary glands and release of milk from the breasts, begins one to three days after childbirth. Until that time, the suckling child receives **colostrum,** a fluid high in protein, minerals, and immunoglobulins that is secreted by the mammary gland for a few days surrounding birth.

Therapeutics

Diseases

Infections are among the most common of the diseases affecting the reproductive system, notable among them being the **sexually transmitted diseases** (STDs). Formerly, STDs were known primarily by the term venereal disease (VD), indicating that they are transmitted during coitus, yet other sexual activity (as well as several other mechanisms) may transmit these infections, so the term STD has become the standard in the medical community. According to the World Health Organization, STDs are the most common communicable diseases in the world and include a large number of etiologic organisms and a variety of symptoms. In the United States, many of the STDs must legally be reported to health officials, as must several other contagious diseases. Statistics are maintained for these **reportable diseases** by the Centers for Disease Control, and state and local officials usually investigate and "track" cases to find and treat other individuals who are infected.

Gonorrhea is the most common of the reportable STDs, resulting from infection with *Neisseria gonorrhoeae*. The acute infection generally affects the epithelium of the urethra, cervix, ovaries, and rectum, although the infection can become disseminated. The infection acquired from orogenital contact, called **gonococcal pharyngitis**, affects the pharynx. Women are often asymptomatic carriers of the organism for weeks or months after infection, and males may also be asymptomatic. The most common symptoms are a purulent, yellowish green urethral discharge in men; dysuria and frequency of micturition in both sexes; and vaginal discharge. Gonorrhea can become disseminated, resulting in such infections as **gonococcal endocarditis** in the heart and **gonococcal meningitis** in the central nervous system. And an infant born to a mother with gonorrhea can develop an eye infection called **gonococcal ophthalmia neonatorum**. Complications of gonorrhea include **salpingitis** (also called **pelvic inflammatory disease** or PID), which is infection and inflammation of the **salpinx** (Greek for "tube") **uterina**, more commonly known as the uterine tube.

Although the most frequent pathogen involved in salpingitis is *N. gonorrhoeae*, gram-negative bacilli, gram-positive cocci, *Mycoplasma* species, and viruses are frequently implicated. Although PID specifically refers to salpingitis, some use the term "pelvic inflammatory disease" more generally to include infection of the cervix (**cervicitis**), uterus (**endometritis**), or ovaries (**oophoritis**) since all those structures are in the pelvic region. PID should not, however, be used to describe all types of pelvic pain of unknown etiology since the result can easily be confusion in communication. Salpingitis can be acute and even life-threatening, or it may lead to chronic complications. A tubal **abscess** can form, which may drain spontaneously, or it may rupture into the peritoneum, an acute event that can cause shock and death within an hour. One or both tubes may also become filled with pus, creating the condition of **pyosalpinx** (*pyo-* = pus). In the end stage of pyosalpinx, the tube may become occluded and fill with fluid (**hydrosalpinx**), which often causes infertility.

Similar in presentation to gonorrhea but caused by a different organism is **nongonococcal urethritis** (NGU), which is most frequently, but not exclusively, associated with *Chlamydia trachomatis*. Its name is derived from its symptoms, which are essentially the same as the urethritis caused by gonorrhea, but it is nongonococcal in origin.

Another sexually transmitted infection is **syphilis** (also called **lues**), which is caused by the spirochete *Treponema pallidum*. After initial infection, the primary **chancre** develops at the site of inoculation, definitive of the primary stage of syphilis. The secondary stage occurs in untreated patients about six weeks after infection and includes more widespread skin eruptions. Both primary and secondary syphilis are called **infectious syphilis**. Latent syphilis includes untreated seropositive patients with no clinical manifestations. Tertiary syphilis is a late stage involving skin, bones, the central nervous system, or the cardiovascular system. The site of infection changes both the symptomatology and the name; for example, **neurosyphilis** affects the cerebrospinal fluid, and **meningovascular neurosyphilis** principally involves the cerebral cortex, although the infection is originally sexually acquired. **Congenital syphilis** is acquired in utero. Other STDs include **trichomoniasis, genital candidiasis, genital herpes, genital warts (condyloma acuminata), chancroid, lymphogranuloma venereum** (LGV), and several others.

Colporrhagia, vaginal hemorrhage, is pathologic and distinct from uterine bleeding. Bleeding from the uterus via the vagina may be physiologic, occurring with normal menstruation and, in some women, at the time of ovulation. There are, however, numerous uterine bleeding disorders.

Amenorrhea (*a-* = without; *men* = month; *rhein* = flow) is the absence of menstruation and may be either primary or secondary. Primary amenorrhea is a lack of **menarche** (the normal beginning of menstruation at puberty) in a woman at least 16 years old, while secondary amenorrhea is the cessation of menses in a woman who has previously had her menarche. Primary amenorrhea is a symptom rather than a disease and may be nothing more than a physiologic delay of menarche; it can, however, also be indicative of underlying pathologies. Anatomic causes of amenorrhea include absence of the vagina, uterus, or ovaries or some obstruction to menstrual flow such as a transverse vaginal septum or imperforate hymen (lack of the normal opening in the hymen; literally, unperforated). If the flow is obstructed, other menstrual symptoms may occur, but the menstrual fluid will be prevented from escaping, a condition called **cryptomenorrhea** (*crypt-* = hidden). Primary amenorrhea may also be due to endocrine disorders such as pituitary dysfunction, ovarian diseases like polycystic ovarian disease, or disorders of other endocrine systems. The most frequent cause of primary amenorrhea is chromosomal abnormalities; physiologic function also can be disturbed enough by crash dieting, obesity, anorexia nervosa, emotional stress, and severe illnesses to delay or prevent menarche.

Amenorrhea after menarche is physiologic during pregnancy and lactation, and menstrual periods are commonly irregular in the first few years after menarche. Pathologic secondary amenorrhea may be anatomic, endocrine, or psychogenic in nature. **Oligomenorrhea** (from *oligos*, the Greek for "little"), also called **relative amenorrhea,** is a reduced frequency of menstruation.

Other abnormalities of menstrual bleeding are also only symptoms of other underlying pathologies, and the terms describe the symptom. **Dysmenorrhea** is painful menstruation, and the term is often modified to indicate the etiology. For example, **congestive dysmenorrhea** is accompanied by congestion of the uterus; **essential dysmenorrhea** or **primary dysmenorrhea** has no apparent cause; **mechanical dysmenorrhea** is caused by mechanical obstruction, such as from clots or uterine flexion; and **psychogenic dysmenorrhea** is caused by psychological factors.

Because the suffix *-algia* normally indicates pain, one might assume that **menorrhalgia** is synonymous with dysmenorrhea, but it is not. Menorrhalgia describes distress associated with menstruation, including dysmenorrhea, premenstrual tension, and pelvic vascular congestion. **Epimenorrhea** (also called **polymenorrhea**) denotes that the period of flow is abnormally frequent, and **hypermenorrhea** or **menorrhagia** indicates that the amount of flow is greater than usual but the period is normal; thus **epimenorrhagia** is the term applied to a flow that is both abnormally frequent (*epi-* prefix) and excessive (*-agia* suffix), although the term *menorrhagia* is also sometimes used instead of epimenorrhagia. If the flow of uterine bleeding is normal in amount but occurs at completely irregular intervals, the bleeding is called **metrorrhagia.**

Dysfunctional uterine bleeding (DUB) is any abnormal uterine bleeding not associated with tumor, inflammation, or pregnancy. Ironically, it is also called **functional uterine bleeding** because it appears to be caused by some body function rather than an external source such as a tumor. Such bleeding is often due to endometrial hyperplasia from excessive estrogen, either from an estrogen-producing ovarian tumor, polycystic ovaries, or liver disease, which interferes with estrogen metabolism.

Menopause or **climacteric** (frequently called "change of life") is a transitional phase in women in which menstruation ceases, usually occurring about age 50, although the age is extremely variable. Not pathologic, menopause nonetheless may be symptomatic, causing hot flushes and sweating, nervousness, depression, and other symptoms; these symptoms are caused by estrogen deficiency and vasomotor responses, so they are often treated with exogenous estrogen. **Premature menopause** refers to cessation of ovarian function before age 40, and **artificial menopause** follows any medical procedure that "artificially" ends endogenous estrogen production, such as **ovariectomy** (removal of the ovaries; also called **oophorectomy**), irradiation of the ovaries, or radium implantation in the uterus.

For some reason, menopause is often referred to in nearly mythic ways and is often called "the menopause," even in medical literature. Inclusion of the article "the" is so nearly universal in some circles that some medical editors automatically add it to any published work on the subject. Menopause is not a single entity that is passed from one woman to another, as "the menopause" might indicate, and no linguistic reason exists to require inclusion of the article. Pharmacists should be aware of this usage, however, since they may hear someone say she has "recently reached the menopause."

Several neoplastic disorders affect the female reproductive organs, the most frequent being **cervical carcinoma**. Cervical carcinoma is closely associated with a history of early and frequent coitus and multiple sex partners, and trauma from viral and bacterial infections is thought to be related to the neoplastic process. On the continuum from normal to invasive cancer, minimal cervical **dysplasia** is the first histologic change seen, indicating abnormal cell proliferation in the lower third of the epithelium, most of such lesions reverting to normal. Severe dysplasia is abnormal proliferation in two-thirds of the epithelium, and it is felt that most severe dysplasias progress to carcinoma in situ.

The second most common malignancy of the female reproductive organs is **endometrial carcinoma**, which is usually postmenopausal. Other malignancies include **ovarian carcinoma**, carcinoma of the vulva, **vaginal carcinoma**, and carcinoma of the fallopian tube.

Inflammation of the vulva (**vulvitis**) has numerous causes, including mechanical and chemical irritation, urinary or fecal contamination, allergic reactions, infections, or simple hygienic neglect. Acute vulvitis presents with marked edema and erythema of the vulva and may cause pain so severe that the patient cannot sit or walk; chronic vulvitis, on the other hand, is less severe.

Leukorrhea (*leuko-* = white) is characterized by a distressing, often whitish discharge from the genital tract. Also simply called **vaginal discharge,** leukorrhea is a symptom rather than a disease, and the term should only be applied to an abnormal discharge. Common causes include chronic **cervicitis, cervical eversion** (turning inside out), and infections with organisms such as *Trichomonas vaginalis, Candida,* and *Haemophilus vaginalis.* If the discharge is due to inflammation of the vagina, it is called **vaginitis.**

Premenstrual syndrome (PMS or **premenstrual tension)** is characterized by nervousness, irritability, emotional instability, depression, headaches, generalized edema, and breast tenderness. PMS occurs during the 7 to 10 days before menstruation and is caused by fluctuations in estrogen and progesterone.

In men, the most common disorders of the reproductive organs are the infections previously discussed. Also, bacterial infections beneath the foreskin may cause **balanoposthitis,** generalized inflammation of the glans penis and foreskin. The prefix *balano-,* like glans, is from a word meaning ''acorn'' and refers to the glans penis or glans clitoridis; *posth* is from the Greek for ''prepuce.'' This inflammation predisposes to **meatal stricture,** a stenosis of the meatus; **phimosis,** constriction of the prepuce, which prevents it from being retracted; or **paraphimosis,** constriction of the prepuce, which prevents it from being reduced over the glans.

Priapism is a persistent and painful erection of the penis in the absence of sexual arousal, and it may be caused by diseases and injuries to the spinal cord or secondary to obstruction of the outflow of blood from the penis.

Peyronie's disease is a fibrous hardening (**induration**) of the cavernous sheaths of the penis, eventually causing contractures that pull the penis to the involved side. The cause is unknown.

The most common intrinsic mass within the scrotum is **hydrocele** (*hydro-* = water; *-cele* = hernia), a condition characterized by excessive accumulation of normal fluid within the **tunica vaginalis testis** (the peritoneal covering of the testis) resulting from inflammation or reduced resorption. **Hematocele** is an accumulation of blood in the tunica vaginalis. **Spermatocele** (also called **spermatic cyst**), unlike hydrocele and hematocele, occurs in the epididymis, not the tunica vaginalis, and it contains sperm; an

epididymal cyst also occurs in the epididymis, but it differs from a spermatic cyst in that it contains clear fluid rather than sperm.

Neoplastic disorders affecting the male reproductive organs include penile, testicular, and prostatic cancer. In the penis, carcinoma is the predominant type; **adenocarcinoma** is more common in the prostate; and the testes are prone to a variety of malignant tumors.

Infertility, whether relative or absolute, affects perhaps 5% of married men. Interference with spermatogenesis, transit of sperm through the seminal tract, or deposition in the vagina will cause infertility. **Varicocele,** a varicose condition of the venous plexus in the scrotum, can increase testicular temperature sufficiently to inhibit sperm production, resulting in **azoospermia** (absence of sperm in the semen) or **oligospermia** (lowered sperm density). Further, congenital anomalies, **orchitis** (inflammation of the testis), **epididymitis** (inflammation of the epididymis), **vasitis** (inflammation of the vas deferens), **prostatitis** (inflammation of the prostate), **seminal vesiculitis** (inflammation of the seminal vesicles), **urethritis** (inflammation of the urethra), or **urethral stricture** all can obstruct the seminal tract. Such an obstruction can lead to infertility by causing **aspermia,** the absence of ejaculate. Other causes of infertility include hormonal disorders, including **hypothyroidism** and **hypogonadism**.

Impotence (also called erectile dysfunction), which is the inability to achieve or maintain an erection, is most frequently psychogenic, although several physical disorders such as diabetes mellitus and hypothyroidism may be involved as well.

Although pregnancy is not a disease, there are several disorders that are specific to pregnancy and childbirth. **Abruptio placentae** is the premature separation of the placenta from the uterus, and it is often associated with maternal systemic reactions such as shock and diminished urine output. Escape of the amniotic fluid is called **amniorrhea,** and **amniorrhexis** denotes rupture of the amniotic membrane. If the childbirth process is abnormal or difficult, it is referred to as **dystocia,** a combination of the prefix *dys-* and the Greek root for birth, *-toc.*

Toxemia of pregnancy is characterized by hypertension, edema, and proteinuria. Clinically, the syndrome is divided into the stages of **preeclampsia** and **eclampsia.**

Early fetal death and abortion may be caused by incompatibility of the ABO blood groups between the mother and infant, involving antigens and antibodies of the red cells.

The complexity of the reproductive system in both sexes necessarily gives rise to a large number of diseases and conditions. A few of the more common disorders are listed in Table 10.1; abbreviations associated with the reproductive system are listed in Table 10.2.

Diagnosis and Therapy

The pelvic examination is an essential part of routine annual gynecological examination and begins with a visual inspection of the external genitalia and, after insertion of the speculum, of the cervix and vaginal wall. During the exam, a cervical smear is taken for the **Papanicolaou test (Pap test)** to detect abnormal cells indicative of cervical cancer. Pap smear reports are grouped into four categories. A Class I result indicates no abnormal cells; Class II contains atypical cells that are usually caused by inflammation; cells suspicious of carcinoma are found in Class III; and carcinoma cells are present in Classes IV and V. Any suspicious lesion is generally biopsied, and a **cervical punch biopsy** and **endocervical curettage** are used to diagnose invasion. **Cold knife cone**

Table 10.1—Common Disorders of the Reproductive System	
Gynecologic:	acute salpingitis
	carcinoma of the vulva
	cervical carcinoma
	endometrial carcinoma
	fibromyoma
	membranous dysmenorrhea
	ovarian cyst
	tubal abscess
Pregnancy:	anemia
	erythroblastosis fetalis (Rh disease)
	habitual abortion
	hyperemesis gravidarum
	missed abortion
	placenta previa
	premature labor
	septic abortion
Breast:	carcinoma of the breast
	chronic cystic mastitis
	fibroadenoma
	gynecomastia
	lipoma of the breast
Female sexual disorders:	dysfunction of arousal and orgasm (frigidity)
	dyspareunia
	vaginismus
Male sexual disorders*:	erectile dysfunction (impotence)
	premature ejaculation
	sexual ennui (low sex drive)

*See Chapter 11—"The Urinary System and Its Disorders" for other common disorders of the male reproductive system.

biopsy can confirm the diagnosis and remove the lesion, which is sometimes sufficient treatment. Biopsy is also the primary diagnostic procedure for most other malignancies, although **laparoscopy** (insertion of and examination with a **laparoscope**) is needed for examination and biopsy of some organs.

Infections are generally diagnosed by standard culture techniques or serologic tests. Serologic tests for syphilis include both screening and specific tests for antitreponemal antibodies. The screening tests most frequently used are the Venereal Disease Research Laboratory (VDRL) test, complement fixation tests, and the Rapid Plasma Reagin (RPR) test.

Table 10.2—Abbreviations Associated with the Reproductive System

Ab	abortion		**FAST**	fetal acoustical stimulation test
ADS	anonymous donor's sperm		**FDIU**	fetal death in utero
AID	artificial insemination donor		**FBM**	fetal breathing movements
AIH	artificial insemination with husband's sperm		**FBP**	fetal biophysical profile
ARM	artificial rupture of membranes		**FHR**	fetal heart rate
			FHS	fetal heart sounds; fetal hydantoin syndrome
AROM	artificial rupture of membranes		**FM**	fetal movements
A-Z test	Ascheim-Zondek test		**FPAL**	full term, premature, abortion, living
BB	breakthrough bleeding		**FT**	full term
BC	birth control		**FTLFC**	full-term living female child
BCP	birth control pills		**FTLMC**	full-term living male child
BOW	bag of waters		**FTND**	full-term normal delivery
BTB	breakthrough bleeding		**FUB**	functional uterine bleeding
BTL	bilateral tubal ligation		**G**	gravida
BVL	bilateral vas ligation		**GIFT**	gamete intrafallopian transfer
BW	birth weight		**G/P**	gravida/para
CAN	cord around neck		**GPMAL**	gravida, para, multiple births, abortions, and live births
CB	Caesarean birth		**Gyne**	gynecology/gynecologist
CD	Caesarean delivery		**HCG**	human chorionic gonadotropin (test)
C & D	curettage and desiccation			
CDC	calculated day of confinement		**HPL**	human placental lactogen
CMC	chronic mucocutaneous moniliasis		**HRT**	hormone replacement therapy
			IMB	intermenstrual bleeding
COC	combination oral contraceptive		**IUCD**	intrauterine contraceptive device
CPID	chronic pelvic inflammatory disease		**IUD**	intrauterine device
			IVF	in vitro fertilization
CST	contraction stress test		**IVF-ET**	in vitro fertilization, embryo transfer
CVS	chorionic villus sampling			
D & C	dilatation and curettage		**LAVH**	laparoscopic-assisted vaginal hysteroscopy
D & E	dilatation and evacuation			
DFMC	daily fetal movement count		**LGV**	lymphogranuloma venereum
DFU	dead fetus in uterus		**LMP**	last menstrual period
DGI	disseminated gonococcal infection		**LNMP**	last normal menstrual period
			LTL	laparoscopic tubal ligation
DGM	ductal glandular mastectomy		**MPR**	multifetal pregnancy reduction
DLMP	date of last menstrual period		**NFTD**	normal full-term delivery
DLNMP	date of last normal menstrual period		**NGU**	nongonococcal urethritis
			NSD	normal spontaneous delivery
DUB	dysfunctional uterine bleeding		**NSFTD**	normal spontaneous full-term delivery
EDC	estimated date of confinement/conception			
			NST	nonstress test
EDD	estimated date of delivery		**NSU**	nonspecific urethritis
EFW	estimated fetal weight		**NSV**	nonspecific vaginitis
EGA	estimated gestational age		**NSVD**	normal spontaneous vaginal delivery
EPT	early pregnancy test			
ERP	estrogen receptor protein		**NVD**	normal vaginal delivery
ERT	estrogen replacement therapy		**Pap test**	Papanicolaou smear
ETO	estimated time of ovulation		**PECHO**	prostatic echogram
EUS	endoscopic ultrasonography		**PET**	pre-eclamptic toxemia
EWB	estrogen withdrawal bleeding			
F & C	foam and condom			

PGU	postgonococcal urethritis	**SRBOW**	spontaneous rupture bag of waters
PID	pelvic inflammatory disease	**SROM**	spontaneous rupture of membranes
PIH	pregnancy-induced hypertension		
PMB	postmenopausal bleeding	**STD**	sexually transmitted disease
PME	postmenopausal estrogen	**STS**	serologic test for syphilis
PMP	previous menstrual period	**SUB**	Skene's urethra and Bartholin's glands
PMS	premenstrual syndrome		
PMT	premenstrual tension	**SVD**	spontaneous vaginal delivery
PMTS	premenstrual tension syndrome	**SVE**	sterile vaginal exam
		TA	therapeutic abortion
PNV	prenatal vitamins	**TAB**	therapeutic abortion
POC	product of conception	**TAH**	total abdominal hysterectomy
POL	premature onset of labor	**TH**	total hysterectomy
PPD	postpartum day	**TL**	tubal ligation
PPH	postpartum hemorrhage	**TOP**	term of pregnancy
PPROM	prolonged premature rupture of membranes	**TSS**	toxic shock syndrome
		TURP	transurethral resection of the prostate
PPS	postpartum sterilization		
PPTL	postpartum tubal ligation	**UCI**	urethral catheter in
PROM	premature rupture of membranes	**UCO**	urethral catheter out
		UPT	urine pregnancy test
PSRBOW	premature spontaneous rupture bag of waters	**USG**	ultrasonography
		VBAC	vaginal birth after Caesarean
PTL	pre-term labor	**VD**	venereal disease
PU	pregnancy urine	**VDG**	venereal disease—gonorrhea
RPR	rapid plasma reagin (test)	**VDRL**	Venereal Disease Research Laboratory
RRA	radio receptor assay		
SAVD	spontaneous assisted vaginal delivery	**VDS**	venereal disease—syphilis
		VH	vaginal hysterectomy
SIT	sperm immobilization test	**VIP**	voluntary interruption of pregnancy
SPROM	spontaneous premature rupture of membranes		
		V & V	vulva and vagina
		ZIFT	zygote intrafallopian transfer

Roentgenographic techniques such as CT scans can be used to detect masses and other anomalies in reproductive organs, but they are used much less frequently than in other systems because of the sensitivity of the gonads, sperm, and ova to the chromosomal effects of radiation.

Several common surgical procedures are specific to the reproductive system, most notably those used for sterilization. In the female, infertility is induced permanently by **tubal ligation**, commonly called a "tubal" or "tying the tubes." With tubal ligation, the uterine tubes are constricted by the application of a ligature; additionally, the tubes are usually severed or crushed to prevent the restoration of fertility if the ligatures fail. In the male, **vasectomy** (removal of all or part of the ductus deferens) is used to induce sterility. Both tubal ligation and vasectomy are surgically reversible in certain instances.

Abortion applies to both intentional and unintentional termination of an existing pregnancy by expelling the products of conception from the uterus. A **spontaneous abortion** occurs naturally and may result from either fetal or maternal abnormalities, infection, or other diseases. **Induced abortion** (also called **artificial abortion**) may be induced by the administration of an abortifacient drug or surgically by dilating the cervix and scraping the uterine lining, a procedure known as dilation and curettage (D&C). A D&C is also used to remove excess endometrium in several bleeding and endometrial disorders. If the abortion is performed to medically benefit the mother, it is usually termed a **therapeutic abortion**.

Diagnostic tests for pregnancy include the **chorionic gonadotropin** (HCG, or human chorionic gonadotropin) tests and the **radio receptor assay** (RRA).

Prenatal diagnosis by **amniocentesis** involves percutaneous withdrawal of amniotic fluid. The **amniocytes**, cells in the fluid, are studied for their chromosomal makeup or for levels of specific enzymes. Screening for Down's syndrome is a primary indication for the procedure. Other methods of diagnosis include **fetoscopy** for direct observation of malformations and for fetal blood sampling. **Ultrasonography** permits visualization of some malformations using ultrasound radiation. The **alpha-fetoprotein** test is the fetal equivalent of serum albumin and is elevated in some congenital disorders.

Besides surgical induction of infertility, several other methods of contraception are available. In females, administration of estrogen–progestin combinations known commonly as birth control pills or oral contraceptives can prevent ovulation. Other medications for contraception include continuous low doses of progestins, available as daily oral doses known commonly as "mini-pills," surgically implanted progestin dosage forms for continuous release, and even as a component in an intrauterine device. Other drugs prevent conception by reducing sperm motility or killing spermatozoa (spermicides). Several mechanical methods of contraception are also available, including the cervical cap, intrauterine device (IUD), diaphragm, condom, and vaginal condom.

Besides preventing conception by inducing male infertility, vasectomy is also performed in association with **prostatectomy** (removal of the prostate), usually when removing a tumor rather than benign hypertrophic tissue. For the removal of a tumor, a prostatectomy may be performed through an incision through the peritoneum, but the more common procedure for benign prostatic hypertrophy is currently a **transurethral resection** of the prostate (TURP).

Pronouncing Glossary

Root	Meaning	Example	Pronunciation
andro-	male	androgen	ann drow JEHN
colpo-	vagina	colporrhaphy	coal PORR oh fee
galact-	milk	galactocele	gul AKT oh seal
gravi-	pregnant	gravida	GRAV eh dah
gyneco-	woman	gynecology	gyn ee KOLL oh jee
hyster-	uterus	hysterectomy	his terr EK toh mee
masto-	breast	mastoplasty	MAST oh plas tee
meno-	menses	menorrhagia	men oh RAY jah
metro-	uterus	metrorrhagia	met troh RAY jah

Root	Meaning	Example	Pronunciation
oo-	egg	oocyte	Uwo site
oophor-	ovary	oophorectomy	uwo for EKT omee
orchi-	testis	orchiocele	ORK eeh oh seal
para-	to bear	multipara	mull TIP or ah
salpingo-	fallopian tube	salpingocele	sal PENG oh seal
thel-	nipple	thelitis	th eye LI tis
toc- tok-	childbirth, labor	oxytocia tokodynograph	ox ee TOSH eeh ah to ko DIEN oh graff
trachel-	neck (of uterus)	trachelitis	trak el I tis

Glossary

abruptio placentae—the premature separation of the placenta from the uterus

amniorrhea—escape of amniotic fluid

amniorrhexis—rupture of the amniotic membrane

breech presentation—position of the fetus at delivery with the buttocks approaching the cervix

cephalic presentation—position of the fetus at delivery with any part of the head directed toward the cervix

colporrhaphy—the procedure of suturing the vagina; denuding and suturing the vaginal wall to narrow the vagina

corpus luteum—postovulatory ovarian follicle, in some species with a yellow color imparted by the accumulation of lipid, giving the term its name

dyspareunia—pain with intercourse

dystocia—abnormal or difficult childbirth

eclampsia—convulsions and coma in a pregnant woman associated with hypertension, edema, and/or proteinuria

epimenorrhagia—menstrual flow that is both abnormally frequent and excessive

epimenorrhea—menstrual flow that is abnormally frequent but of normal amount

external urethral meatus—opening of the urethra at the surface of the body

face presentation—position of the fetus at delivery with the face directed toward the cervix

fertilization—the act of rendering a gamete capable of further development; fusion of a spermatozoon and an ovum, which stimulates the completion of the maturation of the ovum

follicle—a sac or pouch-like cavity; specifically, ovarian follicle, the egg and its encasing cells at any stage of development

gamete—a reproductive cell; ovum or sperm

gonad—organ that produces gametes; testis or ovary

hypermenorrhea—menstrual flow that is of greater than usual amount but of normal frequency

inguinal—pertaining to the groin or junctional region between the abdomen and thigh

isthmus—a narrow connection between two larger bodies or parts; specifically, the narrow part of the uterus

ligature—any substance, such as catgut or silk, used to tie a vessel or strangulate a part, as in a tubal ligation

menorrhagia—hypermenorrhea

menorrhalgia—distress associated with menstruation, including dysmenorrhea, premenstrual tension, and pelvic vascular congestion

metrorrhagia—menstrual flow of the normal amount but at completely irregular intervals

multiparous—having given birth to more than one child

nulliparous—never having given birth to a viable infant

orchiocele—hernial protrusion of a testis; scrotal hernia; tumor of a testis

orifice—an opening

placenta previa—the placenta is obstructing the opening of the cervix

polycystic ovary—condition in which one or both ovaries contain or are made up of many cysts

polymenorrhea—epimenorrhea

preeclampsia—a toxemia of late pregnancy characterized by hypertension, edema, and proteinuria

primitive or primordial follicle—an ovarian follicle consisting of an egg encased by a single layer of cells

salpingocele—hernial protrusion of a uterine tube

spermatogenesis—process of the formation of sperm

toxemia (of pregnancy)—a group of metabolic disturbances in pregnant women characterized by preeclampsia and fully developed eclampsia

trachelitis—inflammation of the uterine neck

transverse presentation—position of the fetus at delivery with the shoulder or any other part of the trunk directed toward the cervix

vertex presentation—position of the fetus at delivery with the vertex of the head directed toward the cervix

CHAPTER 11

The Urinary System and Its Disorders

The urinary system functions to remove waste products that are dissolved in the plasma of circulating blood and carry these products out of the body. The upper urinary tract consists of the **kidneys, ureters,** and **bladder** (sometimes referred to by the acronym **KUB**). Excretion of the waste is carried out by the kidneys. The ureters are the primary ducts that carry the urine away from the kidneys and into the bladder, which serves to store the urine until a sufficient volume has accumulated. Then the urine is voluntarily expelled through the **urethra** to an opening at the surface of the external genital organs at the **urethral meatus.**

Anatomy and Physiology

The organs that remove dissolved waste products from the blood are the two kidneys. The kidneys are located on each side of the spinal column high on the posterior abdominal wall behind the peritoneum. Despite this retroperitoneal (''behind the peritoneum'') location, the kidneys are actually covered by the **renal fascia,** extraperitoneal connective tissue attached to the abdominal wall. Many terms related to the kidneys incorporate the terms **renal** (or its combining form *reni-*) or **nephri** (or its combining forms *nephr-* or *nephro-*), which are derived from the Latin and Greek words for kidney, respectively. The term *fascia* is from the Latin for ''band'' and is often applied to any band of connective tissue that covers an anatomic structure. Thus, the renal fascia is connective tissue that covers the kidneys. Within the renal fascia and providing a protective cushion for the organ is a large collection of adipose tissue called the **perirenal fat,** so named because it is around (*peri-* = around) each kidney.

Shaped like a bean, each kidney has a long convex lateral border and a shorter, indented medial border, as shown in Figure 11.1(A). The upper end is topped by the **suprarenal gland,** also called the **adrenal gland;** either name is derived from the gland's position in relation to the kidney since *supra-* means ''above'' and *ad-* indicates ''near.'' The indentation on the medial border of each kidney is called the **hilum** and is the point where the renal artery enters the kidney and the renal vein and ureter leave it.

Although the hilum appears to be a deep indentation in the smooth, fibrous **capsule** covering the kidney, a cross-sectional examination reveals that it actually reaches deep into the center and forms a cavity called the **renal sinus.** The renal sinus is filled with fat and provides the bed for the renal vessels and nerves as well as the ureter. Within the renal sinus, the ureter expands into a funnel-shaped structure, the **renal pelvis,** from which reach tubular projections called the **major calyces** (singular: **calyx,** named for the Greek word *kalyx,* the cup of a flower, like which it is shaped). The major calyces reach

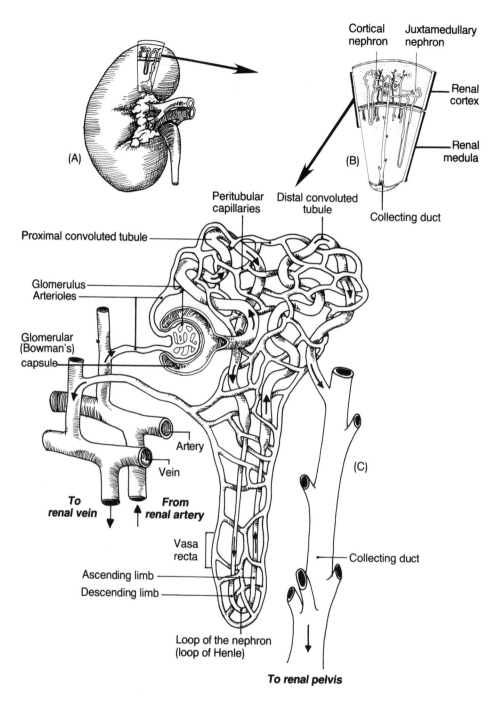

Figure 11.1—The Nephron.
(A) Entire kidney. (B) Enlarged section. (C) A cortical nephron enlarged even further.

toward the glandular part of the kidney, and each divides into several **minor calyces.** Together, the calyces and renal pelvis form the drainage system for urine in its path from the glandular part of the kidney, where it is formed, to the ureter.

The glandular portion of the kidney that surrounds the structures of the renal sinus is divided into the **medulla** and the **cortex** [Figure 11.1(B)]. The medullary portion consists of a series of conical structures called **renal pyramids** with their blunted points facing in toward the renal sinus. The blunted end of each renal pyramid is perforated by the openings of ducts and projects into a minor calyx. The cortex lies between the bases of these pyramids and the capsule or surface of the kidney and projects between the pyramids in the renal columns.

Within the cortex are the **nephrons,** which actually form the urine [Figure 11.1(C)]. At the outer end of each nephron is a sac-like structure of epithelial cells called the **glomerular capsule** (or **Bowman's capsule**). Within the capsule is a knot of capillaries termed the **renal glomerulus,** which is fed by an **afferent arteriole** and drained by an **efferent arteriole**. Together a glomerulus and its surrounding glomerular capsule are called a **renal corpuscle.** Within the corpuscle, the blood in the capillaries is separated from the capsule by only two layers of flat epithelial cells, the capillary wall and the epithelium of the sac. More complex than two cell layers might seem, the separation between capsule and glomerulus consists of **podocytes**—the cells of the capsule that have both foot-like (*podo-* = foot) processes extending from a central cytoplasm and secondary **pedicles** (or "end feet") touching the capillary—and a capillary wall with numerous pores. Because of these pores and pedicles, electrolytes and small molecules pass through this membrane while blood cells, fatty substances, and the large molecules of plasma proteins are retained in the capillary. Thus, the millions of nephrons provide a filtering mechanism for blood, all of which passes through the kidneys about 15 times each hour.

Each glomerular capsule leads into a twisted tubule. The **proximal convolution** (or **proximal convoluted tubule**) twists around in the cortex near the corpuscle. The tubule then straightens into the medulla, turns in a U-shaped curve, and climbs back toward the corpuscle. This loop, called the **loop of Henle,** consists of a narrow descending limb on the proximal side and wider ascending limb on the distal side. As the tubule approaches its own capsule, it twists again into the **distal convolution** (or **distal convoluted tubule**) and then straightens again as it joins the first of a series of **collecting tubules.** The collecting tubules pass through the cortex into the medullary pyramid, collecting the filtrate of other nephrons along the way and joining with other collecting tubules until they make their final junctions into **papillary ducts.** The papillary ducts emerge from the apex of the pyramid into a minor calyx.

After the efferent arteriole leaves the glomerular capsule, it branches into secondary capillary plexuses around both the proximal and distal convolutions before finally reaching the renal vein. Through these capillaries, the circulatory system selectively reabsorbs some of the filtrate from the Bowman's capsule. Ions and glucose are reabsorbed early in the proximal convolution, and other nutrients and much of the water are reabsorbed in the distal convolution, converting glomerular filtrate into urine by the time it reaches the collecting tubules for transport to the renal pelvis.

Besides forming urine, the kidneys also have other functions. Some of the smooth muscle cells of the afferent arteriole are modified by the presence of a well-defined **Golgi complex;** these, together with cells of the adjacent distal convoluted tubule, form the **macula densa,** which secretes **renin.** Renin is a proteolytic enzyme that catalyzes the formation of **angiotensin I** from a plasma protein, which is then transformed to **angiotensin II** by **angiotensin converting enzyme** (ACE). This **juxtaglomerular** (*juxta-* = near) **apparatus,** through the renin–angiotensin system, plays a significant role in controlling plasma volume and blood pressure. The kidneys also produce **renal erythropoietic factor** (REF), which increases erythropoietin output, increasing hemoglobin synthesis. Further, although **prostaglandins** are named for the prostate gland where they were first discovered, some are released by the renal medulla.

The ureters are the excretory ducts that transport the urine from the kidneys to the urinary bladder. At the hilum, the renal pelvis narrows, funneling the urine into the tubular ureters. The muscular walls of the ureter contract in waves, propelling the urine along its length and into the bladder in spurts rather than as a steady flow.

The urinary bladder is a distensible, muscular sac in the pelvis. When empty, the bladder's walls collapse; as it fills, it expands upward. Covered at the top by peritoneum, the bladder is separated from the rectum posteriorly by the **rectovesical pouch** in the male and from the uterus by the **vesicouterine pouch** in the female. The internal floor of the bladder forms a smooth triangular area known as the **urethral trigone** (*trigonon* is Greek for "triangle"). At the posterolateral angles of the trigone, the ureters enter at the uretic orifices; at the front angle is the internal urethral orifice through which the urethra leaves the bladder. The **detrusor uniae** muscles, the muscles of the bladder, stretch when the bladder fills and contract in response to relaxation of the **urethral sphincter** to empty the contents.

Urine passes from the bladder to the surface of the body through the **urethra.** In the female, the urethra passes straight downward and forward through both the pelvic and urogenital diaphragms, becomes fused to the anterior wall of the vagina, and ends at the **external urethral meatus** at the vestibule. In the male, the urethra extends through the prostate gland where it is joined by the ejaculatory duct of the vas deferens, through the pelvic and urogenital diaphragms, and down the length of the penis to the external urethral meatus.

Therapeutics

Diseases of the Urinary System

Pathologies affecting renal function can occur in any part of the urinary tract, and the affected organ or site is often involved in the nomenclature of the disease. For example, diseases of the glomerulus usually include the combining form *glomerulo-* in the name, those involving the pelvis of the kidney often incorporate the combining form *pyelo-* or *pyel-,* and the forms *nephr-* and *nephro-* apply to the entire kidney.

Inflammation of the glomeruli is called **glomerulitis** and involves proliferative or necrotizing changes in the glomerular cells. **Glomerulonephritis,** on the other hand, is an inflammation of the glomerulus and other parts of the nephron. Simple glomerulitis is relatively uncommon, and the latter term is much more frequently encountered to refer to inflammatory diseases involving the glomerulus.

Glomerulonephritis may present with an abrupt onset, often as a result of immune-complex disease following an infection. Termed **acute, postinfectious,** or **poststreptococcal glomerulonephritis** (PSGN), the disorder causes edema, **oliguria** (decreased urine output, technically less than 500 ml per day), **hematuria** (blood in the urine), **proteinuria** (protein in the urine), and even headaches and visual disturbances secondary to hypertension if fluid retention is severe enough. With a more insidious onset is **subacute glomerulonephritis,** also called **rapidly progressive glomerular disease** or **RPGN.** Although fairly rare, subacute glomerulonephritis presents with hematuria, proteinuria, and RBC casts in the urine and often progresses to total, irreversible **anuria** (*an-* = without; *-uria* = urine production: production of less than 100 ml of urine per day) of terminal renal failure. **Chronic glomerulonephritis** is a syndrome characterized by slow, progressive loss of renal function and is often asymptomatic for years before it is detected. Pathologically, chronic glomerulonephritis produces sclerosis of glomeruli; and the clinical presentation includes proteinuria, **cylindruria** (the presence of cylindrical casts in the urine), and usually hematuria.

Some terms describing diseases and syndromes can provide significant confusion. For example, **nephrosis** and **nephrotic** may be used to describe any disease of the kidneys, yet both also have more specific meanings. The term *nephrosis* most commonly refers to degenerative disease specific to the tubules of the nephron, distinguishing it from an inflammatory process (or "nephritis"). The degenerative lesions of a nephrosis are marked by severe proteinuria and decreased serum albumin, symptoms that together are specifically known as the **nephrotic syndrome.** Thus, in one sense the two terms are synonymous; in another, a nephrosis can lead to nephrotic symptoms. Because of the loss of albumin in the urine, nephrotic syndrome leads to hyperlipidemia and edema; the disorder is classified by its cause, including primary nephrotic syndrome for which an underlying cause is not identifiable. To further complicate the terminology, primary nephrotic syndrome is also referred to as **idiopathic nephrotic syndrome,** and the term *idiopathic nephrotic syndrome* is often associated by pediatricians and internists with two different, distinct types of lesions, removing any clarity that may have ever surrounded the term.

Among the more diffuse **nephropathies** (diseases of the kidneys) is **acute pyelonephritis,** named for its abrupt onset and the inflammation (*-itis*) frequently involving the pelvis (*pyelo-*) of the kidney (*nephr-*). Infective in origin, acute pyelonephritis may affect the renal pelvis, the **parenchyma** (functional part of the organ rather than structural elements, a term that applies to any organ), or both; approximately 85% of all cases are caused by infection by *Escherichia coli.* The kidney is usually enlarged, and the acute inflammation may cause extensive parenchymal destruction.

Since stasis allows bacterial invasion through the urinary tract, **urinary stasis** is frequently implicated in acute pyelonephritis, and it may arise from such underlying disorders as ureteral or urethral strictures, **renal calculi** ("kidney stones" formed through the process of **nephrolithiasis**), tumors, prostatic hypertrophy, or **neurogenic bladder.** Symptoms of acute pyelonephritis include fever and chills, vomiting, and bladder irritation from infected urine, causing urgency and frequency of urination (also called **miction** or **micturition**). A more descriptive term for acute pyelonephritis, although one that is less frequently used, is acute infective tubulointerstitial nephritis because it describes the infective nature of the disease and the involvement of the tubules and their interstitial spaces. The term *pyelonephritis* should only be applied to diseases with documented **urinary tract infection (UTI).**

Chronic pyelonephritis is also infective in origin, but low-grade or recurrent infections make the progress of the disease more insidious, and progression to end-stage renal failure occurs commonly in patients with obstruction. Correction of the underlying obstruction is an essential part of effective therapy.

Several vascular disorders affect the kidneys, including renal vein **thrombosis,** renal **infarction,** and **malignant nephroangiosclerosis** (literally, "hardening of the arteries of the kidney"). Malignant nephroangiosclerosis is also called **malignant nephrosclerosis** and **malignant hypertension.** Malignant nephroangiosclerosis is a necrosis of the renal arteries associated with hypertension, and it rapidly progresses to renal failure.

Infection or other irritation of the lower urinary tract is often characterized by **dysuria** (painful or difficult urination). A UTI may also present with numerous changes in the composition of the urine, including the presence of bacteria **(bacteriuria),** blood **(hematuria),** and pus **(pyuria).** Some drugs such as the sulfonamides, which are often used to treat UTIs, are concentrated in the urine, causing the formation of crystals **(crystalluria)** that can injure the kidneys, ureters, and urethra. Other diseases also change urine composition; for example, diabetes mellitus may produce **glucosuria** and **hyperketonuria.** Similarly, several renal diseases exhibit effects on other systems, particularly blood composition since the kidneys filter wastes from the blood. For example, **renal azotemia** (as well as shock, dehydration, excessive protein catabolism, and GI hemorrhage) can increase blood urea nitrogen **(BUN)** levels.

Other urinary symptoms are nonspecific and may arise from numerous causes. Frequency and urgency generally indicate a relative decrease in bladder capacity, which may result from loss of elasticity caused by infection or inflammation or may be related to bladder mucosal injury from stones, tumors, or infections. **Nocturia** (voiding during the night) may reflect early renal disease, may be associated with cardiac or hepatic failure, or may simply result from excessive fluid intake. **Enuresis** (bed-wetting at night) is physiologic during the first two or three years of life but later may be produced by a delay in neuromuscular development or organic disease.

Since the urinary system eliminates such a variety of wastes, alterations in urinary function can quickly alter the composition of the blood. Along with the lungs, the kidneys perform a significant function in maintaining acid–base balance in the body, primarily by tubular reabsorption of filtered bicarbonate and excretion of hydrogen ions released by nonvolatile acids. Thus, the urinary system is involved in **metabolic acidosis** of several types. **Renal tubular acidosis** is **hypokalemic** (abnormally low serum potassium) in nature, while **hypoaldosteronism** can lead to metabolic acidosis, which is **hyperkalemic.** Starvation can lead to **ketoacidosis,** and kidney failure leads to **lactic acidosis.**

The kidneys also regulate osmolality of the blood and help control the concentration of numerous electrolytes in the plasma. As a result, a urinalysis can indicate a variety of electrolyte disturbances, such as **hyponatremia** (excess sodium in the blood), **hypernatremia** (sodium depletion in the blood), **hypocalcemia** (abnormally low serum calcium), **hypophosphatemia** (low phosphate ion in plasma), and so on. Other common diseases of the urinary system are listed in Table 11.1.

Therapy

The most frequently performed laboratory test related to the urinary system is a **urinalysis (UA).** Urinalysis usually includes qualitative evaluation for the presence of protein, glucose, ketones, and blood and determination of urinary pH and osmolarity. Further, microscopic examination of the urinary sediment is an essential component of a UA and allows detection of crystals, cells, and a variety of **casts** (mucoprotein masses

Table 11.1—Common Diseases of the Urinary System

Kidney:	acute noninfective tubulointerstitial nephritis
	diabetic nephropathy
	carcinoma
	chronic tubulointerstitial nephropathy
	hydronephrosis
	lupus nephritis
	toxic tubulointerstitial nephritis
Lower urinary tract:	benign prostatic hypertrophy
	exstrophy of the urinary bladder
	megacystic syndrome
	neurogenic bladder
	penile carcinoma
	prostatic carcinoma
	testicular tumors
	urethral carcinoma
Vascular:	atherosclerosis
	malignant hypertension (malignant nephrosclerosis, malignant nephroangiosclerosis)
	renal infarction
	renal vein thrombosis
Electrolytes:	hypercalcemia
	hypernatremia
	hyperphosphatemia
	hyperuricemia
	hypocalcemia
	hyponatremia
	potassium depletion
Hereditary:	hereditary nephritis
	medullary cystic disease (familial juvenile nephronophthisis)
	polycystic renal disease

that may entrap cellular components or fat droplets). Casts are identified by their components and may aid diagnosis. For example, RBC casts contain red blood cells indicating glomerulonephritis, WBC casts include white blood cells suggestive of pyelonephritis or several other disorders, and bacterial casts are diagnostic of bacterial pyelonephritis. Urinary infections may be diagnosed by **culture and sensitivity** (C&S), which is often performed in relation to a UA.

Renal function may be evaluated by a number of laboratory findings. **Glomerular filtration rate (GFR)** is estimated by endogenous **creatinine clearance, plasma cre-**

atinine, or plasma **urea** concentration or may be measured by the clearance of inulin. Other tests measure **renal plasma flow, proximal tubular transport,** and **distal tubular transport.**

Visualization of renal structures can be accomplished in several ways, depending on the view that is needed. Plain X-ray of the abdomen can display gross anatomy of the kidneys and image some renal calculi in several urinary organs, but **computerized tomography** (CT) scans provide better detail and may overcome obscuring of the kidney by the intestine as well as image other urinary structures. The kidney and lower urinary tract may be visualized with an **excretory urogram** by infusing a triiodinated benzoic acid derivative, which is readily filtered by the kidney and is radiopaque. If renal function is compromised, the radiopaque agent may be introduced directly into the urinary tract via a catheter in a **retrograde pyelogram.** An image of the bladder is a **cystogram,** which is part of a **urogram** or may be performed separately. The urinary system may also be visualized by **ultrasonography.**

Urethroscopy and **cystoscopy** allow the practitioner to view the lumen of the urethra and interior of the bladder, respectively, via fiber-optic techniques. Surgical procedures can be performed using the same technology. For example, **urethrotomy** to repair a stricture may be done with the aid of a **urethroscope** as well as by surgically opening the abdomen.

Urinary stones are often treated only symptomatically with analgesics until they are passed through the urethra, but large stones in the bladder are usually removed surgically **(lithotomy)** or crushed into smaller pieces by sound waves and washed out using a **lithotriptor** through a procedure known either as **lithotripsy** (from the Greek words for "stone" and "to rub") or **litholapaxy** (*lapaxis* = evacuation).

Renal failure may necessitate **dialysis,** from the Greek words *dia* (across) and *lysis* (dissolution). **Peritoneal dialysis (peritoneal lavage)** uses the patient's own peritoneum as a semipermeable membrane to remove dissolved wastes. **Hemodialysis,** on the other hand, cycles the blood from an **arteriovenous shunt** or **fistula** to a synthetic membrane where it contacts the **dialysate** (dialysis solution) for removal of the wastes. **Kidney transplant** may be the necessary outcome.

In patients who should not or are unable to void intentionally, the bladder may be manually drained through a urinary **catheter.** Catheterization is commonly performed pre- and postoperatively or in otherwise debilitated patients suffering from urinary **incontinence.** It is also used simply to void (or fill) the bladder to perform any number of procedures. **Indwelling catheters,** such as a **Foley** catheter, are held in place within the urethra by an inflatable tip placed in the bladder; others are specifically designed to open urethral strictures, dilate the ureter, instill antimicrobial irrigants and other fluids, bypass an enlarged prostate, or serve several other specialized purposes.

Abbreviations commonly encountered in referring to the urinary system are listed in Table 11.2.

Table 11.2—Abbreviations Associated with the Urinary System

ADPKD	autosomal dominant polycystic kidney	**KUB**	kidney, ureter, bladder
AGN	acute glomerulonephritis	**LK**	left kidney
AHC	acute hemorrhagic cystitis	**LRD**	living renal donor
AIN	acute interstitial nephritis	**MCGN**	minimal change glomerular nephritis
APD	automated peritoneal dialysis	**MGN**	membranous glomerulonephritis
APKD	adult onset polycystic kidney disease	**MPGN**	membranoproliferative glomerulonephritis
ARF	acute renal failure	**MSK**	medullary sponge kidney
ATN	acute tubular necrosis	**MSUD**	maple syrup urine disease
BNO	bladder neck obstruction	**NS**	nephrotic syndrome
BNR	bladder neck retraction	**NSN**	nephrotoxic serum nephritis
BOO	bladder outlet obstruction	**ONC**	over-the-needle catheter
BPH	benign prostatic hypertrophy	**PKD**	polycystic kidney disease
BT	bladder tumor	**PNT**	percutaneous nephrostomy tube
BTR	bladder tumor recheck	**PSGN**	poststreptococcal glomerulonephritis
CBD	closed bladder drainage	**RDT**	regular dialysis/hemodialysis treatment
CCPD	continuous cycling/cyclical peritoneal dialysis	**REF**	renal erythropoietic factor
C & D	cystoscopy and dilatation	**RER**	renal excretion rate
CGN	chronic glomerulonephritis	**RK**	right kidney
CIN	chronic interstitial nephritis	**RPGN**	rapidly progressive glomerulonephritis
CMG	cystometrogram	**RPN**	renal papillary necrosis
CMK	congenital multicystic kidney	**RTA**	renal tubular acidosis
C & P	cystoscopy & pyelography	**RUA**	routine urine analysis
CPD	chronic peritoneal dialysis	**SNGFR**	single nephron glomerular filtration rate
CPGN	chronic progressive glomerulonephritis	**SRNS**	steroid responsive nephrotic syndrome
CPKD	childhood polycystic kidney disease	**TIN**	tubulointerstitial nephritis
CPN	chronic pyelonephritis	**TRP**	tubular reabsorption of phosphate
CRD	chronic renal disease	**TUR**	transurethral resection
CRF	chronic renal failure	**TURBN**	transurethral resection of bladder tumor
CRI	chronic renal insufficiency	**TURP**	transurethral resection of prostate
CUG	cystourethrogram	**TURV**	transurethral resection valves
Cysto	cystoscopy; cystogram	**TVC**	triple voiding cystogram
ERPF	effective renal plasma flow	**UA**	urinalysis
ESWL	extracorporeal shock wave lithotripsy	**UCX**	urine culture
EU	excretory urography	**UFR**	uroflowmetry
EX U	excretory urogram	**UG**	urogenital
FSGS	focal and segmental glomerulosclerosis	**UN**	urinary nitrogen
GFR	glomerular filtration rate	**UNA**	urinary nitrogen appearance; urinary sodium
GN	glomerulonephritis	**USI**	urinary stress incontinence
GU	genitourinary	**UTI**	urinary tract infection
HUS	hemolytic uremic syndrome	**UUN**	urine urea nitrogen
INC	incontinent; inside-the-needle catheter		
IPD	intermittent peritoneal dialysis		
IVU	intravenous urography		
KF	kidney function		
KTU	kidney transplant unit		

Pronouncing Glossary

Root	Meaning	Example	Pronunciation
cysto-	bladder, sac	cystitis	sis TI tis
nephro-	kidney	hydronephrosis	hi dro neh FRO sis
pyelo-	pelvis	pyelography	pi el OG ra fee
reni-	kidney	reniform	ray NEE form
uro-	urine	urology	ur OLL o gee
vesico-	bladder	vesicotomy	ves ee KOT oh mee

Glossary

afferent glomerular arteriole—a branch of an interlobular artery of the kidney that conveys blood to the glomerulus

anuria—the suppression of urine formation by the kidney

azotemia—uremia; an excess of urea and other nitrogenous waste in the blood

bacteriuria—presence of bacteria in the urine

Bowman's capsule—the blind sac located at the beginning of the tubular component of a nephron

cast—mold formed in a renal tubule and discharged in the urine, consisting of materials such as albumin, cells, blood, and so on

catheter—a flexible tubular instrument used for the passage of fluid into or out of the body

crystalluria—presence of crystalline (solid) material in the urine

cystitis—inflammation of the urinary bladder

cystogram—X ray of the bladder

cystoscopy—visual inspection of the bladder with an endoscope

dialysis—separation of crystalloid from colloid substances in solution using a semipermeable membrane

dysuria—difficult or painful urination

efferent glomerular arteriole—vessel that carries blood from the glomerular capillaries to the proximal convoluted tubule capillaries

enuresis—involuntary discharge of urine, usually occurring at night or during sleep

erythropoietin—protein secreted by the kidney that stimulates the release of reticulocytes from bone marrow

glomerulitis—inflammation of a glomerulus

glomerulonephritis—inflammation of the glomeruli not caused by infection

glomerulus—tuft or cluster of capillary loops found at the beginning of the kidney tubule

Golgi—referring to the flattened saccules and vesicles near the cell nucleus responsible for formation of secretions

glycosuria—presence of glucose in the urine

hematuria—presence of blood or red blood cells in the urine

hemodialysis—use of a semipermeable membrane to separate soluble substances and water from the blood while being circulated outside the body

hyperketonuria—increased levels of ketone compounds in the urine

incontinence—involuntary excretion of urine or feces

infarction, renal—insufficiency of blood supply to the kidney, resulting in necrosis of tissue

ketonuria—increased number of ketone bodies in the urine

litholapaxy—crushing of a stone in the bladder and washing out the fragments through a catheter

lithotomy—surgical incision for the removal of a stone

lithotripsy—crushing of a stone in the urinary tract

loop of Henle—the U-shaped part of the nephron

macula densa—the group of closely packed cells in the distal tubular epithelium of a nephron

malignant hypertension—severe, rapid, potentially fatal hypertension causing necrosis of arteriolar walls and uremia

meatus, urethral—opening of the urethra in the bladder

micturition—urination

nephritis—inflammation of the kidney

nephrolithiasis—presence of stones in the kidney

nephrosclerosis—hardening of the kidney resulting from vascular disease

nephron—the structural and functional unit of the kidney

nephropathy—disease of the kidney

nephrosis—degenerative disease of the kidney

nephrotic syndrome—nephrosis; a condition including edema, proteinuria, and susceptibility to infections

nocturia—increased urination at night

oliguria—scanty urination in relation to fluid intake

podocyte—an epithelial cell of the renal glomerulus, named for its foot-like radiating processes

polyuria—excessive excretion of urine

proteinuria—presence of protein in the urine

pyelogram—X ray of the renal pelvis and ureter

pyelonephritis—inflammation of the kidney and pelvis due to local bacterial infection

renin—an enzyme that converts angiotensinogen to angiotensin

sphincter, urethral—contracting muscles of the urethra

trigone—the triangular smooth area at the base of the bladder

tubule—a small tube; the collecting tubes of the kidney

uremia—azotemia; excess of urea and nitrogenous wastes in the blood

urethritis—inflammation of the urethra

urethroscopy—visual inspection of the urethra using an endoscope

urethrotomy—surgical incision of the urethra

urinalysis—laboratory analysis of the urine

urogram, excretory—X-ray visualization of the urinary tract using an intravenous contrast fluid

CHAPTER 12

The Nervous System and Its Disorders

The terminology of the nervous system is at once both fairly simple and extremely complex. Its simplicity lies in the fact that most of the cells of the nervous system are physiologically quite similar and function primarily in one of two ways. The complexity, however, is derived from the vast array of functions performed by nerves, the sometimes overwhelming number of nerves in the body, and the myriad of diseases that can affect the nervous system.

Understanding the terminology of the nervous system requires the pharmacist to understand the cellular structure and function of the nerve cell as well as many of the interactions of nerves in the body. The primary function of the nervous system is the transmission from one part of the body to another of electrical impulses that can be interpreted by the brain or used by other nerves to control bodily activities. Some of the information transmitted in the form of electrical impulses is interpreted on the conscious level as thought processes in the brain. Other information is entirely outside the conscious realm but is necessary for control of bodily functions such as arterial pressure, respiration, secretion of substances by the gastrointestinal tract, and many others.

Many body systems are most easily understood by beginning with the gross anatomy; an understanding of the nervous system, however, most readily begins with the nerve cell.

Anatomy and Physiology

The primary functional unit of the nervous system is the **nerve cell**, called a **neuron**, which is the Greek word for nerve. Each neuron consists of several basic components. An enlarged portion forms the **cell body** (also called the **perikaryon**), which contains the **nucleus** and **cytoplasm** (Figure 12.1). From the cell body extend several processes called **dendrites**, which contact other nerves and carry impulses into the cell body. A longer process called the **nerve fiber** or **axon** extends outward and carries impulses away from the cell body. The axon, which contains a gelled substance called **axoplasm** surrounded by a membrane, does not branch except at the nerve ending.

Some axons are surrounded by a **myelin sheath (neurilemma** or **neurolemma)** consisting of the lipid substance **myelin.** The myelin sheath is discontinuous approximately every millimeter at the **neurofibril nodes,** also called the **nodes of Ranvier.** The myelin serves as an electrical insulator, forcing the impulse to jump from one node to another, which functions to increase the speed of conduction in a **myelinated** nerve and decrease the energy required for transmission. Further, the larger a nerve is, the more quickly it can conduct impulses. Because of their speed of conduction, large myelinated nerves are the primary conductors of impulses to skeletal muscles, allowing the rapid responses

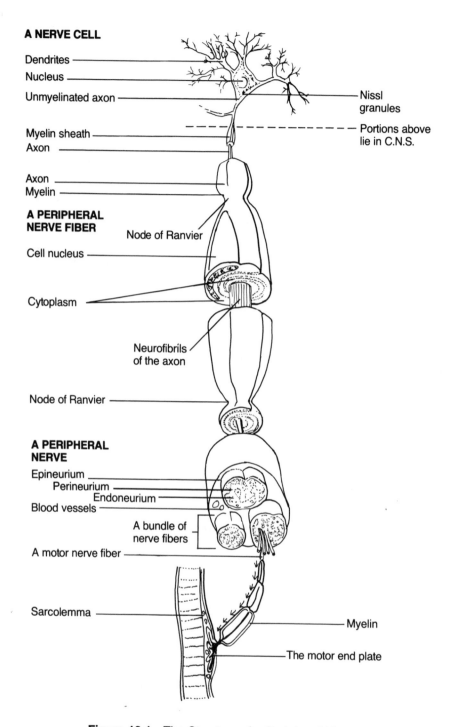

A NERVE CELL

Dendrites

Nucleus

Unmyelinated axon

Nissl granules

Myelin sheath

Axon

Portions above lie in C.N.S.

Axon

Myelin

A PERIPHERAL NERVE FIBER

Node of Ranvier

Cell nucleus

Cytoplasm

Neurofibrils of the axon

Node of Ranvier

A PERIPHERAL NERVE

Epineurium

Perineurium

Endoneurium

Blood vessels

A bundle of nerve fibers

A motor nerve fiber

Sarcolemma

Myelin

The motor end plate

Figure 12.1—The Structure of a Peripheral Nerve.

needed for locomotion. **Unmyelinated** nerves conduct impulses more slowly; thus they often serve functions requiring less prompt response such as controlling blood pressure, crude touch, pain, and emptying of the urinary bladder.

The impulses are conducted along the axon by depolarization of the **membrane potential,** the electronegative potential created inside the fiber as a result of the active transport of sodium ions into the axon and potassium ions to the interstitial fluid. When the nerve is stimulated, the axon depolarizes progressively along its length in a **depolarization wave** or **nerve impulse.** The sheath on myelinated nerves speeds the transmission because the depolarization is forced to "jump" from one node of Ranvier to another in a process called **saltatory conduction.** Unmyelinated nerves simply allow the wave to progress steadily down the axon. Obviously, one possible pathology of the nervous system is loss or lack of the myelin sheath, which can occur both congenitally and later in life, causing a number of diseases discussed later in this chapter.

After a section of nerve has "fired" or become **depolarized,** it must reestablish its membrane potential or **repolarize** before another impulse can be transmitted, so it is refractory to further stimulation. During this **refractory period,** potassium flows outward through the membrane pores to reestablish the potential quickly, and the active transport of sodium continues more slowly to maintain the potential after multiple firings. The refractory period is extremely short, varying in the normal individual from about 1/2500 of a second to 1/250 of a second. The "strength" of a nerve impulse is the combination of the number of firings a second within each nerve cell and the number of nerve cells in a **nerve trunk** (group of nerve cells packed together in a bundle) that are firing.

Transmission of the impulse from a nerve cell to a muscle takes place in the **neuromuscular junction,** the connection between a large myelinated nerve fiber *(neuro-)* and a skeletal muscle fiber *(-muscular).* The **endplate** of the nerve fiber spreads out around an area of the muscle fiber with a small space, the **synaptic cleft,** between the two. When the impulse reaches the endplate, **acetylcholine** is released from vesicles in the nerve, crosses the synaptic space, and stimulates acetylcholine receptors on the muscle fiber. The acetylcholine is then degraded by cholinesterase and re-uptake by the nerve begins.

Transmission from one neuron to another follows a similar course. As an impulse moving down the axon of one neuron reaches the **presynaptic terminal** (the end before [*pre-*] the synapse), a neurotransmitter is released into the synapse so it can attach to a receptor on a dendrite of the next nerve. In the neuromuscular junction, the transmitter is always acetylcholine; between nerves, however, the transmitter can excite the next nerve or inhibit it. In the central nervous system, the primary excitatory neurotransmitter is acetylcholine, so these nerves and those that stimulate muscles comprise what is called the **cholinergic system** (literally, "responding to choline," but actually referring to acetylcholine).

Acetylcholine is not the only neurotransmitter, nor is the cholinergic the only system. Epinephrine, **norepinephrine, dopamine, serotonin,** and several other chemicals also serve as excitatory neurotransmitters in certain parts of the brain as well as in sensory nerves, forming the **adrenergic system,** so named for adrenaline, an earlier term (and now a trade name) for **epinephrine.** Understanding this distinction between neurotransmitters is important to the pharmacist since different drugs act on different receptors. Among the anxiolytics, for example, are inhibitors that are partially specific to either serotonin or dopamine receptors. This specificity helps explain both the differing effects and adverse effects of some of the anxiolytics. Other neurotransmitters, such as **gamma**

aminobutyric acid (GABA), inhibit the firing of the nerve leading away from the synapse.

The nerves of the body are organized in several different ways. To communicate effectively with other health professionals and with patients, pharmacists should understand the organization system being considered. The distinction between adrenergic and cholinergic nerves has already been mentioned and is important in drug therapy, but other classifications affect other therapeutic concerns.

All the nerves may be divided into two physiologic areas, the **central nervous system (CNS)** and the **peripheral nervous system.** The CNS is comprised of the **cerebral cortex,** basal regions of the brain, and the spinal cord. The spinal cord extends down from the **foramen magnum** of the skull to the first lumbar **vertebra** and is surrounded and protected by the vertebral column. It contains two enlargements known as the **cervical** and **lumbosacral enlargements** from which emerge the spinal nerves innervating the upper and lower limbs. The 31 pairs of spinal nerves are named for the vertebrae from which they emerge. For example, the 12 spinal nerve pairs in the thoracic region are referred to as T1 through T12. Similarly, the five **lumbar nerves** are denoted with the letter L, the five **sacrals** with the letter S, and the one **coccygeal** as Co1.

The spinal cord is surrounded by protective membranes called the **meninges,** the plural of the Greek word for membrane (Figure 12.2). The outer layer of the meninges is called the **dura mater** (Latin for "hard mother") because it is tough and fibrous. The middle layer is called the **arachnoid** (Greek for "cobweb-like") since it is delicate and transparent with filaments running to the inner layer. The **pia mater** ("tender mother") is the vascular inner layer attached to the spinal cord. Outside the meninges is the **epidural space,** so called because it is outside (from the Greek *epi,* meaning "upon" or "over") the dura mater. This space is the site of injection for anesthetics for a **saddle block,** a procedure that allows the patient to remain conscious during childbirth or surgery of the pelvic region. The **subdural** space is below (*sub-*) the dura mater and above the arachnoid, an area perhaps of greatest interest to pharmacists when they deal with trauma patients; bleeding into this space produces a **subdural hematoma,** which can cause convulsions and death from increased pressure on the brain or spinal cord. Separating the arachnoid from the pia mater is the **subarachnoid space.** Any number of disorders can affect the meninges, including tumors (**meningioma**) and infections (**meningitis**).

In addition to the protection provided by the vertebrae and the meninges, the **cerebrospinal fluid (CSF)** offers a liquid cushion for the spinal cord. Formed in the brain and drained into the blood, the CSF is involved in the transfer of nutrients and wastes between the blood and neurons. Although similar in composition to plasma, the CSF is distinct and separate from the blood, and it has several diagnostic uses. A **lumbar puncture** or "spinal tap" consists of inserting a needle into the subarachnoid space to detect alterations in cellular and chemical content or pressure. Changes such as increases in white blood cells, protein content, and glucose levels, for example, can indicate viral infections, multiple sclerosis, and bacterial infections, respectively.

Above the spinal cord lies the upper part of the central nervous system, the **encephalon** or, as it is more commonly called, the **brain.** The technical term is derived from the Greek words for "in" (*en*) and "head" (*kephale*) and forms the root of many other medical terms relating to the brain and its diseases (e.g., **encephalitis, encephalopathy,** and **diencephalon**). The brain has four major divisions—**brainstem, cerebellum, cerebrum,** and **diencephalon.**

Immediately above the spinal cord and continuous with it is the **medulla,** or **medulla**

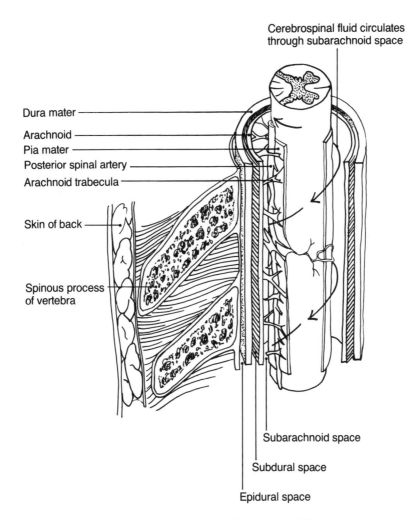

Cerebrospinal fluid circulates
through subarachnoid space

Dura mater

Arachnoid

Pia mater

Posterior spinal artery

Arachnoid trabecula

Skin of back

Spinous process
of vertebra

Subarachnoid space

Subdural space

Epidural space

Figure 12.2—The Structure of the Spinal Meninges.
The Meninges are peeled away to show the meningeal layers and the spaces
between them.

oblongata. The general term *medulla* refers to the marrow or innermost part of an animal; this "oblong medulla" is basic to the human, controls some of the innermost animal functions such as respiration, and is the neural pathway to the rest of the brain. On the ventral surface of the medulla are raised ridges called **pyramids** consisting of motor tracts from the cerebral cortex to the spinal cord. These **pyramidal tracts** cross over in the lower medulla, so each side of the brain controls the opposite side of the body.

Forming a bridge between the medulla and the midbrain is the **pons** (the Latin term for "bridge"), and above that is the **midbrain** or **mesencephalon**. The midbrain helps coordinate movement of the eyeballs and head and regulates focusing and pupil diameter of the eyes. Also located in the midbrain is the **substantia nigra** (literally, "black substance," from its physical appearance), a structure that is involved in Parkinson's disease.

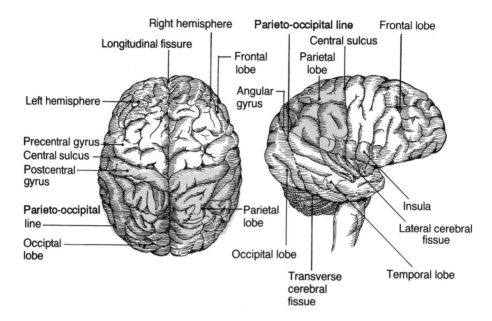

Figure 12.3—Major Structures of the Cerebral Hemispheres.
(A) Superior view. (B) Right lateral view.

Anterior to the midbrain is the **cerebellum** (Latin for "little brain"). The cerebellum is essentially a regulatory structure; it does not consciously perceive sensations or initiate movements, but it coordinates muscle movements and refines body position and balance. Disease of the cerebellum, for example, may result in **ataxia,** although sensory nerve disorders may also be involved. Information from sensory receptors is processed in the cerebellum through connections with the cerebral cortex and other parts of the brain.

The **cerebrum** (Latin for "brain") is the largest and most complex part of the nervous system. Consisting of two hemispheres, the cerebrum is composed of an outer area of grey matter called the **cortex** (the Latin word for "bark"), **white matter,** and **basal ganglia.** The cortex is further divided into six lobes named for their position. The frontal lobe at the front of the skull provides motor control as well as some emotional, moral, and ethical regulation (Figure 12.3). The **parietal lobe,** named for its position relative to the upper rear wall of the skull, is concerned with the evaluation of general senses and taste, providing a general bodily awareness. The **occipital lobe,** so called because it is adjacent to the occiput or rear of the head, contains the visual cortex and the posterior speech area involved in understanding the symbols of written and spoken words. The **temporal lobe** near the ear (from the Latin *tempora,* meaning "temple"; not *tempus,* meaning "time") is important to hearing and memory, especially short-term, as well as some aspects of vision and speech. Damage to the temporal lobe can cause **dyslexia** or **aphasia,** depending on severity. The **limbic lobe** (from the Latin *limbus,* "border") surrounds the central core of the cerebrum and contains the **olfactory cortex,** involved with the perception of odors. Associated with the limbic lobe is the **limbic system,** a group of structures in the cerebrum, diencephalon, and midbrain involved in memory, emotions, and the responses to them. Among these structures are the **hippocampus**

(Greek for "sea horse" because of its S-shape) and **amygdala.** The **insula** (Latin for "island") or **central lobe** is located in the middle of the brain, somewhat like an island. Although little is known about it, the insula seems to be involved in visceral activities.

The surface of the cerebral cortex is a series of raised ridges called **convolutions** or **gyri** (singular is "gyrus," indicating "turning," as in gyroscope) separated by small slit-like depressions called **sulci** (singular: "sulcus"). The effect of these structures is to increase the surface area of the cortex, increasing the proportion of gray matter to underlying white matter. Two deep grooves cross the cortex: the **longitudinal fissure** (from the Latin for "crack"), which separates the two cerebral hemispheres, and the **transverse cerebral fissure,** which separates the cerebrum from the cerebellum.

The **diencephalon** (meaning "between brain") is the deepest part of the cerebrum connecting the midbrain to the cerebral hemispheres. Among other structures, it contains the **thalamus** and the **hypothalamus.** The thalamus receives and decodes sensory input for the cerebrum; influences the motor functions of the cerebral cortex; and helps regulate emotions, thought, and other "human" characteristics through the limbic system. The hypothalamus serves numerous functions, although pharmacists most frequently deal with its control of endocrine functions through the **hypophysis (pituitary gland),** which projects from it.

Outside the CNS is the peripheral nervous system. The peripheral nervous system is further organized into two elements based on the direction of conduction; the sensory system contains **afferent** (from the Latin *ad,* meaning "toward," and *ferre,* "to bring") nerves, which conduct impulses from sensory receptors toward the brain or spinal cord, and the motor system includes **efferent** (*ex,* meaning "away from," and *ferre*) nerves, which conduct impulses away from the CNS to the **effectors** (muscles and glands). The peripheral nervous system may be further divided on a functional basis into the **somatic** and **visceral** systems, each containing both afferent and efferent nerves.

The term *somatic nervous system* is derived from the Greek word *soma,* meaning "body," because the system controls sensations and voluntary movement of the body. Somatic afferent nerves receive and process information from the skin, voluntary muscles, joints, and special sensory organs. This information is conducted to the spinal cord and brain by the spinal and cranial nerves and used by the nervous system at the unconscious level. At the conscious level, this input is perceived as sound, sight, smell, touch, pain, heat, cold, and balance. Somatic efferent pathways descend from the brain through the brainstem and spinal cord to excite skeletal muscles to contract in "voluntary" movement.

The visceral nervous system controls the **viscera,** the Latin term for the internal body organs. Visceral afferent nerves conduct impulses from the cardiovascular, respiratory, digestive, urinary, and reproductive organs to the brain, conveying perceptions such as bladder fullness, intestinal discomfort, and pain. Visceral efferent nerves influence smooth muscles, cardiac muscle, and glands of the skin and viscera. This efferent division of the visceral nervous system is more commonly known as the **autonomic nervous system,** from the same roots as the English word *autonomous,* meaning self-governing.

The autonomic nervous system modulates involuntary visceral activities such as heart rate and secretions of glands. Many visceral activities can be carried out without innervation; heart beat, for example, can continue with no nervous stimulation from outside the heart, which is why a transplanted heart continues to contract. The impulses carried by the autonomic nervous system, however, can increase or decrease both the strength of contraction and the heart rate.

The autonomic system is divided into two complementary subsystems: the **sympathetic** and **parasympathetic.** The term *sympathetic* is derived from the Greek prefix *sym-,* meaning "together," and the root *pathos,* meaning "feeling," the same sources as the word *sympathy.* The sympathetic nervous system stimulates the so-called "fight or flight" phenomenon, an increase in heart rate, cardiac contraction strength, serum glucose, and blood pressure and a concomitant decrease in blood flow to the gastrointestinal tract. "Feeling together" is a fairly reasonable meaning for sympathetic since it controls the "gut response" of fear. The parasympathetic system, on the other hand, conserves and restores body resources by decreasing heart rate and contractility and increasing gastrointestinal activities associated with digestion and absorption of food. The parasympathetic complements the sympathetic as implied by its prefix (*para-* means "beside" or "helping in a secondary way").

The names of specific nerves can be important for the pharmacist in communicating with patients or other professionals. Most are categorized by the areas in which they are located (e.g., thoracic nerves or cranial nerves) and are individually named for the structures they innervate (e.g., the **glossopharyngeal nerve** to the tongue and throat, in addition to a few other structures). The number of individual nerves is overwhelming, so the pharmacist may be wise to use a medical dictionary or anatomy text to identify them as their names arise in practice.

Therapeutics

Diseases

Diseases of the nervous system can result from injury to nerve tissue, infection, anatomical abnormalities, or several other causes. Injury may be severe and affect large areas, such as with a **transection** (severing) of the spinal cord. If a spinal transection occurs between the cervical and lumbosacral enlargements, the result is a **paraplegia,** loss of motor or sensory function in both lower extremities. An injury higher in the spinal cord can cause **quadriplegia,** paralysis of all four limbs and any parts of the body below the injury. Management of the quadriplegic patient is usually much more difficult because of the effects of muscle inactivity on other body systems such as respiration and the cardiovascular system. Damage can also affect only one side, causing **hemiplegia** (or **hemiparesis,** a milder form of paralysis of one side).

Also the result of trauma to the nerve, **sciatica,** is a **neuritis** (nerve inflammation) of the sciatic nerve and its branches, usually causing pain down the back of the leg. Commonly caused by a **herniated** disk causing pressure on the nerve, sciatica may also be caused by a tumor or any other source of damage to the nerve.

Numerous infections can also affect nerve tissue. Caused by a viral infection, **poliomyelitis** is now better known for the vaccine to prevent the infection than for the paralysis it can cause. Also caused by a virus, **shingles** or **herpes zoster** is an acute inflammation of the **dorsal root ganglia.** Usually beginning with fever and a general malaise, shingles progresses to severe deep pain and a rash along the course of one of the spinal nerves. The virus, which causes chickenpox in childhood, may lie dormant in the ganglia of cranial nerves or the ganglia of posterior root nerves; if that virus becomes activated later in life and attacks the root ganglion, shingles results.

Inflammation of the spinal meninges is called **spinal meningitis.** Caused by either a viral or bacterial infection of the meninges, particularly the arachnoid and pia mater, the inflammation increases the amount of cerebrospinal fluid and changes its composition, resulting in the symptoms. The first sign is usually headache, fever, chills, and vomiting; neck rigidity, changes in reflexes, and back spasms are common. Diagnosis is usually made by examination of cerebrospinal fluid collected by lumbar puncture, and antibiotic therapy for the etiologic organism is primary in treatment.

Insufficient blood supply to the brain is another possible insult to the nerves. A **thrombosis,** an **embolism,** or a **hemorrhage** resulting from an **aneurysm** can each cause a sudden decrease in blood flow to the brain, resulting in what is known as a **cerebrovascular accident (CVA)** or **stroke.** The resulting hypoxia may be transient and cause little more than temporary unconsciousness, or it can be of sufficient duration to damage or destroy brain tissue, causing irreversible brain damage or death. Although a single CVA may only infarct a small area of the brain for a short period, several small strokes known as **transient ischemic attacks (TIAs)** can have an additive effect, leading to the memory loss and personality changes of **multi-infarct dementia.**

Many nervous system disorders, however, seem to be unrelated to trauma of any kind and are biochemical in nature. **Epilepsy,** for example, may be traced to a single cause such as a tumor, an abscess, certain poisons, or perinatal brain damage; however, it is more commonly **idiopathic** (with no known cause, literally "self-caused") epilepsy in which brain cells fire unpredictably for no apparent reason. If the motor areas are involved, the disease is often referred to as a **grand mal** (French for "great illness") seizure; although the term is outdated, it is still used frequently. Current terminology refers to such seizures as **generalized tonic-clonic seizures,** which is much more specific and descriptive. The seizures are generalized over large areas of the brain, and the patient initially loses consciousness and falls; then tonic (continuous, from the same source as "tone") contractions occur, followed by a period of clonic seizures (**clonus** refers to alternating contractions and relaxations of muscle fibers).

Absence seizures primarily affect children and result in a brief loss of consciousness. Formerly called **petit mal** (French for "small illness") seizures, they can affect sensory areas without muscle involvement, as in **simple absence seizures,** or they can involve **automatisms** or **myoclonic** jerking, which is categorized as **atypical** or **complex absence seizures.**

Seizures can be limited to one hemisphere of the brain, as in **simple partial seizures,** also called **focal motor seizures;** they can also start as a focal discharge in one hemisphere and spread to partially involve the other hemisphere as with a **complex seizure,** also called **psychomotor** or **temporal lobe seizure.**

Parkinson's disease (also called **Parkinsonism** or **paralysis agitans**) is a motor dysfunction characterized by stiff posture, tremor at rest, difficulty in initiating movements (**bradykinesia**), an expressionless face (**masked faces**), and a shuffling gait. Parkinson's disease results from a shortage of the neurotransmitter dopamine for neurons with their cell bodies in the substantia nigra. As a result of the dopamine deficiency, these brain cells do not perform their usual inhibitory function. Deficiency of a different neurotransmitter, gamma aminobutyric acid (GABA), is associated with Huntington's chorea.

Cerebral palsy (CP) is actually a general term for a group of neuromuscular disorders usually resulting from damage before, during, or shortly after birth. The term *palsy* is a distortion of "paralysis," so "cerebral palsy" simply denotes a paralysis from the brain.

Multiple sclerosis (MS) results from a progressive demyelination of neurons, interfering with the conduction of sensory and motor impulses. If a myelinated nerve is inflamed repeatedly for whatever reason (and the specific cause of MS is unknown), sclerosis or scarring of the myelin sheath takes place. The disease usually progresses slowly with recurring periods of remission. Symptoms include muscle weakness and spasms, urinary infections and bladder incontinence, and severe mood changes.

Alzheimer's disease (AD) is a degenerative dementia resulting in brain atrophy much earlier than usual but with symptoms of anxiety, difficulty with speech, loss of memory, and irrationality as in **senile dementia** (more commonly called **senility**). The degeneration is complex, involving an increased amount of the protein **amyloid** in and around blood vessels, reduced amount of the enzyme **protein kinase C,** and accumulation of **neuritic plaques** and tangled **neurofilaments,** and a loss of cholinergic nerves in parts of the brain. This complexity and the lack of any definitive indicator make diagnosis difficult or impossible in many cases.

Even immune responses cause neural diseases. Within the synaptic space, an autoimmune response of the immune system may produce antibodies to the receptors, making them less responsive to acetylcholine, resulting in a paralysis called **myasthenia gravis** (a grave or severe weakness, *asthenia,* of the muscle, *my-*). Drugs such as neostigmine which inhibit the cholinesterase from destroying the acetylcholine are used to reverse the paralysis.

The etiology of many nervous system disorders is not easily determined. For example, **headache (cephalgia)** may be caused by head injuries, intracranial tumors, severe hypertension, cerebral hypoxia, and infections, or it can occur without any apparent cause. Those with a known cause such as inflammation of pain-sensitive areas are said to have an ''organic etiology,'' but most are without known cause. Headaches can be mild and isolated like the persistent, dull, bilateral pain of a **tension headache,** or they can be severe, throbbing, and recurrent, as in **migraine**. Migraines are associated with **aura** symptoms in about 10% of cases, neurological features that precede or accompany the headache. **Cluster headache** (which is also called **histamine headache**) is named for the pattern or recurrences, which appear in clusters that may be separated by months or even years. Both migraines and cluster headaches are caused by vascular mechanisms, although cluster headache is more likely to be **hemicranial** (affecting only one side of the head).

The names of many of the other diseases, syndromes, and symptoms affecting the nervous system are readily decipherable by those with an understanding of the basic terminology of the system. For example, a **meningioma** is simply a tumor (*-oma*) of the meninges, while a **meningocele** is a protrusion (*-cele*) of the meninges through an opening in the skull or spinal column. **Myelitis** is any inflammation of the spinal cord since *myelo* refers to the spinal cord; similarly, **neuritis** is an inflammation of a nerve. Using the same root, **neuralgia** is pain along the length of a nerve. From the same prefix, one can decipher the meanings of **ataxia** and **aphasia** as indicating a lack (*a-* means ''without'') of ability to properly perform a postural (*-taxia*) or speech (*-phasia*) function. Table 12.1 lists many of these terms.

Diagnosis and Therapy

The terminology that applies to diagnostic and therapeutic procedures related to the nervous system follow the same pattern and terminology of the diseases. For example,

Table 12.1—Common Disorders and Symptoms of the Nervous System	
Focal:	aphasia
	apraxia
	astereognosis
Ischemic:	cerebrovascular accident (CVA)
	hypertensive encephalopathy
	intracerebral hemorrhage
	stroke
	subarachnoid hemorrhage
	transient ischemic attack (TIA)
Memory:	Alzheimer's disease
	anterograde amnesia
	retrograde or posttraumatic amnesia
Consciousness:	coma
	hypersomnia
	narcolepsy
	stupor
Convulsive:	akinetic seizures
	epilepsy
	focal seizures
	grand mal seizures
	petit mal seizures
	psychomotor seizures
	status epilepticus
Symptomatic:	headache
	hiccup (hiccough, singultus)
	migraine
	vertigo
Demyelination:	acute disseminated encephalomyelitis (postinfectious encephalitis)
	multiple sclerosis (disseminated sclerosis)
	optic neuromyelitis
Extra-pyramidal/cerebellar:	Huntington's chorea
	paresis
	Parkinsonism
	tic
Cerebral palsy:	ataxia
	dyskinesis
	hemiplegia

Peripheral nerves:	Bell's palsy
	Guillain-Barré syndrome
	herniated nucleus pulposus (herniated or ruptured disc)
	trigeminal neuralgia (tic douloureux)
Infection:	Meningitis

if myelitis is an inflammation of the spinal cord, a **myelogram** is a picture of the spinal cord. Indeed, a myelogram is obtained by injecting a contrast medium into the subarachnoid space and taking an X ray.

Diagnosis of nervous system disorders often begins with the **neurologic examination,** a systematic exploration of the patient's mental state, cranial nerves, motor system, sensory system, and reflexes. During the initial history and a series of tasks, the examiner can evaluate speech function, intellectual impairment, voluntary movement, abnormal involuntary movements, gait, posture, and balance. Cranial nerves are evaluated by visual field testing, ophthalmoscopic exam, hearing test, examination of other senses and muscles, and attention to facial expression or such apparent indicators as **nystagmus.** Tests for coordination and deep tendon reflexes are used to assess motor function, and a series of tests using a variety of movements and stimuli while the patient keeps his eyes closed assesses sensory function.

A radiographic technique useful in diagnosing nervous system disorders is **computerized tomography,** frequently called a **CT scan** or **CAT scan** (from "computerized axial tomography," the original term for the technique). A major imaging technique for the brain, the CT scan can image tumors, abscesses, alterations in ventricles, changes in blood flow, and numerous other abnormalities. Using ultrasound waves, an **echoencephalogram** can detect changes in brain shape; for example, deviations in the midline of the brain suggest an expanding intracranial lesion, and widening of the distance between the ventricular walls suggests **internal hydrocephalus.** Other cerebral imaging techniques include **cerebral arteriography** (employing a contrast medium to image cerebral arteries) and **pneumoencephalography** (which employs a gas as the contrast medium). A **radioactive brain scan** employs a radioactive isotope to image portions of the brain, and **magnetic resonance imaging (MRI)** uses a strong magnetic field to create the image.

Electroencephalography is the technique for recording the electrical activity of different parts of the brain and converting it into a tracing called an **electroencephalogram (EEG).** The pattern of an EEG reflects the state of the patient's brain and level of consciousness in a characteristic manner. Abnormalities in the EEG allow the practitioner to locate structural abnormalities such as a tumor or diagnose and manage epilepsy and other electrical abnormalities.

Lumbar puncture is used to obtain a CSF specimen for diagnostic study or to administer radiopaque dyes or medications.

If entry into the skull is required for surgical correction of an abnormality, a **craniotomy** (incision into the skull) can provide access to the brain. Similarly, a **craniectomy** involves the surgical removal (-*ectomy* = "removal") of a portion of the skull to provide a wider access, allow drainage of pressure, or correct premature closure of the **sutures** (seams) of the skull.

The suffix found in "craniectomy" is also used in the term **neurectomy,** the surgical removal of a nerve tract. **Cordotomy** (also spelled **chordotomy;** literally "cutting the spinal cord") is the surgical procedure in which the **spinothalamic tracts** (nerve tracts from the spine to the thalamus), which conduct pain sensations to the consciousness, are severed in the cervical area; although seldom employed, the procedure can relieve severe pain in the pelvis and legs.

Another surgical technique known as **cryoneurosurgery** involves the application of extreme cold (*cry-* or *cryo-* denotes cold) with a **cryoprobe** in order to destroy the nerve or an associated tumor or other tissue.

Nonsurgical techniques are often employed in treating nervous system disorders. Passing a low-voltage electric current through tissues can eliminate pain (**electroanalgesia**) or even provide anesthesia (**electroanesthesia**), and **TENS (transdermal electrical nerve stimulation)** units have numerous applications in the relief of pain.

Table 12.2 lists abbreviations used in reference to the nervous system.

Table 12.2—Abbreviations Associated with the Nervous System

AD	Alzheimer's disease	**FAP**	familial amyloid polyneuropathy
ADEM	acute disseminated encephalomyelitis	**FVH**	focal vascular headache
AIE	acute inclusion body encephalitis	**GABA**	gamma-aminobutyric acid
		HIE	hypoxic-ischemic encephalopathy
ANS	autonomic nervous system	**HPM**	hemiplegic migraine
BAEP	brain stem auditory evoked potential	**HSE**	herpes simplex encephalitis
BAER	brain stem auditory evoked response	**ICH**	intracranial hemorrhage
		ICP	intracranial pressure
BEAM	brain electrical activity mapping	**ICVH**	ischemic cerebrovascular headache
BEP	brain stem evoked potentials	**IICP**	increased intracranial pressure
BSE	bovine spongiform encephalopathy (mad cow disease)	**LHL**	left hemisphere lesion
		LHP	left hemiparesis
BSER	brain stem evoked responses	**MBD**	minimal brain damage/ dysfunction
BT	brain tumor		
CBS	chronic brain syndrome	**MCA**	middle cerebral aneurysm/ artery
CH	cluster headache		
CM	common migraine	**MIH**	migraine with interparoxysmal headache
CNS	central nervous system		
CP	cerebral palsy	**MMECT**	multiple monitor electroconvulsive therapy
CPA	cerebellar pontile angle		
CPTH	chronic posttraumatic headache	**MPTR**	motor, pain, touch reflex deficit
CPS	complex partial seizures	**MS**	multiple sclerosis
CSF	cerebrospinal fluid	**NF**	neurofibromatosis
CVA	cerebrovascular accident	**NFL**	nerve fiber layer
CVI	cerebrovascular insufficiency	**NGF**	nerve growth factor
DAI	diffuse axonal injury	**NSE**	neuron-specific enolase
EEG	electroencephalogram	**NVS**	neurologic vital signs
ESAP	evoked sensory (nerve) action potentiation	**PCA**	posterior cerebral artery
		PD	Parkinson's disease

PENS	percutaneous epidural nerve stimulator	**SFC**	spinal fluid count
PHH	posthemorrhagic hydrocephalus	**SFP**	spinal fluid pressure
		SNAP	sensory nerve action potential
PHN	postherpetic neuralgia	**SNCV**	sensory nerve conduction velocity
PNI	peripheral nerve injury		
PNP	progressive nuclear palsy	**SNE**	subacute necrotizing encephalomyelopathy
PNS	partial nonprogressive stroke; peripheral nervous system		
		Sp fl	spinal fluid
PSE	portal systemic encephalopathy	**SSEPs**	somatosensory evoked potentials
PSH	postspinal headache	**TBE**	tick-borne encephalitis
PVE	perivenous encephalomyelitis	**TENS**	transcutaneous electrical nerve stimulation
RCA	radionuclide cerebral angiogram		
		TCVA	thromboembolic cerebrovascular accident
RHL	right hemisphere lesions		
RIND	reversible ischemic neurologic defect	**TGA**	transient global amnesia
		THA	transient hemispheric attack
SAH	subarachnoid hemorrhage	**TIA**	transient ischemic attack
SCI	spinal cord injury	**TIE**	transient ischemia episode
SDH	subdural hematoma	**WEE**	western equine encephalitis

Pronouncing Glossary

Root	*Meaning*	*Example*	*Pronunciation*
cephal-	head	encephalitis	en sef all EYE tis
cerebro- encephalo-	brain	cerebrovascular encephalopathy	sir eeh bro VAS que ler in seff ah LOP ah thee
idio-	self	idiopathic	id eeh oh PATH ik
meningo-	membrane (of spine, brain)	meningocele	men IN go seal
neuro-	nerve	neurogenic	nur oh JIN ik

Glossary

acetylcholine—a nerve transmitter that acts upon an effector organ to achieve a nerve impulse

amygdala—one of the basal ganglia deep in each cerebral hemisphere, which is involved in mood, feeling, and instinct

aphasia—a language disorder affecting the generation and understanding of speech

arachnoid—the middle layer of the meninges covering the brain and spinal cord, located between the dura mater and pia mater

ataxia—shaky movements and unsteady gait caused by the brain's failure to control posture and limb movement

autonomic nervous system—the involuntary nervous system; that part of the nervous system that represents the motor innervation of the internal organs

axon—the nerve fiber that extends outward from a nerve cell and carries impulses away from the cell body

axoplasm—neuroplasm of the axon

bradykinesia—a symptom of Parkinsonism; difficulty in initiating voluntary movements, slowness in executing movements, and inability to make postural changes

cell body—portion of nerve cell that contains the nucleus and cytoplasm

central nervous system—the brain and the spinal cord

cerebellum—the large posterior brain mass lying above the pons and medulla and beneath the posterior portion of the cerebrum

cerebrospinal fluid—a fluid secreted by the choroid plexuses of the ventricles of the brain, filling the ventricles and the subarachnoid cavities of the brain and spinal cord

cerebrum—the largest part of the brain, including practically all parts within the skull, except the medulla, pons, and cerebellum

cervical enlargement—spindle-shaped swelling of the spinal cord extending from the fourth cervical to the first segment, with the maximum thickness opposite the fifth or sixth cervical vertebra

cholinesterase—one of a family of enzymes capable of catalyzing the hydrolysis of acylcholines and a few other compounds

coccygeal nerve—a small nerve, the lowest of the spinal nerves

corpus callosum—the band of nervous tissue connecting the two cerebral hemispheres

cortex—the outer area of the cerebrum

dendrite—one of the two types of branching protoplasmic processes of the nerve cell (the other being the axon)

depolarization—sudden surge of charged particles across the membrane of a neuron or muscle cell that produces an action potential

dura mater—the outer layer of the meninges

endplate—the ending of a motor nerve fiber in relation to a skeletal muscle fiber

epidural space—the space between the walls of the vertebral canal and the dura mater of the spinal cord

frontal lobe—the portion of each cerebral hemisphere anterior to the fissure of Rolando

hemicrania—headache affecting only one side of the head

hydrocephalus—accumulation of fluid within the ventricles of the brain causing increased intracranial pressure

lumbar nerves—five nerves on each side, emerging from the lumbar portion of the spinal cord

lumbosacral enlargement—a spindle-shaped swelling of the cord beginning at the level of the tenth thoracic vertebra and tapering into the conus medullaris, with the maximum thickness opposite the last thoracic vertebra

membrane potential—electrical potential created by the ionic difference between the axoplasm (or cytoplasm) and interstitial fluid at the membrane of a neuron or muscle cell

meninges—one of the membranous coverings of the brain and spinal cord

myelin—protein and phospholipid substance laid down in layers forming a sheath around certain axons

neuralgia—severe burning or stabbing pain that often follows a nerve track

neurilemma (neurolemma)—myelin sheath

neurofibril node—node of Ranvier; one of the gaps that occurs in a myelin sheath between adjacent Schwann cells

nerve fiber—axon; the long, thin process extending from the body of a neuron, which carries nerve impulses

nerve impulse—the action potential of a nerve fiber

neuromuscular junction—the synaptic connection of the axon of the motor neuron with a muscle fiber

neuron—nerve cell

node of Ranvier—short interval in the myelin sheath of a nerve fiber, occurring between each two successive segments of the myelin sheath

nystagmus—rapid involuntary movements of the eyes, which may be side to side, up and down, or rotary

occipital lobe—the posterior, somewhat pyramid-shaped part of each cerebral hemisphere

parietal lobe—the middle portion of each cerebral hemisphere, separated from the frontal lobe by the central sulcus

perikaryon—cell body

peripheral nervous system—nervous system composed of nerves and ganglia

poliomyelitis—an infectious viral disease affecting the CNS, which may cause symptoms varying from stomach upset to muscle paralysis

pons—part of the brainstem between the medulla oblongata and the mesencephalon

presynaptic terminal—the terminal before the synapse

refractory period—the recovery time needed for a nerve cell that has passed a nerve impulse to restore membrane potential and prepare for conduction of another impulse

sacral nerves—five nerves issuing from the sacral foramina on either side

saltatory conduction—the conduction in which the nerve impulse jumps from one node of Ranvier to the next

spinal cord—the elongated cylindrical portion of the cerebrospinal axis or central nervous system.

subarachnoid space—the space between the arachnoidea and pia mater

subdural space—the very narrow interval between the dura mater and the arachnoid

CHAPTER 13

The Special Sense Organs and Their Disorders

Sense organs or receptors function to integrate the body with the outside world, as well as to detect changes within the body. **Taste, smell, hearing, equilibrium,** and **vision** are called the special senses because they originate from sensors in restricted (or special) regions of the head.

Anatomy and Physiology

Taste

The sense of taste or act of tasting is termed **gustation**. The surface of the tongue is covered with small protuberances called **papilla** of three types: filiform (from the Latin word meaning "thread"), fungiform (mushroom-shaped), and circumvallate (from the Latin *vallum*, "wall"). Within the crevices of these papillae are **taste buds,** the receptor organs for the sense of taste. The four basic taste sensations are sweet, sour, salty, and bitter.

Smell

The sense of smell is termed **olfaction, osmesis,** or **osphresis**. The olfactory receptor cells (neurons) are located high in the roof of the nasal cavity in the olfactory epithelium consisting of receptor cells, sustentacular or supporting cells, and basal cells. These neurons end in a bulbous olfactory vesicle or sac from which extend cilia that project through the fluid covering the surface epithelium. The olfactory bulbs connect olfactory nerve fibers to axons of neurons projecting into the olfactory area of the brain (Figure 13.1).

Hearing

The ear consists of two functional units: the **auditory** or **acoustic** apparatus involved with hearing, and the **vestibular** apparatus involving balance and posture. The term *auditory* pertains to the sense of hearing or to the organs of hearing. The components of the auditory apparatus are the external, middle, and inner ear. The external ear is composed of the **auricle** (also called the **pinna** from the Latin "wing") and **external auditory canal.** The middle ear consists of the **tympanic membrane** (eardrum), **tympanic**

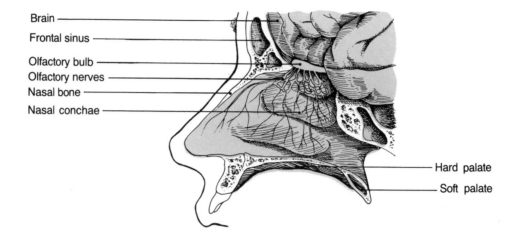

Brain
Frontal sinus
Olfactory bulb
Olfactory nerves
Nasal bone
Nasal conchae

Hard palate
Soft palate

Figure 13.1——Olfactory Receptors.
Olfactory receptive area in the roof of the nasal cavity, medial view.

cavity, auditory or **eustachian tube,** and three **auditory ossicles** or ear bones—the **malleus** (hammer), the **incus** (anvil), and the **stapes** (stirrup). The **round** and **oval windows** are openings in the inner wall of the middle ear. The inner ear or **labyrinth** is composed of the **vestibule,** containing the **utricle** and **saccule; semicircular canals** and **ducts;** and **cochlea,** which contain the **spiral organ of Corti** (Figure 13.2).

Sound waves reach the spiral organ through a sequence of vibrations that begin in the external ear and tympanic membrane and progress through the auditory ossicles to the

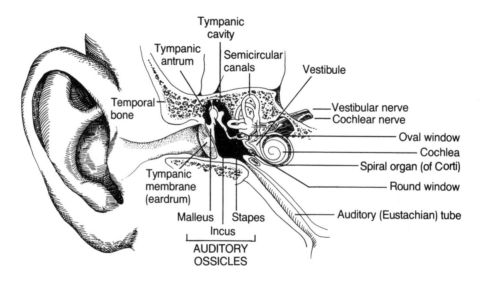

Tympanic
cavity

Tympanic
antrum

Semicircular
canals

Vestibule

Temporal
bone

Vestibular nerve
Cochlear nerve

Oval window
Cochlea
Spiral organ (of Corti)
Round window
Auditory (Eustachian) tube

Tympanic
membrane
(eardrum)

Malleus   Stapes
Incus
AUDITORY
OSSICLES

Figure 13.2——The Ear.
Frontal cutaway view of the right ear, showing the external, middle, and inner ear.
A section of the cochlear duct has been removed to show the spiral organ.

inner ear. Displacement of hair cells in the spiral organ generates nerve impulses in the **cochlear nerve,** where auditory pathways convey the influences to the auditory area of the temporal lobe in the brain.

Equilibrium

The primary receptors for balance or **equilibrium** are the **utricle, saccule,** and **semicircular ducts** in the inner ear. Impulses affecting equilibrium are also received from the eyes and from some sensory end organs in the skin and joints. The purpose of the vestibular system is to signal changes in the motion of the head (**dynamic** equilibrium) and in the position of the head with regard to gravity (**static** equilibrium).

Hair cells, arranged in clusters called **hair bundles,** are specialized receptor cells of the vestibular sense organs. These hair cells convert a mechanical force into an electrical signal that is sent into the brain via the vestibular nerve. **Statoconia,** also called **otoconia** because of their location (*oto-* = ear), are calcium carbonate crystals in the inner ear that respond to gravity and cause the hair cells to stimulate the nerve fibers and eventually produce posture changes, keeping the person erect (*stato-* = standing).

The utricles and saccules are organs of gravitation, responding to movements of the head in a straight line. The **crista ampullaris** of the semicircular ducts responds to changes in the direction of head movements, including rotating and bending. Hair cells in the cristae project into a gelatinous flap called the **cupula.** When the head rotates, the **endolymph** in the semicircular canals causes action potentials to be sent to the neural centers in the brain, signaling certain muscles to respond in maintaining the body's equilibrium.

Vision

The primary organ of vision is the **eyeball.** The wall of the eyeball consists of three layers of tissue: the outer supporting layer, the vascular layer, and the inner retinal layer. The supporting layer is composed mostly of the **sclera** (the ''white'' of the eye), which gives the eyeball its shape and protects the inner layers. In front of the sclera is the transparent **cornea,** through which light enters the eye. The middle coat of the eye is referred to as the **uvea** or **uveal tract,** a vascular layer that contains many blood vessels. The posterior two-thirds of the uvea is a thin membrane called the **choroid,** and the front thickened portion is the **ciliary body.** The anterior extension of the choroid is a muscular layer called the **iris,** the colored part of the eye. The **pupil** is an adjustable opening in the center of the iris that opens and closes in response to the amount of light available. The **lens,** an elastic body, changes shape to focus light onto the retina. The **retina,** or innermost portion of the eyeball, contains a layer of nervous tissue (**neuroretina**) that receives light rays and processes the effects into nerve impulses that are carried along two **optic nerves** and converted into visual perceptions in the brain. An additional pigmented layer lies behind the neural layer and absorbs light not utilized by the **rods** and **cones,** the photoreceptor nerve cells (*photo* = light). Rod cells function in dim light and peripheral vision; the color-sensitive cone cells are located primarily in the center of the retina in an area called the **fovea centralis.**

The hollow eyeball is divided into three cavities: the **anterior chamber** located between the iris and cornea; the **vitreous chamber,** the space behind the lens that contains the **vitreous humor;** and the **posterior chamber** between the iris, lens, and vitreous

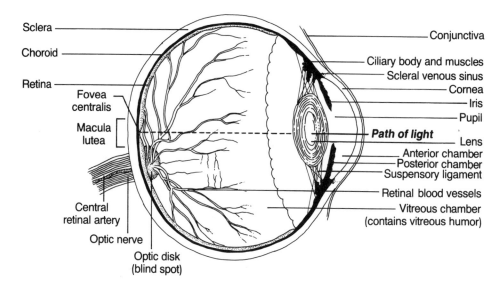

Figure 13.3——The Eye.
Horizontal section through the eye.

chamber. The other chambers of the eye are filled with **aqueous humor,** which is secreted by the **ciliary processes** and reabsorbed into the venous system through the **canal of Schlemm** (Figure 13.3).

Accessory structures of the eye that function primarily as protective and supportive devices are the **eyelids, eyelashes, eyebrows, conjunctiva** (mucous membrane covering the anterior surface of the eyeball and lining the lids), **bony orbits** (orbital cavity), **ocular muscles** that act on the eyeball and eyelid, and **lacrimal** (tear) **ducts.**

Disorders of the Special Senses

Taste

Loss of the sense of taste is termed **ageusia,** meaning "without gustation," while a lesser loss resulting in a blunting of the sense of taste is called **hypogeusia.** A **gustatory hallucination** is the perception of a taste that is not actually present.

Diseases of the tongue can affect the sense of taste. **Glossopathy** (the combining form *glosso-* from the Greek word meaning "tongue") is a general term for any disease of the tongue, and the same combining form occurs in many more specific terms. **Glosson-cus** refers to any swelling involving the tongue and is derived from the same source as the word *oncology.* Similarly, **glossolysis** or **glossoplegia** indicates paralysis of the tongue, and **glossitis** is an inflammation of the tongue. **Glossodynia** is a condition characterized by a painful or burning sensation of the tongue.

Taste sensation may also be altered by dental problems, psychiatric disorders, nutritional deficiencies, neurologic problems, and the normal aging process, as well as changes in the ability to smell. Several drugs have been reported to cause taste disorders, usually by decreasing taste acuity. Drugs can also interfere with the ability to sense sweet or sour taste and increase sensitivity to bitterness.

Smell

Parosmia and **parosphresia,** from the Greek words *osme* and *osphresis* (meaning smell or smelling), refer to any disorder of the sense of smell, especially the subjective perception of odors that do not exist. Loss of the sense of smell is termed **anosmia** (also, **olfactory anesthesia** or **smell blindness**). The types of anosmia, according to their cause, are **essential** or true, due to lesion of the olfactory nerve; **mechanical** or respiratory, due to obstruction of the nasal fossae; **reflex,** due to disease in some other location; and **functional,** without any apparent cause. Nasal congestion ("stuffy nose") caused by allergic rhinitis, bacterial or viral inflammation, or anatomical defects will also interfere with the sense of smell.

Hearing

Problems with any of the structures involved in sound transmission from the body surface to the brain may impair hearing. **External otitis** is an inflammation of the outer ear and may block the progress of sound waves. Impacted **cerumen** is an accumulation of cerumen or earwax that blocks the ear canal and prevents sound waves from reaching the tympanic membrane. Inflammation of the tympanic membrane is known as **myringitis** or **tympanitis** and may prevent the tympanic membrane from vibrating appropriately. **Eustachian tube dysfunction** is a general term used to describe any condition in which the ability of the eustachian tube to equilibrate ambient and middle ear pressure is impeded.

Otitis media is an inflammation of the mucous membranes of the middle ear and tympanic membrane that involves eustachian tube dysfunction and viral or bacterial infection. Types of the disorder are classified according to duration and complications: acute/chronic suppurative otitis media; acute bacterial otitis media; purulent otitis media; and secretory, nonsuppurative, serous otitis media.

Nerve deafness, also called perceptive or sensorineural deafness, is caused by to disease of the cochlea or of the cochlear division of the eighth cranial nerve. **Conductive deafness** results from disease of the middle ear such as otosclerosis, chronic otitis media, or from occlusion (closure) of the external auditory canal or eustachian tube. **Otosclerosis** (*oto + sclerosis,* Greek word meaning hardening) is the term for new formation of spongy bone about the stapes, preventing proper vibration of the bones, which prevents transmission of sound waves to the inner ear, resulting in progressively increasing deafness.

Ototoxicity is defined as the condition of having a toxic or poisonous effect upon the ear. A number of drugs can result in hearing loss because of their ototoxicity. Aminoglycoside antibiotics have a high degree of ototoxicity, possibly because of their high concentrations in the inner ear fluids that are retained for long periods of time. This can result in both auditory (hearing) and vestibular (equilibrium) effects. Auditory effects are manifested by high-frequency hearing loss.

Equilibrium

Dizziness is a nonspecific term that is used to describe symptoms that may include **vertigo** (a sense of spinning or rotating), lightheadedness (a sense of floating), impending **syncope** (fainting), **ataxia** (unsteadiness in standing), or **diplopia** (double vision). **Oscillopsia** is a sense that the environment is moving back and forth. **Vertigo** can be classified as physiological, which indicates that it is caused by external stimuli (e.g., motion sickness, height/visual vertigo); pathological, or caused by disease of the vestibular apparatus; or benign paroxysmal positional vertigo **(BPPV)**, which is related to changes in posture and often due to an undetermined cause.

Labyrinthitis, or inflammation of the inner ear, can cause hearing loss along with vertigo and other types of dizziness. In **peripheral vestibulopathy,** also called acute labyrinthitis or **vestibular neuronitis,** vertigo is acute, severe, and often associated with nausea, vomiting, and nystagmus.

Idiopathic symptomatic endolymphatic hydrops or **Meniere's disease** is another disorder of the inner ear that produces hearing impairment, dizziness, and **tinnitus** (ringing or whistling in the ears). The disease is thought to be caused by an excess of **endolymph,** the inner ear fluid, and dilation or stretching of the labyrinth. Most patients progress to some baseline hearing loss and to bilateral disease.

Excessive stimulation of the labyrinthine receptors of the inner ear produces **motion sickness** with its symptoms of nausea, vomiting, pallor (paleness), and cold sweats. Vestibular disorders also result from drug toxicity, blood dyscrasias (hemorrhage into the labyrinth), and lesions of the eighth cranial nerve.

Vision

Inflammation of several parts of the eye can impair vision. Redness, itching, and tearing of the eyes can be caused by bacteria, viruses, foreign particles, or environmental pollutants. **Conjunctivitis** is an inflammation of the conjunctiva which causes reddened eye (sometimes called "pink eye") and purulent or serous discharge with itching, smarting, stinging, or a scratching sensation. Allergic conjunctivitis is an inflammation resulting from allergens (such as ragweed, grass, or tree pollen) that irritate the conjunctiva and cause mast cells to release chemicals that interact with the allergen.

Inflammation of the other parts of the optic system are denoted by the suffix *-itis,* as in **retinitis** (retina), **scleritis** (sclera), **keratitis** (cornea), **uveitis** (uvea), **iritis** (iris), and **blepharitis** (eyelid).

Other diseases can also impair vision. **Glaucoma** is characterized by an increase in intraocular pressure (IOP). Most cases of primary glaucoma are of the open-angle type **(primary open-angle glaucoma** or **POAG),** where IOP may fluctuate but the aqueous humor outflow is consistently decreased. **Angle-closure** or **narrow-angle** glaucoma occurs when the anterior chamber angle is blocked by the root of the iris, causing severe pain and loss of vision along with the increase in IOP. Complications include cataracts, atrophy (tissue wasting) of the retina and optic nerve, and blindness **(amaurosis, typhlosis).**

Cataract formation, in which the lens becomes opaque, causes progressive vision loss, possibly resulting in total blindness. Types include senile, congenital, traumatic, and toxic, depending on the cause.

Achromatopsia (*kroma,* color + *ope,* vision) denotes complete color blindness.

Amblyopia, also called "lazy eye," is the term for dullness of vision resulting from lack of use of an eye. **Anopia** denotes the lack of vision, particularly in one eye.

Muscular and neural abnormalities may also affect vision. **Esotropia,** in which the eyeball turns inward, is also called **convergent strabismus** or **"crosseye"** and is an involuntary deviation of the eyes from the normal position caused by a muscular defect or weakness in coordination. **Exotropia,** also called **divergent strabismus** or **"walleye,"** is a lateral deviation or outward turning of the eyeball, resulting in **diplopia** (double vision). Dysfunction of the eye muscles or their innervation (nerve supply) can cause a defect in ocular movement called **ocular paralysis. Cycloplegia** results from temporary paralysis of the ciliary muscle and zonules, causing decreased accommodation and blurred vision; cycloplegia can be caused by anticholinergic agents. **Ametropia** (from the Greek word *ametros,* "without measure") is an inability of the eye to focus images correctly on the retina, resulting in a refractive disorder such as diplopia, **myopia** (near-sightedness), **hyperopia** (farsightedness), astigmatism, or **presbyopia** ("aging eye").

Disorders of light perception include **photopsia, photophthalmia, photophobia, nyctalopia,** and **photonosus.** Ocular emergencies include **chemical burns** and corneal trauma from **abrasion** or **foreign bodies.**

Disorders of the special sense organs are summarized in Table 13.1; abbreviations commonly encountered are listed in Table 13.2.

Diagnosis

Smell

If a patient is suspected of having a decrease in the sense of smell, the degree of sensibility of the olfactory organ may determined by **olfactometry** using an **olfactometer,** a device for estimating how keen the sense of smell is. Study of the sense of smell is known as **olfactology.**

Equilibrium

The clinical sign of a vestibular abnormality is **nystagmus,** also called **ocular ataxia,** a rhythmical jerky or pendular oscillation of the eyeballs. Precipitation or exacerbation of sensations of imbalance by head movements is considered evidence of vestibular involvement. **Tandem walking** (heel to toe) intensifies ataxia and simulates the sensation of disequilibrium. Other tests to simulate symptoms of vestibular vertigo include the **Barany rotation maneuver, caloric** tests, and **positional tests. Electronystagmography** (ENG), electrical recording of eye movement with the eyes closed, is used to identify and localize lesions of the vestibular system. The **glycerol dehydration test, acetazolamide testing,** and **electrocochleography** (measurement of the electrical potentials generated in the inner ear) are used in diagnosis of Meniere's disease. CAT scans, myelograms, and tomograms are used to detect possible eighth cranial nerve tumors.

Hearing

Hearing impairment can result from a number of causes: high fevers from viral infections that damage the inner ear; extreme accumulation of earwax (**ceruminosis**); dete-

Table 13.1—Common Disorders of the Special Sense Organs

Taste:

ageusia
glossoncus
glossolysis/glossoplegia
glossodynia
hypogeusia

Smell:

anosmia
parosphresia/parosmia

Hearing:

acoustic neuroma
cholesteatoma
conductive deafness
external otitis
myringitis/tympanitis
nerve deafness
otitis media
otosclerosis
ototoxicity

Equilibrium:

labyrinthitis
Meniere's disease/endolymphatic hydrops
vertigo
vestibular neuronitis

Vision:

achromatopsia
amaurosis/typhlosis
amblyopia
ametropia
anopia
cataracts
cycloplegia
diplopia
esotropia
exotropia
glaucoma
hordeolum
inflammations: conjunctivitis, retinitis, scleritis,
    keratitis, uveitis, iritis, blepharitis
macular degeneration
papilledema
photopsia
photophthalmia
photophobia
photonosus
refractive: myopia, hyperopia, astigmatism, presbyopia
retinitis pigmentosa
strabismus
trauma: chemical burns, abrasion, foreign body;
    retinal detachment

Table 13.2—Abbreviations Associated with the Special Senses

A/C	anterior (eye) chamber; air conduction
ACD	anterior chamber diameter
ACTSEB	anterior chamber tube shunt encircling band
AD	right ear
AM	myopic astigmatism
AMD	age-related macular degeneration
AOM	acute otitis media
AS	left ear
AsM	myopic astigmatism
AST	astigmatism
AU	both ears
BC	bone conduction
MT	bilateral myringotomy tubes
BOM	bilateral otitis media
BPV	benign paroxysmal vertigo
BPPV	benign paroxysmal positional vertigo
BSOM	bilateral serous otitis media
CM	cochlear microphonics
CS	conjunctiva-sclera
CSC	cornea, conjunctiva, sclera
CSOM	chronic serous otitis media
CT	corneal thickness
DEVR	dominant exudative vitreoretinopathy
EAC	external auditory canal
EAM	external auditory meatus
ECCE	extracapsular cataract extraction
EENT	eyes, ears, nose and throat
EKG	epidemic keratoconjunctivitis
Em	emmetropia
EMP	extraocular muscle paresis
ENG	electronystagmography
EOG	electro-oculogram
EOM	extraocular movement/ muscles
EOMI	extraocular muscles intact
ERA	evoked response audiometry
ERG	electroretinogram
ET	esotropia
EWSCL	extended wear soft contact lens
GVF	good visual fields
HA	hearing aid
HAE	hearing aid evaluation
HCL	hard contact lens
HD	hearing distance
HDLW	hearing distance for watch in left ear
HDRW	hearing distance for watch in right ear

HFHL	high-frequency hearing loss
HH	hard of hearing
HL	hearing level
HOH	hard of hearing
IAC	internal auditory canal
IAM	internal auditory meatus
IHS	iris hamartomas
IO	intraocular pressure
IOF	intraocular fluid
IOFB	intraocular foreign body
IOL	intraocular lens
IOP	intraocular pressure
KID	keratitis, ichthyosis, deafness
LMEE	left mid ear exploration
LOM	left otitis media
LOV	loss of vision
LPC	laser photocoagulation
LPO	light perception only
LR	light reflex
M	myopia
MEE	middle ear effusion
My	myopia
NAG	narrow angle glaucoma
NRC	normal retinal correspondence
NVG	neovascular glaucoma
O	eye
O2	both eyes
OD	right eye; doctor of optometry
OKAN	optokinetic after nystagmus
OKN	optokinetic nystagmus
OM	otitis media
OME	otitis media with effusion
OMSC	otitis media secretory/ suppurative chronic
ORL	otorhinolaryngology
OS	left eye
OTO	otology
OU	both eyes
PCIOL	posterior chamber intraocular lens
PCL	posterior chamber lens
PD	interpupillary distance
PDR	proliferative diabetic retinopathy
PERL	pupils equal, reactive to light
PERR	pattern evoked retinal response
PERRLA	pupils equal, round, reactive to light and accommodation
PET	pressure equalizing tubes
PK	penetrating keratoplasty
PL	light perception
POAG	primary open angle glaucoma

PPL	pars planus lensectomy	**SMD**	senile macular degeneration
PRRE	pupils round, regular, equal	**SOM**	serous otitis media
PRVEP	pattern reversal visual evoked potentials	**SPK**	superficial punctate keratitis
		TKP	thermokeratoplasty
PSC	posterior subcapsular cataract	**TMB**	transient monocular blindness
		Tn	normal intraocular tension
PVD	posterior vitreous detachment	**TORP**	total ossicular replacement prosthesis
PVR	proliferative vitreoretinopathy		
RA	right auricle	**TRD**	traction retinal detachment
RAPD	relative afferent pupillary defect	**TTY-TDD**	teletypewriter for the deaf
		UGH	uveitis, glaucoma, hyphema
RE	right eye	**VA**	visual acuity
RK	radial keratotomy	**VAS**	visual analogue scale
RMEE	right middle ear exploration	**VASC**	Visual-Auditory Screen Test for Children
RP	retinitis pigmentosa		
RPE	retinal pigment epithelium	**VDA**	visual discriminatory acuity
RPICCE	round pupil intracapsular cataract extraction	**VF**	vision field
		VISC	vitreous infusion suction cutter
RRE	round, regular and equal		
RRRN	round, regular, react normally	**VKC**	vernal keratoconjunctivitis
RTL	reactive to light	**VOD**	vision right eye
RVO	retinal vein occlusion	**VOR**	vestibular ocular reflex
SCL	soft contact lens	**VOS**	vision left eye
SISI	short increment sensitivity index	**VOU**	vision both eyes
		VRA	visual reinforcement audiometry
SLE	slit lamp exam		
SLK	superior limbic keratoconjunctivitis	**VVOR**	visual-vestibulo-ocular reflex
		XT	exotropia

rioration due to aging (**presbyacusia**); dietary deficiencies that restrict nutritional maintenance of the specialized tissues in the inner ear; environmental noise; or congenital (birth) defects.

The general term for any disease of the ear is **otopathy,** which contains the combining form *oto-* that is used in many terms referring to ear disease. For example, **otoneuralgia** is an earache of neuralgic origin, and **otorrhagia** denotes bleeding from the ear. Symptoms of infection, as in otitis media, include a deep throbbing pain or pressure that is perceived as coming from the ear (**otalgia, otodynia**), **otorrhea** or discharge from the ear, fever, and possible hearing loss. Examination (**otoscopy**) of the tympanic membrane with an **otoscope** may show a bulging, erythematous (red and inflamed) membrane. Visualization of bony landmarks may be impaired due to **opacification** (imperviousness to light) and edema or swelling. Reduced mobility and **effusion** (fluid from the middle ear) may also be noted on otologic exam.

Material for cultures may be obtained by performing a **tympanocentesis,** which involves piercing the eardrum with a sterile needle and collecting fluid from the middle ear.

Evaluation of hearing can be done with several tests using a **tuning fork** to distinguish between nerve deafness and conductive deafness and using an **audiometer,** which provides an **audiogram** to reveal the range of hearing. Other diagnostic procedures associated with hearing evaluation include **tympanometry** (impedance testing), visual reinforcement audiometry (**VRA**), electroacoustic evaluation, and a short increment sensitivity index (**SISI**).

Vision

Initial diagnostic evaluation of vision would include history, general observation, and external ocular and adnexal examination. Visual loss may be preceded by **halos** seen around illuminated lights and by pain in the eye. High intraocular pressure (IOP) is associated with ring or annular **scotomas** or dark areas in the visual field and a deeply cupped optic disc. **Retinal detachment** causes distortion of visual images and is identified by irregularities seen in the retina on examination, which also detects other disorders causing visual symptoms. An **ophthalmoscope** is the instrument used to inspect the optic disc; the procedure is called ophthalmoscopy. **Accommodation** (the process that brings images to exact focus on the retina) causes the pupils to constrict rapidly. Contraction of the pupil is referred to as miosis, from the Greek meaning ''lessening.'' **Argyll Robertson pupils** are small, unequal, irregular, and fixed to light. During eye examination, visual acuity is assessed in both the right **(OD)** and left eyes **(OS).** Unless contraindicated, pupils of both eyes **(OU)** are inspected after administration of a mydriatic/cycloplegic agent to temporarily dilate the pupil and prevent accommodation; this is termed mydriasis.

Gonioscopy is the examination of the angle of the anterior chamber with a **gonioscope** (lens) or a contact prism lens and beam illumination from a **slit lamp.** This procedure is used to detect retinal or optic nerve disease. **Applanation tonometry** is used to measure intraocular pressure in millimeters of mercury (mmHg). If diagnosis is still in doubt, provocative procedures such as a water drinking test, darkroom test, or mydriatic tests are employed. Other diagnostic procedures may include gross visual fields and basic motor exam, fluorescent **angioscopy** (examination of the capillary vessels), slit lamp examination, **keratometry, ophthalmodynamometry,** needle **oculo-electromyography,** electro-oculography **(EOG),** and **retinoscopy.**

Treatment

Taste

Treatment of taste disorders involves treatment of the disease causing the dysfunction and/or discontinuation of the offending drug.

Smell

A specialist in diseases of the nose is a **rhinologist.** If the specialty is combined with treatment of the ear and larynx, the specialist is called an **otorhinolaryngologist.** Treatment of nasal congestion with **decongestants** will result in improvement of the sense of smell in many cases (see Chapter 9 for discussion of the treatment of respiratory disorders).

Equilibrium

Treatment of vertigo may involve bedrest, vestibular exercises, **antiemetics, anticholinergics,** and **antihistamines.** A number of drugs are utilized in treatment of Meniere's disease, including **diuretics, antihistamines, sedatives, vasodilators,** and **bioflavonoids.** **Anticholinergics** and **antihistamines** are the agents used most often for prevention of motion sickness. Less traditional modalities for treatment of Meniere's disease and otitis media include nutritional and homeopathic therapies, helium-neon laser treatments, and exercise therapy.

Surgical terms relating to the treatment of Meniere's disease and incapacitating vertigo include middle fossa **vestibular nerve section,** trans-labyrinthine **labyrinthectomy,** retrolabyrinthine vestibular **neurectomy,** sac incision, endolymphatic subarachnoid/mastoid **shunting,** and cochleo-endolymphatic shunt.

Hearing

An **otologist** is a specialist in treating disorders of the ear. This specialty is often combined with treatment of the upper respiratory tract (**otolaryngology**), and the patient may be referred to an **otolaryngologist** for hearing disorders. **Antimicrobial** drugs are used in treatment of otitis media to eradicate the pathogen, shorten the period of illness, and prevent suppurative (pus) complications. **Myringotomy,** incision into the tympanic membrane, is a procedure utilized for drainage of the middle ear. A **tympanoplasty** or **myringoplasty** is performed to repair perforations of the tympanic membrane that do not satisfactorily heal spontaneously.

Pharmaceutical services for the hearing impaired can be expedited with use of a Teletypewriter for the Deaf (TTY, TDD), which permits communication by transmission of messages over telephone lines to a visual monitor.

Vision

Disorders of the visual senses are usually referred to a specialist in treating eye disorders. An **ophthalmologist** or **oculist** is a physician who specializes in diseases and surgery of the eye. An **optometrist** is qualified to examine the eyes for vision problems and eye disorders and to prescribe lenses and other optical aids. The specialist who fills prescriptions for lenses, dispenses the eyeglasses, and makes and fits contact lens is an **optician.** Radial **keratotomy** (*kerat* = cornea, *-otomy* = incision) is a commonly used corrective surgical technique. A newer method utilizes a laser device and is referred to as photoreflective keratotomy. A **keratoplasty,** sometimes called a corneal transplant, involves replacing a section of diseased cornea with a normal one.

Treatment of glaucoma varies with the type and extent of the disease. Medical treatment involves increasing the ability of fluid to leave the eye, decreasing the amount of fluid entering the eye, or dehydration by hypertonic solutions. Pharmacologic agents used most often include **miotics** (cause contraction of the pupil), **mydriatics** (cause dilation of the pupil), beta-blockers, and carbonic anhydrase inhibitors. Surgical terms include peripheral **iridectomy, goniotomy, goniopuncture,** laser **trabeculectomy, iridencleisis, cyclodialysis, cyclodiathermy, cyclocryotherapy** and **sclerectomy.**

Ophthalmic **decongestants** are used to relieve redness of the eyes due to minor irritation. Treatment of ocular allergies involves removal of the offending allergen and possible use of topical antihistamines to relieve symptoms and vasoconstrictors to whiten the eye by constricting the conjunctival blood vessels. Cromolyn sodium and topical corticosteroids may be employed for more severe cases.

Ophthalmic **antibiotic** drops or ointments are utilized in treatment of infections.

Treatment for cataracts varies from frequent changes in eyeglasses to compensate for gradual vision loss, to surgery in which the lens is removed and replaced with an artificial lens. Removal of the entire lens is termed an **intracapsular extraction,** while extracapsular extraction denotes retention of the posterior portion of the lens capsule. **Phacoemulsification** is a technique utilizing ultrasonic vibration to disintegrate the lens for aspiration. A combination of the artificial lens and bifocal glasses or contact lenses is used to restore focusing ability. Refractive errors and unilateral **aphakia** (absence of the crystalline lens) can also be treated with **corneal contact lenses.**

Photocoagulation by laser beam and **cryosurgery** can successfully reattach layers of the retina in treatment of diabetic retinopathy and macular degeneration of blood vessels in the eye. Cataracts, glaucoma, and macular degeneration have also been treated with vitamins, minerals, botanical medicines, transcendental meditation (TCM), biofeedback, and nutritional therapies as prophylaxis.

Pronouncing Glossary of Roots

Root	Meaning	Example	Pronunciation
audio-	hearing	audiometry	ah de OM eh tree
auri-	ear	auriform	OR ee form
blephar-	eyelid	blepharoptosis	blef ar TOW sis
cilio-	eyelid, cilia	cilioretinal	sil ee oh RET en al
core-	pupil	corelysis	kor ee LIE sis
cyclo-	circle, cycle (ciliary body)	cycloplegia	si klo PLAY ja
dacry-	tear duct, tears	dacryocystocele	dak re oh SIS toe seal
glosso-	tongue	glossitis	glah SI tis
irido-	iris	iridectomy	er ed EK to mee
kerato-	cornea	keratectasia	ker ah TEK ay shuh
lacri-	tears	lacrimation	lak ree MA shun
linguo-	tongue	lingual	LING gwal
myringo-	eardrum	myringoplasty	mi RIN go plas tee
naso-	nose	nasolacrimal	NA zo LAK ri mal
ocul- ophthal-	eye	oculist ophthalmic	OK u list off THAL mik
optico- opto-	vision, sight	opticociliary optometry	op tee ko SIL ee ar ee op TOM eh tree
osmo- osphresio	smell	osmology osphresiology	os MOLL oh jee os FREZ e ol o jee

Root	Meaning	Example	Pronunciation
oto-	ear	otodynia	oto DEN ee ah
phaco-	lens	phacocele	FAK o seel
photo-	light	photophobia	fo to FO bee ah
rhino-	nose	rhinology	rin OHL o jee
scoto-	darkness	scotoma	sko TOH mah
tympano-	eardrum, middle ear	tympanocentesis	tem pan o sen TEE sis
typhlo-	blind	typhlosis	ti fill OH sis

Glossary

accommodation—adjustment of the eye for seeing at various distances

achromatopsia—complete color blindness; monochromatism

acoustic—relating to hearing or the perception of sound

ageusia—loss of the sense of taste

amaurosis—blindness, especially that occurring without apparent change in the eye itself

amblyopia—dimness of vision

ametropia—an error of refraction in which images are not focused properly on the retina

angiography—procedure to detect lesions in the macular area of the retina

anosmia—absence of the sense of smell

anterior chamber—portion of the eyeball located between the iris and cornea

aqueous humor—the watery fluid that fills the anterior and posterior chambers of the eye

astigmatism—defective curvature of the lens or cornea

audiogram—a recording of results of tests of hearing at various frequencies against decibels of sound intensity

audiometer—an electrical instrument for measuring the threshold of hearing for various frequencies of sound waves

auditory—pertaining to the sense or to the organs of hearing

auricle—the external ear

biomicroscopy—examination of the cornea, aqueous and vitreous humor, lens and retina by use of a slit lamp combined with a binocular microscope

blepharitis—inflammation of the eyelids

canal of Schlemm—a vein in the sclera that encircles the cornea

cataract—a loss of transparency or clouding of the lens of the eye, or of its capsule

cerumen—earwax

ceruminosis—excessive formation of earwax

cholesteatoma—presence of cyst-like masses within the middle ear

choroid—the middle vascular layer of the eye between the retina and sclera

ciliary body—thickened portion of the eye between the choroid and the iris

ciliary process—portion of the eye that secretes the aqueous humor

cochlea—the essential organ of hearing, forming one of the divisions of the labyrinth or internal ear

cone—one of the visual receptors in the retina

conjunctiva—the mucous membrane covering the anterior surface of the eyeball and lining the lids

conjunctivitis—inflammation of the conjunctiva

cornea—the transparent membrane, forming the anterior outer coat of the eyeball

crista ampullaris—an elevation on the inner surface of the ampulla of each semicircular duct

cryosurgery—utilization of extreme cold to destroy tissue

cyclocryotherapy—application of a freezing probe to the sclera in the region of the ciliary body in treatment of glaucoma

cyclodialysis—establishment of a communication between the anterior chamber of the eye and the suprachoroidal space in order to relieve intraocular pressure in glaucoma

cyclodiathermy—destruction of a portion of the ciliary body by diathermy or heating of the tissues

cycloplegia—loss of power in the ciliary muscle of the eye

deafness, conductive—hearing impairment caused by a defect of the sound-conducting apparatus

diplopia—double vision; the perception of two images of a single object

electrocochleography—measurement of the electric potentials generated by the eighth cranial nerve in response to sound stimulation

electronystagmography—a procedure using electrodes to register eye movements

electro-oculography—a sensitive electrical test for detection of retinal pigment epithelial dysfunction

electroretinography—recording and study of the retinal action currents

endolymph—the fluid contained within the membranous labyrinth of the inner ear

equilibrium—the condition of balance between forces

esotropia—cross eye; interval or convergent squint

exotropia—external squint, divergent strabismus

glaucoma—a disease of the optic disk caused by increased intraocular pressure, resulting in damage to the retina and optic nerve

glossitis—inflammation of the tongue

glossodynia—burning or pain of the tongue

glossoncus—any swelling involving the tongue

glossopathy—any disease of the tongue

goniopuncture—a surgical procedure in which a puncture is made in the filtration angle of the anterior chamber, used in treating glaucoma

gonioscope—an optical instrument for examining the anterior chamber of the eye

gonioscopy—use of a gonioscope or contact prism lens and beam illumination from the slit lamp to examine the angle of the anterior chamber

goniotomy—surgical opening of Schlemm's canal used in treating glaucoma

gustation—the act of tasting; the sense of taste

halo—the colored circle seen around a light in glaucoma

hordeolum—a suppurative infection of a marginal gland of the eyelid

hydrops—abnormal accumulation of clear, watery fluid in the tissues or cavities of the body

hyperopia—a hypermetropia; farsightedness

hypogeusia—blunting of the sense of taste

iridectomy—excision of part of the iris

iridencleisis—surgical incarceration of a portion of the iris in a wound of the cornea to facilitate aqueous drainage

iris—the circular, colored part of the eye behind the cornea, perforated in the center by the pupil

iritis—inflammation of the iris

keratitis—inflammation of the cornea

keratotomy—surgical incision into the cornea

labyrinth—the internal or inner ear, composed of the semicircular ducts, vestibule and cochlea

labyrinthectomy—excision of the labyrinth

labyrinthitis—inflammation of the inner ear or labyrinth

lacrimal duct—tear duct

lens—a transparent biconvex body of cells lying between the iris and the vitreous body of the eye

macula—part of the retina responsible for fine vision

Meniere's disease—a disease characterized clinically by vertigo, nausea, vomiting, tinnitus, and progressive deafness

miotic—an agent that causes contraction of the pupil

mydriatic—an agent that dilates the pupil

myopia—shortsightedness; nearsightedness

myringitis—inflammation of the tympanic membrane

myringoplasty—operative repair of a damaged tympanic membrane

myringotomy—incision of the tympanic membrane

nerve deafness—deafness due to dysfunction or disease in the auditory pathway or nerve

neuroma, acoustic—benign tumor arising from the eighth cranial nerve producing tinnitus, vertigo, and decreased hearing

neuronitis, vestibular—degenerative inflammation of vestibular nerve cells

nyctalopia—night blindness; poor vision in faint light or at night

nystagmus—involuntary rhythmical oscillation of the eyeballs in a horizontal, rotary, and/or vertical direction

oculist—ophthalmologist

oculo-electromyography—record of the electrical currents generated in the ocular muscles

olfaction—the sense of smell

olfactory—relating to the sense of smell

olfactology—study of the sense of smell

olfactometer—a device for testing the keenness of the sense of smell

olfactometry—determination of the degree of sensibility of the olfactory organ

ophthalmodynamometry—measurement of blood pressure in the retinal vessels

ophthalmologist—a specialist in diseases and refractive errors of the eye

ophthalmoscope—a device for studying the interior of the eyeball through the pupil

optic nerve—part of the nervous system that conveys light impulses from the eye to the brain

optician—one who fills prescriptions for ophthalmic lenses and products

optometrist—a specialist in the examination of the eyes and related structures to determine the presence of vision problems, eye disease or other abnormalities

orbital cavity—the eye socket, the bony cavity containing the eyeball and its associated vessels, nerves and muscles

oscillopsia—the subjective sensation of stationary objects swaying

osmesis—olfaction; relating to the sense of smell

osphresis—relating to the sense of smell

ossicle—one of the bones of the tympanic cavity or middle ear

otalgia—earache

otitis media—inflammation of the middle ear or tympanum

otoconia—statoconia; ear crystals

otodynia—earache

otologist—a specialist in diseases of the ear

otolaryngologist—a physician who specializes in diseases of the ear and larynx, often including the upper respiratory tract

otoneuralgia—earache of neurologic origin, not caused by inflammation

otopathy—any disease of the ear

otorhinolaryngologist—a specialist in diseases of the ear, nose and larynx

otorrhagia—bleeding from the ear

otorrhea—a discharge from the ear

otosclerosis—formation of spongy bone about the stapes, resulting in progressively increasing hearing loss

otoscope—an instrument used for examining or auscultating the ear

otoscopy—inspection of the ear, especially of the drum membrane

ototoxicity—the property of having a toxic action upon the organs of hearing

papilla—any small nipple-like process or elevation

papilledema—edema of the optic disk sometimes caused by increased intracranial pressure

parosmia—any disorder of the sense of smell

parosphresia—parosmia

photocoagulation—use of an intense light beam directed to the interior of the eyeball to produce localized clotting

photonosus—any disease caused by prolonged exposure to intense light

photophobia—abnormal visual sensitiveness to light

photophthalmia—the inflammatory reaction caused by short-waved light (ultraviolet, snowblindness) on the external parts of the eye

photopsia—a subjective sensation of lights, sparks, or colors due to retinal or cerebral disease

posterior chamber—part of the eyeball between the lens, iris and vitreous chamber

presbyacusia—loss of ability to perceive or discriminate sounds that occurs with aging

presbyopia—defect of vision in advanced age

pupil—the circular opening in the center of the iris, through which light rays enter the eye

retina—nervous tunic of the eyeball

retinitis—inflammation of the retina

retinitis pigmentosa—inherited disorder of progressive retinal sclerosis, pigmentation and atrophy with scarring of the retina

retinopathy—disease of the retina

retinoscopy—inspection of the eye to detect errors of refraction by rotation of a mirror to detect movement of the retina

rhinologist—a specialist in diseases of the nose

rod—one of the photosensitive cells in the external granular layer of the retina

saccule—smaller of the two membranous sacs in the vestibule of the labyrinth

sclera—the white of the eye

sclerectomy—excision of a portion of the sclera

scleritis—inflammation of the sclera

scotoma—an isolated area of varying size and shape of absent or depressed vision within the visual field

statoconia—crystalline particles of calcium carbonate and a protein found in the utricle and saccule of the ear

strabismus—a constant lack of parallelism of the visual axes of the eyes; squint

syncope—temporary partial or complete loss of consciousness due to lack of blood flow in the cerebral arteries

tinnitus—ringing (noise) in the ears

tonometry—the measurement of intraocular tension

trabeculectomy—surgical excision of a portion of the trabecular meshwork as a treatment for glaucoma

tympanitis—inflammation of the tympanic membrane

tympanocentesis—puncture of the tympanic membrane to collect fluid from the middle ear

tympanoplasty—surgical reconstruction of a damaged middle ear

typhlosis—blindness

utricle—vestibular organ; the larger of the two membranous sacs in the vestibule of the labyrinth

uvea—the iris, choroid, and ciliary body comprising the middle coat of the eye

vertigo—a subjective or objective sensation of irregular or whirling motion

vestibule—the central, oval cavity of the bony labyrinth

vestibulopathy—disease of the vestibula

vitreous body—transparent gel filling the inner portion of the eyeball between the lens and retina

vitreous chamber—part of the eyeball in the space behind the lens containing the vitreous humor

vitreous humor—fluid portion of the vitreous body

CHAPTER 14

Psychiatric Disorders

The terminology of psychiatric disorders is rampant in the language of lay society, and many pharmacists feel quite comfortable with their understanding of commonly used terms. The medical community uses many of the same terms, but the reference is usually much more specific. A clear understanding of the exact medical meaning of psychiatric terms is useful for the pharmacist who must discuss a patient's condition with other health care providers and apply that information when dealing with the patients themselves.

Although a study of psychiatric terminology, of necessity, includes symptomatology, the intent is not for the student to become a diagnostician. Instead, symptoms are often the definitive criteria. Since the etiology of many psychiatric disorders is not clearly elaborated and no underlying pathologies of anatomy or physiology are evident, symptoms are often the only way of approaching the terminology.

General Considerations

An initial distinction should be recognized between **psychology** and **psychiatry.** The broader of the two terms, psychology is the science of behavior and concerns itself with mental and emotional development, emotional states, and both normal and abnormal reactions to life. Even clinical psychology, which is in many ways similar to psychiatry and may deal with psychiatric disorders, also assesses and treats patients with mental states well within the norm but may require assistance in coping with certain situations, e.g., emotional reactions to a handicap, disease, loss, or other difficulty. Psychiatry, on the other hand, is a specialty within medicine that deals with mental disorders or diseases and their diagnosis, management, and prevention. Thus, psychiatry is a much more specific term.

It should be remembered, however, that psychiatry is certainly not the only medical specialty to address psychiatric disorders. Indeed, psychological factors may contribute directly or indirectly to a number of physical disorders; some physical disorders such as a lesion involving neural or endocrine organs may produce psychiatric symptoms, and psychological symptoms such as depression and anxiety are common reactions to physical illness. In its broadest sense, the term **psychosomatic** illness encompasses all these possibilities. In a narrower sense, psychosomatic illnesses are those in which psychological factors are of etiologic significance or exacerbate the condition. According to this definition, therefore, many chronic or recurrent disorders are at least in part psychosomatic since their progress is intimately affected by psychological and social stress; hypertension, myocardial infarction, diabetes mellitus, malignancies, and rheumatoid arthritis are but a few examples.

Closely related to psychosomatic illness is **Munchausen's syndrome,** in which the patient goes from hospital to hospital for treatment of a fabricated but convincing illness. Although the illnesses, usually acute and dramatic, are either mimicked or physically self-induced (and thus not truly psychosomatic by the narrow definition), the underlying cause is of a complex psychiatric nature and should be treated as such.

Therapeutics

Disorders

Psychiatric disorders are commonly viewed as falling into one of two groups: neuroses and psychoses. Often viewed by the lay public as merely differing degrees of psychiatric illness, they are actually much more distinct in definitions. The term **psychotic** does not have a precise meaning in clinical and research practice; however, it is applied to major distortions of reality having either delusions or hallucinations. It most commonly refers to severe impairment of social/personal functioning, with a marked qualitative departure from normal behavior. The psychotic person's perception of reality is distorted, and even bizarre behaviors are perceived as appropriate or normal by the individual. The term **neurosis** is no longer used in classifications of mental disorders, although the term is still found in the literature. It has come to mean a chronic or recurrent nonpsychotic disorder characterized mainly by anxiety. Neuroses are disorders in which the psychologic and physiologic responses to ordinary stress are exaggerated, usually more severe, and of longer duration. Perception of reality is undisturbed for the neurotic patient; the morbid character of the neurotic behavior remains apparent to the patient, even if it is beyond conscious control. Neurosis appears as a symptom such as a phobia, compulsion, obsession, or a sexual dysfunction.

Cognitive and mental disorders include **delirium, dementia,** and **amnesia.** All have signs and symptoms that indicate underlying abnormalities of neuroanatomy, neurochemistry or neurophysiology. These may include disorders of mood, anxiety, personality, reality testing, intoxication, and withdrawal.

Amnestic disorders have an impairment of memory as the single or predominant cognitive defect. **Retrograde amnesia** refers to the loss of memory of events that took place prior to the onset of the illness. **Anterograde amnesia** is the reduced ability to recall current events. **Korsakoff's syndrome** is an amnestic syndrome caused by thiamine deficiency.

Dementias, organic and global deterioration of intellectual functioning, may present in a variety of forms. **Alzheimer** type involves severe loss of intellectual functioning with an unknown cause. **Pick's disease** refers to an atrophy of the lobes of the brain, also from an unknown cause. Other eponyms reflecting psychiatric disorders are **Huntington's disease, Creutzfeldt-Jakob disease,** and **Mad Hatter syndrome. Neurosyphilis** (general paresis) is a chronic dementia and psychosis caused by the tertiary form of syphilis.

Delirium refers to a restless, confused, and disoriented state associated with fear and hallucinations. **Delirium tremens** (DTs) refers to a marked autonomic hyperactivity occurring three to four days after withdrawal from alcohol. **Intoxication** is defined as a syndrome that follows the recent ingestion and the presence in the body of a substance identified by maladaptive behavior. Idiosyncratic alcohol intoxication is a syndrome of marked intoxication with subsequent amnesia for that period.

Schizophrenia encompasses a group of disorders in which the patient withdraws from reality into his/her own personal world (autism). The term *schizophrenia* literally means "split head," which may account for the popular misuse of the term to indicate dual personality (which is actually a dissociative state categorized as a hysterical reaction.) The somewhat archaic term *dementia praecox* is Latin for "early madness," perhaps a less confusing term, but one that is also much less commonly used. Other designations for types of schizophrenia include disorganized type, paranoid type, and undifferentiated type. The **catatonic** type involves **cataplexy** or other type of marked disturbance in motor function, manifested in muscular rigidity and immobility. Catatonia is marked by the extreme in autism—withdrawal to the point of constant unresponsiveness. Whatever the subtype, the patient with chronic schizophrenia tends to have a blunted affect, loss of drive, and incoherence.

Terms that may be encountered for other psychotic disorders include schizophreniform disorder, schizoaffective disorder, delusional disorder, and postpartum psychosis.

The two major mood disorders are **major depressive disorder** and **bipolar I disorder** (formerly manic-depressive disorder). Disorders related to depression include **dysthymic** disorder, minor depressive disorder, recurrent brief depressive disorder, and premenstrual **dysphoric** disorder. Related to bipolar I disorder is **bipolar II disorder** (recurrent major depressive episodes with hypomania) and **cyclothymic** disorder.

A major depressive disorder reflects a severe **dysphoric** (from the Greek-*phore*, meaning "a carrier") mood and personal loss of interest in usual activities. The sense of unhappiness is characterized by the patient as more than normal sadness and cannot be shaken off when the situation improves. Thus, the affect (emotion, although the term also means "emotional presentation") is intense and enduring, while the patient's mood does fluctuate. The depression tends to worsen in the evening, which may interfere with sleep. The primary somatic symptom is fatigue, and hysterical features may occur.

The term **endogenous depression** may be used to refer to a psychotic depression, reflecting a patient's response to a distorted perception of reality. This disorder has a rapid onset and progression and may be described as an emptiness or apathy. The patient may also deny feelings of depression. This type of depression is termed endogenous ("arising from within") because it lacks a realistic external reference. Endogenous depression may be only the depressive phase of manic-depressive illness.

The bipolar disorders are characterized by pathologic mood swings, spontaneous recoveries, and a tendency to recur. A bipolar disorder involves cyclic **mania** and depression. Less common than depression, the manic phase of the bipolar form is a pathologic mood elevation leading to grandiose ideas, delusions, and total loss of insight. This abnormal or exaggerated sense of well-being may be described as **euphoria**. After a manic phase, two-thirds of patients enter a depressive phase. Milder and more common than mania is **hypomania,** a moderate mood elevation with heightened activity and irritability but without the delusional convictions of mania.

Anxiety disorders include those such as panic disorder, agoraphobia and other phobias, obsessive-compulsive disorder, posttraumatic stress disorder, seasonal affective disorder (SAD), general anxiety disorder, hypochondriasis, and somatization disorder. The anxiety disorders, sometimes called anxiety reactions or phobic states, are characterized by exaggerated fear and anxiety that are long lasting and inappropriate to the situation.

Simple anxiety states include both the psychic and physical symptoms of tension, irritability, sleep difficulties, impaired appetite, impotence and other difficulties with sexual relations, diarrhea when anticipating stress, frustration, tachycardia, and fatigability. **Hyperventilation syndrome** (overbreathing) may lead to tingling skin, numbness in extremities, and dizziness. Pessimism and despondency are common, and patients often have difficulty making decisions.

Phobic states are often characterized by the same symptoms, and an anxiety neurosis will often evolve into a phobic state after added stress. Phobic states can have numerous themes. **Agoraphobia** is characterized by anxiety elicited by the patient's leaving the familiar surroundings of home. Literally a fear of open spaces, agoraphobia occurs most frequently in women, with symptoms beginning in the third decade of life. Similarly, the anxiety in social phobic states is aroused by the presence of others. Socially phobic patients often seek relief in alcohol or drugs. Monosymptomatic phobias are related to a specific theme, including a fearful aversion to death (thanatophobia), high places (acrophobia), night (nyctophobia), light (photophobia), or particular animals such as spiders (arachnophobia), snakes (ophidiophobia), or dogs (cynophobia). Simple lifestyle modifications that avoid the feared object may be successful enough for the patient to avoid any medical treatment. Patients with an underlying phobia, particularly agoraphobia, may experience sudden attacks of severe anxiety called **panic attacks** or **anxiety attacks** when faced with successful situations. This panic disorder may be diagnosed and treated separately, but the phobia may remain unchecked.

Obsessive-compulsive disorders, also called obsessional states, are a group of neuroses characterized by recurrent thoughts or impulses (obsession) and repetitive acts (compulsion) to which the patient feels a strong resistance. Although the patient realizes that the thoughts and actions are irrational, they cannot be controlled because of the overwhelming anxiety created when they are avoided. The most common themes of obsession concern contamination, often associated with the compulsion or obsessive ritual of hand washing. Other common obsessive themes include preoccupation with unlikely dangers; for example, the patient may be obsessed with the possibility of an iron or cigarette causing the house to burn down; repeated trips home to check do not calm the fears. Also common is a preoccupation with violence and death, often with the associated compulsion of hiding or checking weapons or frequent monitoring of family who are believed to be "in danger."

Dissociative disorders include dissociative amnesia or fugue, formerly called psychogenic amnesia; dissociative identity disorder, formerly called multiple personality disorder; depersonalization disorder; and transient global amnesia. In the dissociative states, the patient dissociates himself from the stressful event through a **fugue** or multiple personality. *Fugue* is from the Latin for "flee" and is also used for a musical form that may be viewed as a flight. A fugue is a massive amnesia allowing the patient to flee all memory of the stressful event, but it often leaves the patient wandering aimlessly. Double or multiple personality also allows the patient to dissociate from the event by creating one or more separate identities with no ties to the stress.

Patients with hysterical neuroses present with multiple somatic symptoms affecting any number of body systems and often involving medical and surgical treatment over long periods. Several unsuccessful surgeries for back pain, multiple gynecologic procedures, and repeated abdominal explorations are not uncommon. Similar to conversion symptoms, multiple somatic symptoms convert the psychological to the physical. Some of these patients are at least partly conscious that they are imitating symptoms, particularly those characterized as having **Munchausen's syndrome.**

Hypochondriasis refers to an excessive morbid anxiety about one's health. This may result in a condition termed **somatization disorder,** also known as **Briquet's syndrome,** with recurrent and multiple physical complaints without apparent physical cause. Other somatoform disorders include conversion disorder and body dysmorphic disorder.

Additional disorders falling into the realm of this area include eating disorders such as anorexia nervosa and bulimia (which are discussed in the chapter on nutrition); sleep disorders such as **Kleine-Levin syndrome** (recurrent periods of prolonged sleep), **hypersomnia** (excessive sleeping), **narcolepsy,** and **somniloquy** (sleepwalking); and compulsive behaviors such as **kleptomania** (stealing) or **pyromania** (setting fires).

Personality disorders may present with symptoms similar to other psychiatric disorders; these refer to usually long and fixed patterns of behavior that dominate an individual's personality. These are usually viewed by the person as normal but may manifest in a variety of generally unacceptable social manners. **Hysterical personality,** also called histrionic personality from the Latin term *histria* (actor), is characterized by attention-seeking behavior, excitability, and emotional instability. The person tends to be manipulative, repress unpleasant experiences, and blame others for failures and misfortunes. **Paranoid personality** may be viewed as the opposite of the hysterical in that the person projects his own hostilities as delusions that others are hostile towards him. A person with paranoid personality finds hostile intent in others' innocent actions, may then behave in a manner intended to prove his own adequacy by belittling others, and in return be rejected, thus "proving" the validity of the initial feeling of paranoia. **Obsessive-compulsive personality** is characterized by a conscientiousness and drive toward perfection, but these individuals may not be satisfied with their achievements.

Dependable and methodical, the obsessive-compulsive personality is also rigid and unable to adapt to changing circumstances. The **schizoid personality** is introverted and concerned with his own feelings, often unable to experience closeness. About 40% of schizophrenic patients exhibit this personality type before they become ill. Other personality disorders include the **cyclothymic** (marked by rhythmic mood changes with no apparent external cause), **psychopathic** or **sociopathic** (who act out their aggressions without regard to social rules or apparent sense of morality), **passive-aggressive** (manifesting initially as inefficiency and sullenness, later aggressive and undermining activity), and the **inadequate personality** in which responses to any form of stress are unsuitable to the situation.

Similar in presentation to the paranoid personality are paranoid states and paranoid psychoses. All **paranoias** are characterized by a general tendency to self-reference and to project one's own feelings and thoughts to others. The common usage of "paranoid" meaning exhibition of feelings of persecution is actually a fairly common symptom, although paranoid states range from a somewhat limited delusional system, which may be almost imperceptible, to the complete disorganization of paranoid schizophrenia. A brief paranoid state may be extremely intense, but it is usually a reaction to an event or situation such as a physical handicap. Paranoid psychosis is typified by a more elaborate delusional system that is self-perpetuating. For example, the patient may believe that he is discriminated against because of some minor deformity, real or imagined, and facial expressions and remarks from others are misinterpreted to reinforce the delusion. Delusions may take numerous forms, including injustices that "demand" litigation, pathological jealousy (Othello complex, named for Shakespeare's title character), or messianic beliefs. The delusions may even include hallucinations and disorganization of thought process, and in some patients a paranoid psychosis may progress to the point of frank schizophrenia. Conditions called **catalepsy** (*cata,* meaning "down") occur in psychological disorders and under hypnosis.

Psychoactive substance use disorders are characterized by symptoms and changes in behavior associated with continuing use of psychoactive substances that affect the central nervous system. **Dependence** may be psychological (compulsion) or physical, characterized by onset of withdrawal symptoms when the substance is abruptly discontinued. A feature of dependence is **tolerance,** or declining effect of the drug. Psychoactive substances that may produce these results include alcohol, amphetamines, cannabis, cocaine, hallucinogens, opioids, and sedatives.

Sexual disorders include dysfunctions and the general term **paraphilias** (*para* meaning "abnormal," *philia* meaning "attraction to/love"), which involves disorders such as pedophilia, fetishism, and masochism.

Of particular note in the terminology of psychiatric disorders is that the terms may be used in many different combinations; e.g., paranoid personality, paranoid psychosis, and paranoid schizophrenia actually differ, as do paranoid schizophrenia and schizophrenia. The reason is that these terms actually identify syndromes or groups of symptoms rather than a distinct pathophysiology with a distinct etiology. Since they identify symptoms, they are often combined to denote the specific set of symptoms or level of difficulty the patient is experiencing. For example, paranoid personality, paranoid psychosis, and paranoid schizophrenia all include symptoms of paranoia with its projections of aggression, but one indicates a lifelong reaction to stress, the second a primary disorder, and the third a set of symptoms accompanying a schizophrenic reaction. Thus, the pharmacist who learns the specific meanings of numerous psychiatric terms should not become disconcerted when physicians, even psychiatrists, occasionally use them in unexpected contexts.

Partly because of the variations possible in the diagnosis of psychiatric disorders, the list of recognized disorders and syndromes is quite extensive. Some of the more commonly encountered terms are listed in Table 14.1.

Diagnosis

The diagnostic process in psychiatry generally begins with the psychiatric interview. Similar to any other medical interview or the process of taking a medical history, the objective is to gather the information needed for an accurate diagnosis and the determination of effective treatment. Questioning, however, usually takes an open-ended approach, eliciting from the patient those aspects that seem relevant, since the relationship of ideas and events may have some bearing on diagnosis. Included in the interview is a careful history, but the focus is primarily on the psychiatric difficulty and the symptoms it expresses. Care should be taken to avoid many of the medical terms of psychiatry or to use them in the sense that the patient may (mis)understand, since the terminology is broadly used in society with sometimes very different meanings than in medicine.

Like a medical history, the psychiatric history should include the presenting problem and the history of present illness as well as the previous medical history. Of concern, certainly, may be family history since many psychiatric disorders rely in part on

Table 14.1—Common Psychiatric Disorders		

Cognitive and Mental Disorders:

Amnestic disorders:	Korsakoff's syndrome
	retrograde amnesia
	anterograde amnesia

Dementias:	Alzheimer type
	Pick's disease
	Huntington's disease
	Creutzfeldt-Jakob disease
	neurosyphilis
	Mad Hatter syndrome
	catatonia

Deliriums:	delirium tremens
	idiosyncratic alcohol intoxication
	intoxication

Schizophrenia:
- paranoid type
- disorganized type
- catatonic type
- undifferentiated type
- residual type

Other Psychotic Disorders:
- schizophreniform disorder
- schizophrenic affective disorder
- delusional disorder
- brief psychiatric disorder
- shared psychiatric disorder
- postpartum psychosis
- Capgras' syndrome

Mood Disorders:
- major depressive disorder
- bipolar I disorder
- dysthymic disorder
- cyclothymic disorder
- bipolar II disorder

Anxiety Disorders:
- panic disorder
- agoraphobia
- phobias
- obsessive-compulsive disorder
- posttraumatic stress disorder
- seasonal affective disorder
- general anxiety disorder
- hypochondriasis
- somatization disorder

Somatoform Disorders:
    somatization disorder (Briquet's
    syndrome)

Dissociative Disorders:
    dissociative amnesia
    dissociative fugue
    dissociative identity disorder
    depersonalization disorder
    transient global amnesia

Other Disorders:
    personality disorders
    factitious disorders: Munchausen's syndrome
    eating disorders
    sleep disorders: Kleine-Levin syndrome
                                hypersomnia
                                somniloquy

    kleptomania
    pyromania
    syphilis

---

hereditary factors, but personal history and personality prior to the illness are also important since they may have etiologic or diagnostic significance.

Part of the interview usually consists of a mental status examination (MSE), which includes assessment of such factors as appearance, **mood** (the sustained emotion that colors perception of the world), **sensorium,** intelligence, and **thought content,** a group of factors sometimes identified by the acronym **AMSIT,** along with **affect** (inferred from the facial expression), and **cognition.** Emotions may be referred to as labile or shallow, with **euphoria** or **apathy** predominating. **Sundowning** is observed in both demented and delirious patients. It is characterized by drowsiness, confusion, ataxia and accidental falls, all of which occur near bedtime. Automatisms such as lip-smacking, rubbing, chewing, or **echolalia** (repetition of the interviewer's words or actions) may be noted. Other patient descriptors encountered in diagnostic assessment may include terms such as narcissistic, impulsive, or hyper-vigilant. **Narcosynthesis** (e.g., sodium amobarbital interview), also called narcoanalysis, may be utilized for diagnostic and therapeutic purposes. Abbreviations listed in Table 14.2 are some of those that might be encountered in relation to psychiatric evaluation.

Brain-imaging technologies include computerized tomography (CT), magnetic resonance imaging (MRI), magnetic resonance spectroscopy (MRS), single photon emission computer tomography (SPECT), positron emission tomography (PET), and echoencephalography (ECHO). The term **polysomnography** (PSG) may appear in an order for a diagnostic procedure for sleep apnea. This consists of an electroencephalogram (EEG), electrocardiogram (ECG) and electromyelogram (EMG). A dexamethasone depression test (DST) is useful in making the diagnosis of major depressive disorder with melancholic features. A number of standard tests are utilized to evaluate various aspects of an individual's mental health and intelligence. These are represented in Table 14.3.

Table 14.2—Psychological Evaluations		
Type of Test	*Name*	
IQ	WAIS	Wechsler Adult Intelligence Scale
	WISC	Wechsler Adult Intelligence Scale for Children
	WPPSI	Wechsler Preschool & Primary Scale of Intelligence
		Stanford-Binet Intelligence Scale
Personality		Rorschach test
	TAT	Thematic Apperception test
	DAPT	Draw-A-Person test
	SCT	Sentence Completion test
	MMPI	Minnesota Multiphasic Personality Inventory
Diagnostic, Other	SOFAS	Social & Occupational Functioning Assessment Scale
	GAF	Global Assessment of Functioning (Scale)
		Alfred Binet

Therapy

Psychotherapy is a general term meaning the treatment of mental disorders. Psychological, rather than physical, methods are used with the goal of assisting the patient's personal development and self-understanding in general rather than to remove specific symptoms. An underlying principle is that the symptoms of a psychiatric disorder will lessen or disappear if the patient becomes able to deal with problems effectively. The term **cognitive therapy** is sometimes used to denote standard psychotherapy. **Psychoanalysis** refers to systematic review of the thought processes of an individual. Techniques may involve use of terms such as **free association** (voicing thoughts consecutively without censorship), dream interpretation, or **transference.** Other terms likely to be encountered with reference to diagnosis and treatment of mental disorders include various types of therapy such as crisis intervention therapy, family therapy, group therapy, milieu therapy, reality-oriented therapy, and sex therapy.

Psychosurgery involves the treatment of mental disorders by using surgical techniques. Perhaps the best-known psychosurgical procedure was the prefrontal lobotomy of popular literature, although it is atypical of current procedures. Current procedures use **stereotaxy,** a term derived from the Greek *stereos,* meaning "solid" (thus, three-dimensional) and *taxis,* which means "arrangement," as in "taxidermy" or "taxonomy." Stereotaxy is a technique using precise three-dimensional measurements to determine the position of the tissue and "cutting" it with a cryoprobe, electric cautery, or other technique to make selective lesions in smaller areas of the brain. The procedure is useful in relieving intractable pain, severe depression, obsessional neurosis, and chronic anxiety, usually without adverse effects. The terminology applied to other psychosurgical procedures generally follows the same pattern, usually relying on the root for structure and the suffix for the procedure. For example, cingulectomy refers to excision of the

Table 14.3—Abbreviations Associated with Psychiatric Disorders

AD	Alzheimer's disease	**HDRS**	Hamilton Depression Rate Scale
ADHD	attention deficit hyperactivity disorder	**HID**	headache, insomnia, depression
AMSIT	appearance, mood, sensorium, intelligence, thought process	**IC**	individual counseling
		MA	mental age
APE	acute psychotic episode	**MD**	manic depression
BAD	bipolar affective disorder	**MDD**	manic/major depressive disorder
BDI SF	Beck's Depression Index—Short Form	**MHC**	mental health center
BO	behavior objective	**MID**	multi-infarct dementia
BPRS	brief psychiatric rate scale	**MQ**	memory quotient
CSF	cerebrospinal fluid	**MRI**	magnetic resonance imaging
CST	convulsive shock therapy	**MRS**	magnetic resonance spectroscopy
CT	computerized axial tomography (useful in diagnosis of cognitive disorders)	**MSE**	mental status examination
		MT	music therapy
		NP	neuropsychiatric
CUS	chronic undifferentiated schizophrenia	**NREM**	non-rapid eye movement
		OCD	obsessive-compulsive disorder
DAT	dementia of the Alzheimer type	**PPP**	postpartum psychosis
DST	dexamethasone suppression test	**PSG**	polysomnography (diagnostic procedure for sleep apnea)
DT	delirium tremens	**PTSD**	posttraumatic stress disorder
ECT	electroconvulsive therapy	**QEEG**	quantitative electroencephalogram
EEG	electroencephalogram (used in diagnosis of seizure disorders)	**REM**	rapid eye movement
		SAD	seasonal affective disorder
FAST	functional assessment staging (of Alzheimer's disease)	**SAPD**	self-administration of psychotropic drugs
		SD	senile dementia
GAD	generalized anxiety disorder	**SZ**	schizophrenic
GAT	group adjustment therapy		

cingulum, the bundle of nerve fibers in each cerebral hemisphere surrounding the corpus callosum, which joins the two hemispheres. Similarly, amygdalectomy is the surgical excision of the amygdala, which is involved in mood, feeling, and memory of recent events.

Electroconvulsive therapy (ECT) is also useful in the treatment of severe depression and occasionally for schizophrenia and mania. In ECT, a convulsion is produced by passing an electrical current through the brain. By first administering a muscle relaxant and anesthetic, the convulsion is modified to produce only a few muscle twitches.

Numerous drugs can be effective in treating mental disorders. The **neuroleptic** or **psychotropic** agents, termed thus because they alter mood or literally "turn the mind," refer to antidepressants, monoamine oxidase inhibitors, stimulants, tricyclic antidepressants, lithium, and phenothiazines. **Anxiolytics,** formerly called minor tranquilizers and typified by the benzodiazepines, relieve anxiety and **hypnotics** induce sleep. Each of these agents acts somewhat selectively on certain neurotransmitters or receptors; terminology of **psychoactive** drugs needs little review for pharmacists.

Alternative approaches to treatment of mental disorders such as depression, insomnia, panic disorders, and phobias being used in conjunction with psychotherapy include acupuncture, botanical therapies, homeopathic remedies, nutritional therapies, vitamin and mineral therapies, lithium, hormone therapy, sleep therapy, biofeedback and relaxation, massage therapy, and deep breathing exercises. **Somatotherapy** (*somato*, meaning body) is a general term for the biological treatment of mental disorders. Hypnotherapy or **hypnosis** may be used as a supportive approach and to directly combat anxiety. Another technique known as **systematic desensitization** involves exposing the patient serially to a predetermined list of anxiety-provoking stimuli.

Pronouncing Glossary

Root	Meaning	Example	Pronunciation
anxi	anxious, uneasy	anxiolytic	ang zi oh LIT ik
auto-	self	automatism	aw TOM ah tizm
hypno-	sleep, hypnosis	hypnotism	HIP nah tizm
idio-	self	idiopathic	id ee oh PATH ik
narco-	stupor	narcolepsy	NARK oh lep see
philo-	affinity for	homophilic	ho mo FIL ik
phore-	carrier	heterophoria	het er oh FOR ee ah
phreno-	mind	phrenotropic	fren oh TROP ik
psycho-	mind	psychotherapy	si ko THER ah pee
schizo-	split, divide	schizophrenia	skitz oh FREN ee ah
somato-	body	somatogenic	so mah to JEN ik
thymia-	condition of mind	cyclothymia	si klo THI me ah

Glossary

acrophobia—a morbid dread of heights

affect—emotional feeling tone and mood attached to a thought, including its external manifestations such as fear, depression, panic, or elation

agoraphobia—a type of anxiety reaction characterized by anxiety produced outside of familiar or secure surroundings

apathy—absence of emotions; lack of emotional involvement

autism—lack of response to others

bipolar—describing a form of manic-depressive reaction involving cyclic mania and depression

Capgras' syndrome—delusional belief that a person known to the schizophrenic patient has been substituted for by an impostor

catalepsy—weakness and temporary loss of muscle tone precipitated by a variety of emotional states

catatonia—an abnormal mental state characterized by a syndrome of motor abnormalities involving excitement or inhibition

cognition—the quality of knowing that includes perceiving, recognizing, conceiving, judging, sensing, reasoning, and imagining

compulsion—uncontrollable urge to repeatedly perform an act

conversion—unconscious defense mechanism of converting anxiety into a physical symptom

Creutzfeldt-Jakob disease—rare degenerative brain disorder caused by a slow virus

cyclothymic—pertaining to marked swings of mood representing a personality disorder

delusion—false idea or belief that cannot be changed by logical reasoning or evidence

dissociation—separation of uncomfortable feelings from their real object in order to avoid mental distress

dysphoria—sadness; hopelessness

hallucination—a false perception by any of the senses involving a compulsive sense of the reality of the object or event

Huntington's disease—produces major atrophy of the brain with extensive degeneration of the caudate nucleus

hypomania—a mild degree of mania

hysteria—a neurosis consisting of emotional instability, repression, dissociation, vulnerability to suggestion and physical symptoms

idiopathic—denoting a disease of unknown cause or one that arises spontaneously

labile—unstable; rapidly undergoing emotional change

lobotomy—leukotomy; a surgical procedure interrupting the pathways of the white nerve fibers within the brain

Mad Hatter syndrome—disorder caused by inhalation of mercury nitrate vapors

mania—an emotional disorder characterized by excessive cheerfulness and increased activity

mutism—nonreactive state; stupor

narcissism—state in which the individual regards everything in relation to self, not other persons or things

narcolepsy—a sudden uncontrollable tendency to fall asleep in quiet or monotonous surroundings

neurosis—a mental disorder in which insight is retained but symptoms involve anxiety, depression, obsessions, phobias, or physical complaints

obsession—involuntary persistent idea or emotion

paranoia—a mental disorder characterized by the presence of systematized delusions, often involving a feeling of persecution

phobia—a pathologically strong fear of a specific object or occurrence

postpartum psychosis—acute disorder involving depression, delusions, and thoughts of harm to new mother or infant following childbirth

psychiatry—the study and/or diagnosis, treatment, and prevention of mental disorders

psychoanalysis—a method of treating mental disorders based on the teachings of Sigmund Freud

psychology—the science concerned with the behavior of man and animals

psychopath—an individual whose behavior is antisocial with little or no guilt and limited capacity for forming emotional relationships with others

psychosis—a severe mental disorder involving loss of contact with reality

psychosomatic—relating to or involving both the mind and body

psychosurgery—operative procedures involving the brain for the purpose of relieving mental and psychic symptoms

psychotherapy—use of psychological, rather than physical, methods for the treatment of mental disorders

psychotropic—referring to mood-altering drugs

schizoaffective disorder—disorder involving disturbance of emotional feeling, tone, and mood with external manifestations

schizophreniform disorder—mental disorder characterized by the appearance of symptoms of schizophrenia, but lasting less than six months

schizoid—similar in presentation or symptomatology to schizophrenia

schizophrenia—a severe mental disorder characterized by disintegration of emotional response, contact with reality and the thinking process

sociopath—referring to an individual with a personality disorder where aggressions are acted out without regard to social or moral implications

stereotaxy—a surgical procedure on the brain performed after determination of the precise area using three-dimensional measurements

transference—set of expectations, beliefs, and emotional response that a patient brings into the doctor–patient relationship

unipolar—describing a form of manic-depressive reaction involving endogenous depression

CHAPTER 15

The Endocrine System and Its Disorders

The endocrine system is composed of a number of glands located throughout the body (Figure 15.1). The term **endocrine** means to secrete internally, and these glands produce **hormones** (from the Greek, meaning "to set in motion") that are transported to various parts of the body by blood, lymph, and extracellular fluids.

The hormones of the endocrine glands act in general to regulate the body's metabolism. **Metabolism** simply means change, and the term usually refers to any of the chemical and physical changes that occur in body tissues. These changes regulate the maintenance of normal growth, development, and functions of the body. There are over fifty hormones found in humans. These are categorized as **peptides** or peptide derivatives, **steroids,** and **amines.** Additionally, the **prostaglandins** play a "second messenger" role in affecting the secretory activity of endocrine glands and the functions of their target tissues.

Anatomy and Physiology

By producing hormones that are transported to various parts of the body, the endocrine system exerts what may be called a chemical remote control over the target organs or tissues. Previously believed to function independently, this system is now known to coordinate its actions with the nervous system in affecting the rates of individual metabolic pathways.

Because tissues that synthesize hormones generally have a limited storage capacity, most hormones are released into the circulation in the steady state as a passive reflection of the rate of formation. Therefore, the regulation of a hormone's activity in the plasma is accomplished by regulation of its synthesis; fluctuation in hormone levels in a normal person is determined primarily by changes in production. Production of each hormone is regulated directly or indirectly by a metabolic activity of the hormone itself.

Metabolic clearance of hormones is accomplished by various means. Degradation and inactivation can take place in target, as well as nontarget, tissues, and transformations often facilitate excretion of the hormone by causing its solubility in urine or bile.

The **hypothalamus** is a small specialized area at the base of the brain lying above and behind the optic chiasm and above the pituitary gland. It serves as the highest integrative center for the two systems regulating the body's metabolic activities. Hypothalamic endocrine activity is influenced by events recorded in the brain and in the central and autonomic nervous systems. Interaction at the cellular level involves polypeptide

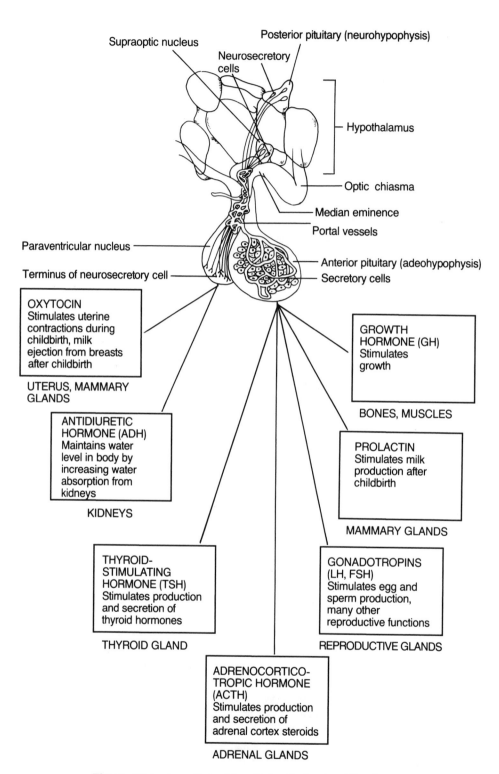

Supraoptic nucleus

Neurosecretory cells

Posterior pituitary (neurohypophysis)

Hypothalamus

Optic chiasma

Median eminence

Portal vessels

Paraventricular nucleus

Terminus of neurosecretory cell

Anterior pituitary (adeohypophysis)

Secretory cells

OXYTOCIN
Stimulates uterine contractions during childbirth, milk ejection from breasts after childbirth

UTERUS, MAMMARY GLANDS

GROWTH HORMONE (GH)
Stimulates growth

BONES, MUSCLES

ANTIDIURETIC HORMONE (ADH)
Maintains water level in body by increasing water absorption from kidneys

KIDNEYS

PROLACTIN
Stimulates milk production after childbirth

MAMMARY GLANDS

THYROID-STIMULATING HORMONE (TSH)
Stimulates production and secretion of thyroid hormones

THYROID GLAND

GONADOTROPINS (LH, FSH)
Stimulates egg and sperm production, many other reproductive functions

REPRODUCTIVE GLANDS

ADRENOCORTICO-TROPIC HORMONE (ACTH)
Stimulates production and secretion of adrenal cortex steroids

ADRENAL GLANDS

Figure 15.1—Location of the Major Endocrine Glands.

hormones, adenylate cyclase, cyclic adenosine monophosphate (called "cyclic AMP" but written "cAMP"), and calcium ions. The hypothalamus and pituitary glands regulate growth; lactation (production of milk); function of the thyroid, adrenals, and gonads; and hydration (taking in of water) in the body.

The **pituitary** gland or **hypophysis** is located in a small cavity in the floor of the skull behind the bridge of the nose. It is about the size of a pea, consisting of two lobes secreting different hormones, and is connected to the hypothalamus by the pituitary stalk. Functions of the anterior (**adenohypophysis**) and posterior pituitary (**neurohypophysis**) are regulated by the hypothalamus, which also regulates thirst, appetite and caloric intake, sleep-wake behavior, emotions, autonomic balance, and cognition (a knowing or recognition).

The anterior pituitary hormones under hypothalamic control are **thyrotropic hormone** (thyroid stimulating hormone or **TSH**), **adrenocorticotropic hormone (ACTH), gonadotropins** (both follicle stimulating hormone or **FSH** and luteinizing hormone or **LH**), **somatotropic hormone** (growth hormone or **GH**), **melanocyte stimulating hormone (MSH)** and **prolactin (Pr),** each regulated by a feedback mechanism (Figure 15.2). These regulate the productivity of the other glands of the endocrine system. The suffix -*tropic* contained in many of these terms denotes a turning toward or having an affinity for something, while the root portion reflects the location or function; for example *thyro* = thyroid, *gonado* = *gonads*, and *somato* = body.

The posterior (rear) lobe of the pituitary produces **antidiuretic hormone (ADH)** or vasopressin, which exerts its primary effect on excretion of urine by the kidney. **Oxytocin** in the female is also produced by the posterior lobe. These are synthesized in the hypothalamus and then stored in the posterior pituitary until released by nerve impulses from the hypothalamus.

Located in the front part of the neck, the **thyroid** gland consists of two lateral lobes joined in front by a narrow band of tissue. The hormones secreted by the thyroid gland are **thyroxin, triiodothyronine,** and **calcitonin.** Its function is to regulate the rate of metabolism of the body cells. The thyroid gland also absorbs ingested iodine from the bloodstream for use in producing thyroxin.

Located in or near the lobes of the thyroid gland are the four **parathyroid** glands. (The prefix *para-* means alongside or near). Each is approximately the size of a pea and produces **parathormone,** which acts on calcium in the body. Parathormone acts primarily on the bones (to move calcium out into the blood and body tissues) and in the kidneys (to remove the calcium from the blood by excretion). Since most of the body's phosphorus is found in combination with calcium in the bones and teeth, phosphorus metabolism is also affected by the parathyroid.

The two **adrenal** glands are located above the kidneys. The inner portion of these glands (the adrenal medulla) secretes **epinephrine** (also called **adrenaline**) and **norepinephrine (noradrenaline).** These are produced in response to strong emotions and prepare the body to meet an emergency by increasing mental alertness, serum glucose, blood pressure, and heart rate. The hormones secreted by the outer layer of adrenals (the adrenal cortex) are known as the **adrenal corticosteroids.** Their primary functions are regulation of salt and carbohydrate metabolism. Those that primarily affect carbohydrates are termed **glucocorticoids,** the most potent being hydrocortisone. Blood sugar levels, fat deposits and white blood cells, as well as several other vital body activities, are affected by glucocorticoids. The hormones that exert their effect primarily on salt metabolism are known as **mineralocorticoids,** the most potent of which is **aldosterone.** These affect

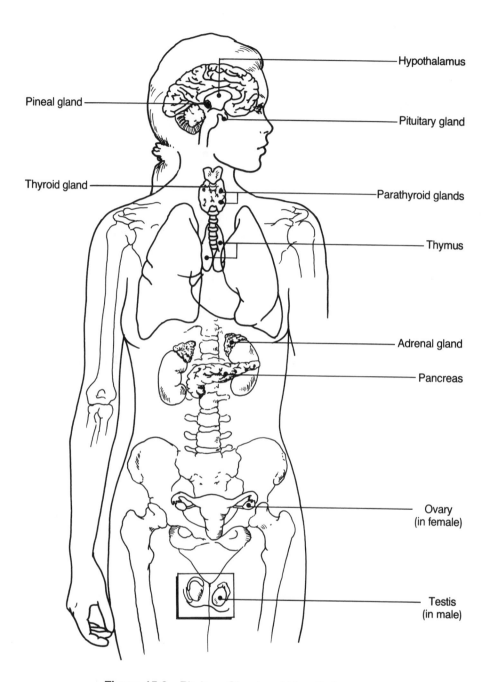

Figure 15.2—Pituitary Gland and Hypothalamus.
Pituitary hormones are indicated with their actions. Target areas for each hormone
are shown under the relevant box.

electrolyte distribution, water balance, and blood pressure. The adrenal cortex also secretes sex hormones (androgens, estrogens, progestins) identical to those secreted by the sex glands, although they are significantly less potent.

Endocrine functions of the **pancreas** are performed by the **Islets of Langerhans,** named after a German anatomist. These secrete insulin, needed at the cellular level for carbohydrate metabolism, and glucagon, which causes conversion of glycogen to glucose.

The sex glands of the body are known as **gonads** (from the word *gone,* meaning seed). In the male, the **testis** (plural, **testes**) produces the male sex hormones called **androgens.** The primary hormone is **testosterone,** which stimulates development of the male secondary sex characteristics and is responsible for **libido,** or sexual/creative energy. Male sex hormones also perform an exocrine (*exo-*= outside) function in the production of sperm cells. In the female, the **ovaries** produce **progesterone** and **estradiol,** which control libido, onset of menstruation, and other secondary sex characteristics. **Androgens** are believed to increase libido and muscular strength and to promote a positive nitrogen balance. The exocrine function of the ovaries is the development and expulsion of the ovum. Sex hormones are discussed in more detail in Chapter 10.

Therapeutics

Diseases

Disorders of the endocrine system are usually caused by "underfunctioning" (designated by the prefix *hypo-*) or "overfunctioning" (with the prefix *hyper-*), inflammation, or tumors of the glands.

Pituitary hypersecretion of the growth hormone somatotropin during the period of skeletal development results in **giantism,** an abnormal increase in the length of skeletal structures causing unusually large body size (hence the name). **Acromegaly** (*acro* = extremity, plus *megaly,* large), a form of gigantism that affects adults, is often caused by a pituitary tumor that produces excess growth hormone after skeletal development is normally complete. Rather than affecting skeletal length, its effects are seen as thickening of cartilage and bone with widening of the jaw, hands, feet, eyebrow ridges, and soft tissue. Conversely, hyposecretion of somatotropin results in **dwarfism,** the condition seen in dwarfs and midgets. Dwarfism can also result from a deficiency in thyroid hormones.

A condition called **diabetes insipidus** results from hyposecretion of vasopressin by the pituitary gland. The disorder in which there is continual release of ADH unrelated to plasma osmolality is known as the syndrome of inappropriate diuretic hormone **(SIADH).** This occurs in association with several clinical disorders, particularly malignant tumors such as oat-cell carcinoma of the lung. Symptoms include weight gain, weakness, lethargy, mental confusion, and progression to convulsions and coma.

An excess of thyroid hormone in the body (**hyperthyroidism**) is termed **Hashimoto's disease,** which may be reflected by an abnormally high metabolic rate. Among the symptoms are nervousness, irritability, weakness, weight loss, and increased blood pressure and heart rate. The **exophthalmos** ("protruding eyeballs") also seen is partly caused by increased fluid behind the eyes. The most common form of this disorder is **thyrotoxicosis** or **Grave's disease.** Conversely, decreased production of thyroid hormone, with resultant slowing of the metabolic rate, is known as **hypothyroidism.** This may be caused by a lack of iodine in the system or by disease of the thyroid. If this occurs in the fetus after the first trimester of pregnancy, **cretinism** results with mental retardation and irregular development of bones and muscles. Occurrence during adulthood produces **myxedema** with swollen facial features, dry skin, fatigue, low basal metabolic rate, cold intolerance, and possible mental retardation. This reduced activity of thyroid hormone is often associated with enlargement of the thyroid, known as a **goiter,** which may be described as toxic, nodular, or diffuse.

Abnormally low activity of the parathyroid glands or **hypoparathyroidism** most commonly is caused by an adenoma or by surgical drainage or removal of the glands. Since parathormone affects calcium and associated phosphorus in bone, low serum calcium (hypocalcemia) and excessive serum phosphorus levels then result with increased muscular and nervous irritability, cramping, convulsions, and possible paralysis of the respiratory system, a condition known as tetany. **Hyperparathyroidism** is most commonly caused by an adenoma and can result in excessive elimination of mineral salts and weakening of bones with eventual kidney and circulatory collapse.

Hyperactivity of the adrenal cortex, or **hyperadrenalism,** produces **Cushing's disease** and adrenogenital syndrome. Both are related to a cortical tumor. Adrenal insufficiency, the inverse of hyperadrenalism, can be divided into two categories: hypoadrenalism associated with a primary inability of the adrenal to produce sufficient hormone and hypoadrenalism associated with a secondary failure of ACTH. **Primary adrenocortical deficiency,** also called **Addison's disease** or chronic glucocorticoid deficiency, results from progressive adrenocortical destruction. Anemia, weakness, fatigue, increased potassium, and decreased sodium levels in the blood are common symptoms. **Secondary adrenocortical insufficiency** is caused by a pituitary deficiency in ACTH production. **Hypoaldosteronism** results from an isolated aldosterone deficiency.

Hypoactivity of the pancreas results in **diabetes mellitus,** the most common of the serious metabolic diseases. Since the beta cells do not produce sufficient insulin, glucose accumulates in the blood (**hyperglycemia**) and then is excreted in the urine without entering the cells. Ketosis occurs when production of ketone bodies is increased; their presence in the urine is called **ketonuria.** Common symptoms are excessive urination (**polyuria**), excessive thirst (**polydipsia**), and excessive appetite (**polyphagia**). Diabetics are also at risk of developing two major acute metabolic complications: **diabetic ketoacidosis** and **hyperosmolar nonketotic coma.** Late complications of diabetes include circulatory abnormalities, retinopathy (disease of the retina), nephropathy (disease of the kidney), neuropathy (disease of the nervous system), disorders of fat metabolism (e.g., lipoatrophy, lipodystrophy), and diabetic foot ulcers. Conversely to diabetes, excessive production of insulin causes **hypoglycemia** or lowered concentrations of glucose in the blood. A combined episode of reactive hyperglycemia followed by hypoglycemia is known as the **Somogyi effect.**

Abnormalities of testicular function can result in **viral orchitis** or **infertility, prostatic hypertrophy,** and **cancer of the prostate.** Ovarian hypofunction can manifest in a number of ways, including **gonadal dysgenesis, autoimmune disorders,** and premature **menopause.** Hyperfunction of the ovary can produce **tumors** or **cysts.**

The most commonly encountered disorders of the endocrine system are summarized in Table 15.1.

Diagnosis

A number of techniques are useful in measuring endocrine status. **Plasma levels** of a hormone are useful when obtained by chemical, radioreceptor, and radioimmunoassay

Table 15.1—Common Disorders of the Endocrine System

Thyroid:	exophthalmic goiter (thyrotoxicosis)
	adenoma
	toxic nodular goiter
	toxic diffuse goiter (Grave's disease)
	nontoxic goiter
	endemic goiter
	subacute thyroiditis
	primary hypothyroidism
	Hashimoto's thyroiditis
	medullary carcinoma (MCT)
	cretinism
	myxedema
Hypothalamus-Pituitary:	hypopituitarism
	hypogonadism
Pituitary:	diabetes insipidus
	syndrome of inappropriate antidiuretic hormone (SIADH)
	acromegaly
	giantism
	dwarfism
	panhypopituitarism
Pituitary-Adrenal:	ACTH deficiency
	neoplasms
Adrenal:	aldosteronism
	hypoaldosteronism
	virilism
	Cushing's syndrome
	congenital adrenal hyperplasia
	primary adrenocortical deficiency (Addison's disease)
	pheochromocytoma
Pancreas:	diabetes mellitus
	hypoglycemia
	insulinoma
	hyperinsulinism
	neoplasms
Testis:	viral orchitis
	infertility
	prostatic hypertrophy
	cancer of the prostate

Ovaries:	gonadal dysgenesis
	autoimmune disorders
	17a-hydroxylase deficiency
	feminizing tumors
	masculinizing tumors
	corpus luteum/follicle cysts
	Stein-Leventhal syndrome
	choriocarcinoma
	struma ovarii
	carcinoid

methods, providing information about the patient's current hormonal state. Measuring the excretion of a hormone or metabolite in urine may be advantageous since it quantifies average levels of the hormone over a period of time, which may be a better estimate of function. Measuring the rate of secretion of a hormone into the circulation may be useful in some patients; however, such measurements involve administration of a radioactive hormone followed by determination of the dilution of that hormone, therefore requiring specialized facilities that are not available in many institutions. **Stimulation tests** are useful in clarifying the meaning of tests on the borderline of being low, helping to assess hormone status when precise quantification is difficult or not totally accurate and to distinguish primary from secondary causes of endocrine failure. **Suppression tests** can diagnose hyperfunction since, by definition, the hyperfunctioning gland does not operate under normal control mechanisms. **Measurement of hormone receptors** is useful in diagnosis of partial hormone resistance states (e.g., hyperglycemia and insulinemia associated with insulin resistance). These are generally performed only in research laboratories. Although an ideal parameter, measurement of the end result of hormone action in the target tissue is often difficult to perform and/or is influenced by outside factors.

The basic screening tests used in initial evaluation of thyroid function include TT_4 by radioimmunoassay (**RIA**), resin T_3 uptake (**RT$_3$U** or **RT$_4$U**), free thyroxine index (**FT$_4$I**), thyroid-stimulating hormone (**TSH**) measurement, and free serum thyroxine (**FT$_4$**). The term **thyroid scan** is often encountered, referring to administration of a radioactive compound and visualized by a scanner device. These procedures are often supplemented by a number of additional tests available for assessment of thyroid functions. For example, an **exophthalmometer** is used to measure the extent of protrusion of the eyeball. Thyroglobulin, the colloid protein secreted by the thyroid gland, is elevated when the thyroid is inflamed or enlarged; this can be measured in the serum by radioimmunoassay. **Cholesterol** levels can also be measured to determine a possible association with thyroid disorder.

Hypopituitarism is evaluated by various provocative tests to examine the adequacy of hypothalamus-pituitary response to stress, releasing factors and blockade of feedback inhibition. **Twenty-four-hour urine** collections for measurement of gonadotropins or steroid secretion are useful for evaluation over a period of time. Other types of evaluation include tests for **prolactin deficiency, growth hormone reserve, LH** and **FSH** reserve, **thyrotropin** (TSH) reserve, and **ACTH deficiency.** Diabetes insipidus is demonstrated by a **dehydration** test, assessing the relationship of plasma to urine osmolality.

Adrenal function can be evaluated by a number of laboratory tests. ACTH and angiotensin II can be measured by **radioimmunoassay;** however, the majority of renin-angiotensin activity involves plasma determinations, as do cortisol and aldosterone levels. Urinary tests determine **excretion measurements. Suppression testing** for cortisol hypersecretion involves suppression of ACTH release to evaluate hypersecretion of adrenocortical hormone.

Diagnosis of diabetes mellitus is generally based on the presence of hyperglycemia along with symptoms of an osmotic diuresis. Laboratory determinations most often utilized are the two-hour **plasma glucose concentration, oral glucose tolerance test (GTT),** and fasting plasma glucose. Urine testing shows elevation of glucose levels (**glucosuria, glycosuria**) and the presence of ketones (**ketonuria**).

The plasma testosterone level is the primary measure of functioning of the testes. Dihydrotestosterone can also be measured by **radioimmunoassay,** as can the plasma luteinizing hormone. Responses to **gonadotropin stimulation** and luteinizing hormone-releasing hormone (**LHRH**) are also utilized to test integrity of the pituitary-testicular axis. **Semen analysis** measures motility and volume in evaluating infertility.

Ovarian dysfunction can be diagnosed by laboratory determination of serum or urinary estrogen levels or by measurement of total urinary **estrogen excretion.** The luteinizing hormone (LH) urine test detects the presence of LH in the urine, thus impending ovulation. **Endometrial biopsy** documents the occurrence of ovulation. **Ultrasonography** can distinguish between single and multiple follicular growth.

Treatment

Hypothyroidism is treated with natural (e.g., desiccated thyroid, thyroglobulin) or synthetic (e.g., L-thyroxine, L-triiodothyronine, thiotrix) thyroid hormones in an effort to attain and maintain a euthyroid (normal) state. The three major approaches to treatment of hyperthyroidism are use of **thioamides** to block conversion of T_4 to T_3, **radioactive iodine (RAI)** to destroy the gland, and **surgery** to remove the gland. Removal of the thyroid gland is known as **thyroidectomy** (-*ectomy* = excision). Adjunctive agents include iodinated contrast dye, iodides, adrenergic antagonists, prednisone, and lithium to block conversion or release the thyroid hormone.

Patients with hypopituitarism are treated with **hormone replacement,** depending on the degree of deficiency and on the type and extent of the lesion. Those patients with space-occupying lesions are candidates for surgery and/or irradiation. Pituitary hormone hypersecretion occurs with adenomas, causing hyperprolactinemia that may be treated with microsurgery, irradiation, or dopamine agonists. Growth hormone excess, manifested in acromegaly, may require both **surgery** and **irradiation** to control tumor growth. Medical treatment has limited success; however, dopamine agonists may be useful adjuncts to treatment. ACTH excess, caused by pituitary adenomas, is preferably treated with microsurgery. Diabetes insipidus can be treated by hormone replacement (vasopressin) or by nonhormonal agents such as chlorpropamide, clofibrate, or carbamazepine. SIADH treatment involves fluid restriction, IV saline to increase serum sodium levels, furosemide to reduce cardiac load, and attention to the underlying cause. Drugs are not presently available for clinical use in suppressing ADH release from the system or from a tumor.

Major components of treatment for diabetes mellitus are **diet, exercise, insulin,** and **oral hypoglycemic agents.** Diet and exercise are indicated for all patients with diabetes mellitus, regardless of type. Insulin is indicated for Type I diabetes and in Type II during times of stress or illness or when symptoms cannot be controlled by diet or oral agents.

Use of oral sulfonylureas and other hypoglycemic agents is reserved for patients with Type II diabetes whose symptoms cannot be controlled with diet and exercise.

Androgen replacement therapy is utilized in males with gonadal hypoactivity when virilization is the goal. Treatment with gonadotropins is utilized to establish or restore fertility in patients with secondary hypogonadism from all causes. **Estrogen and progesterone replacement** therapy in varying sequences is used for ovarian hypofunction.

Abbreviations commonly encountered with reference to the endocrine system are listed in Table 15.2. A number of eponyms reflect disorders of the endocrine system; these are included in Table 15.3.

Table 15.2—Abbreviations Associated with the Endocrine System

ACH	adrenal cortical hormone	**FTI**	free thyroxine index
ACTH	adrenocorticotropic hormone	**GCIIS**	glucose control insulin infusion system
ADH	antidiuretic hormone		
ADX	adrenalectomy	**GD**	Graves disease
AHT	autoantibodies to human thyroglobulin	**GDM**	gestational diabetes mellitus
		GGE	generalized glandular enlargement
AODM	adult onset diabetes mellitus		
ATD	autoimmune thyroid disease; antithyroid drug	**GH**	growth hormone; glycosylated hemoglobin
ATgA	antithyroglobulin antibodies	**GHD**	growth hormone deficiency
BDR	background diabetic retinopathy	**GnRH**	gonadotropin-releasing hormone
BG	blood glucose	**GSD**	glycogen storage disease
BGM	blood glucose monitoring	**GSD-1**	glycogen storage disease, type 1
BHI	biosynthetic human insulin		
BS	blood sugar	**HBGM**	home blood glucose monitoring
CIDS	continuous insulin delivery system		
		HH	hypogonadotropic hypogonadism
CPD	chorioretinopathy and pituitary dysfunction	**HHNK**	hyperglycemic hyperosmolar nonketotic (coma)
DFR	diabetic floor routine		
DK	diabetic ketoacidosis	**HPA**	hypothalamic-pituitary-adrenal (axis)
DKA	diabetic ketoacidosis		
DMKA	diabetes mellitus ketoacidosis	**HPG**	human pituitary gonadotropin
DMOOC	diabetes mellitus out of control	**HPT**	hyperparathyroidism
		IADH	inappropriate antidiuretic hormone
DPN	diabetic peripheral neuropathy		
		IDDM	insulin-dependent diabetes mellitus
DR	diabetic retinopathy		
DU	diabetic urine	**IGT**	impaired glucose tolerance
FB	fasting blood sugar	**IHH**	idiopathic hypogonadotropic hypogonadism
FPG	fasting plasma glucose		
FSH	follicle stimulating hormone	**IHT**	insulin hypoglycemia test
FSHRF	follicle stimulating hormone releasing factor	**IIT**	intensive insulin therapy
		IST	insulin shock therapy; insulin sensitivity test
FT4	free thyroxine		

IVGTT	intravenous glucose tolerance test	**NSILA**	nonsuppressible insulin-like activity
JODM	juvenile onset diabetes mellitus	**OGTT**	oral glucose tolerance test
KA	ketoacidosis	**OHA**	oral hypoglycemic agents
KDDM	kidney disease of diabetes mellitus	**PDR**	proliferative diabetic retinopathy
LATS	long-acting thyroid stimulator	**PGH**	pituitary growth hormone
LH	luteinizing hormone	**PHPT**	primary hyperparathyroidism
LHRH	luteinizing hormone-releasing hormone	**PPBG**	postprandial blood glucose
MDII	multiple daily insulin injection	**PPBS**	postprandial blood sugar
MEN (II)	multi-endocrine neoplasia (type II)	**PPPG**	postprandial plasma glucose
MODY	maturity onset diabetes of youth	**Pr**	prolactin
MSH	melanocyte stimulating hormone	**RAI**	radioactive iodine
MUDPIES	methanol, uremia, diabetic ketoacidosis, paraldehyde, idiopathic, ethylene glycol, salicylate (cause of metabolic acidosis)	**RAIU**	radioactive iodine uptake
		RT3U	resin triiodothyronine uptake
		SIADH	syndrome of inappropriate antidiuretic hormone
		T-7	free thyroxine factor
		TBG	thyroxine-binding globulin
		TBPA	thyroxine-binding prealbumin
		TH	thyroid hormone
MULEPAK	methanol, uremia, lactic acidosis, ethylene glycol, paraldehyde, aspirin, diabetic ketoacidosis (cause of metabolic acidosis)	**TRab**	thyroid-receptor antibody
		TRH	thyrotropin-releasing hormone
		TSH	thyroid-stimulating hormone
		TSI	thyroid-stimulating immunoglobulins
		TT3	total serum triiodothyronine
		TT4	total thyroxine
NIDDM	noninsulin dependent diabetes mellitus	**T3UR**	triiodothyronine uptake ratio
		UGDP	University Group Diabetes Program
NKHS	nonketotic hyperosmolar syndrome		

Table 15.3—Eponyms Associated with the Endocrine Sytem

Addison's disease	Grave's disease
Anderson's disease	Gull disease
Basedow disease	Hashimoto's disease
Conn's syndrome	McArdle's disease
Cushing's syndrome	Plummer's disease
De Quervain disease	Pompe's disease
Forbes disease	Simmonds disease
Fröhlich's syndrome	Stein-Leventhal syndrome
Gierke's disease	Von Gierke's disease

Pronouncing Glossary

Root	Meaning	Example	Pronunciation
aden-	gland	adenoma	add en OH ma
adren-	adrenal gland	adrenalopathy	a dre na LOP a thee
amylo-	starch	amylophagia	amee low FAY jah
andro-	masculine	androgen	AN dro jen
gluco-	sugar, sweet	glucosuria	glu ko SUR ee ah
glyco-		glycosuria	gli ko SUR ee ah
gonad-	gonads	gonadotropic	GON a do TROP ik
pancreat-	pancreas	pancreatitis	PAN kre a TI tis
thyro-	thyroid gland	thyrogenic	thi ro JEN ik

Glossary

acromegaly—progressive enlargement of the hands, feet, and face caused by excessive production of growth hormone by the pituitary gland

adenoma—a benign tumor of epithelial origin derived from glandular tissue

adrenal—located on or near the kidney

adrenogenital syndrome—hormonal disorders resulting from abnormal steroid production by the adrenal cortex

aldosterone—a steroid hormone synthesized and released by the adrenal cortex that acts on the kidney to regulate salt and water balance

aldosteronism—overproduction of aldosterone by the adrenal cortex

androgen—a male steroid hormone that affects growth of secondary sex characteristics

cortisol—a steroid hormone, the major glucocorticoid synthesized and released by the adrenal cortex

Cushing's disease—the condition resulting from excess amounts of corticosteroid hormones in the body

diabetes insipidus—condition of chronic excretion of large quantities of dilute urine accompanied by excessive thirst

diabetes mellitus—a disorder of carbohydrate metabolism in which sugar is not oxidized to produce energy in the body due to lack of or resistance to insulin

dwarfism—condition of being markedly undersized

dysgenesis—defective embryonic development of an organism

endocrine—the internal or hormonal secretion of a ductless gland

euthyroid—having a normally functioning thyroid gland

exophthalmometer—an instrument used for measuring the distance between the anterior cornea and a reference point

exophthalmos—abnormal protrusion of the eyeballs

giantism—abnormal size of all or parts of the body

glucocorticoid—referring to any steroid-like compound capable of affecting metabolism, such as cortisol

glucosuria—urinary excretion of large quantities of glucose

glycosuria—glucosuria; urinary excretion of carbohydrates

goiter—enlargement of the thyroid gland, not caused by tumor

gonad—a male or female reproductive organ

gonadotropin—a hormone synthesized and released by the pituitary gland that stimulates the testes or ovaries (gonads) to produce sex hormones and either ova or sperm

hormone—a chemical substance produced in one part of the body and carried to another organ or tissues where it acts to modify structure or function

hyperadrenalism—overactivity of the adrenal gland

hyperglycemia—excess glucose in the bloodstream

hyperinsulinism—condition resulting from an excessive secretion of insulin by the islets of Langerhans

hyperosmolar nonketotic coma—an unconscious state in which blood glucose concentration is increased without the presence of ketone bodies in the plasma

hyperparathyroidism—overactivity of the parathyroid glands

hyperprolactinemia—elevated levels of prolactin hormone in the blood

hyperthyroidism—overactivity of the thyroid gland

hypoadrenalism—reduction of adrenocortical function

hypoaldosteronism—diminished secretion of aldosterone by the adrenal cortex

hypoglycemia—a deficiency of glucose in the bloodstream

hypophysis—the pituitary gland

hypopituitarism—subnormal activity of the pituitary gland, particularly the anterior lobe

hypothalamus—the region of the forebrain in the floor of the third ventricle, linked with the thalamus above and the pituitary gland below

hypothyroidism—subnormal activity of the thyroid gland

insulinemia—insulin in the circulating blood, usually abnormally large concentrations

insulinoma—an insulin-producing tumor of the beta cells in the islets of Langerhans of the pancreas

ketoacidosis—diabetic acidosis caused by increased production of ketone bodies

ketonuria—enhanced urinary excretion of ketone bodies

ketosis—elevated levels of ketone bodies in the body tissues

libido—the sexual drive

metabolic—referring to the changes occurring in body tissues

myxedema—hypothyroidism accompanied by a number of symptoms, including dryness and loss of hair, hoarseness, muscle weakness, and edema of subcutaneous tissue

orchitis—inflammation of the testes

panhypopituitarism—state in which secretion of all anterior pituitary hormones is inadequate or absent

parathyroid—pairs of small glands located near the thyroid concerned primarily with the metabolism of calcium and phosphorus

pheochromocytoma—a usually benign neoplasm derived from cells in the adrenal glands

pituitary—referring to the master endocrine gland, a pea-sized body attached beneath the hypothalamus at the base of the skull

prolactin—a hormone secreted by the pituitary gland that stimulates the secretion of milk

prostaglandins—a group of naturally occurring fatty acids present in a variety of tissues and body fluids

radioimmunoassay—the technique of using radioactive tracers to determine levels of specific antibodies in the blood

somatotropin—growth hormone; produced by the anterior pituitary gland

steroid—one of a group of compounds having a common structure that consists of three six-member carbon rings and one five-member carbon ring

struma ovarii—an ovarian tumor with a predominance of thyroid tissue, often associated with hyperthyroidism

thyroid—denoting the large endocrine gland situated in the base of the neck

thyroidectomy—surgical removal of the thyroid gland

thyroiditis—inflammation of the thyroid gland

thyrotoxicosis—the condition resulting from excessive amounts of thyroid hormone in the bloodstream

ultrasonography—use of high-frequency or ultrasonic waves to determine the location or measurement of deep structures within the body

virilism—the development of mature masculine characteristics in a female

CHAPTER 16

The Hematologic System and Its Disorders

The circulatory system is composed of the heart and vessels, which circulate blood, and the skeletal system consists of bone and its connective tissues. Yet these two are intimately related to the hematologic system, the system of the body that, largely within the bone marrow, forms the cells circulated in the blood. The hematologic system is responsible for the formation of red blood cells (RBC) that transport oxygen, white blood cells that protect the body from bacteria and other foreign invaders, and platelets involved in blood coagulation. In addition to bone marrow, the liver, spleen, and lymphatic system also produce hematologic constituents.

Anatomy and Physiology

Hematology is the study of the blood and its constituents. The term incorporates the combining form *hema-,* which means blood (as do the forms *hem-, hemo-,* and *hemat-*). Almost all the cells in the blood are red blood cells (RBCs) or **erythrocytes** (*erythro-* = red, and *-cyte* = cell). Normally numbering more than 5 million in each cubic millimeter in the male and slightly less in the female, red blood cells differ from all other cells in that they have no **nucleus;** thus, they can no longer multiply after entering the bloodstream. Erythrocytes consist of a thin cellular membrane and a thick solution of **hemoglobin,** in addition to small quantities of a number of other components. Some of these are proteins like **stromatin** and **elinin** or lipids like **lecithin** and **cholesterol;** the proteins and lipids make up the physical structure of the cell, including both the membrane and internal structures. Other components include enzymes and minerals involved in cell metabolism.

The primary role of red blood cells is to transport oxygen from the lungs to the tissues. The hemoglobin molecule contains an iron atom that loosely binds with the oxygen (O_2) absorbed from the lungs into the blood. When the erythrocyte reaches tissue cells that need O_2, the O_2 is released to the tissue.

The life of a red blood cell is about 120 days, during which time some metabolic processes continue to occur. Some of the enzymes in the **cytoplasm** release energy to maintain cell integrity, but eventually the erythrocyte becomes fragile and breaks as it passes through a capillary. The fragments of the cell structure are engulfed by **reticuloendothelial** cells lining the capillaries of some organs, primarily the liver and spleen. These digest the fragments and release the dissolved components into the circulation. The hemoglobin molecules soon diffuse through the capillary walls and are engulfed by tissue reticuloendothelial cells. Digestion of hemoglobin releases the breakdown products iron and **bilirubin**. The iron combines with a **globulin** to form **transferrin,** the form in which it is carried throughout the body for storage and reuse. In the liver, iron combines with **apoferritin** to form **ferritin,** conserving the iron for future use. The bilirubin is excreted through the liver into the bile.

Erythrocytes are formed in bone marrow, but erythrocyte production varies among different bones. Membranous bones such as vertebrae, ribs, ilia, and the sternum form more red blood cells than long bones. In the fetus, however, red blood cells are formed in the yolk sac, the liver, and the spleen as well as in bone marrow, although marrow assumes the full role by the time of birth.

Regulation of erythrocyte production is controlled by tissue oxygenation. Oxygen deficiency stimulates the production of **erythropoietin** by the kidneys and, to a lesser degree, the liver. Erythropoietin reaching the bone marrow then stimulates all stages of red cell production, but mainly the initial stage, the formation of **hemocytoblasts** from hemopoietic **stem cells.**

The process of erythrocyte production is termed **erythropoiesis,** which is a form of **hemopoiesis** (or **hematopoiesis**), which literally means "formation of blood" and refers to the production of any blood cells. In the process of erythropoiesis, hemocytoblasts (*hemo-* = blood; *cyto-* = cell; *-blast* = formative cell; therefore, "cells that form blood cells") develop in stages into erythrocytes. The second and third stages are **erythroblasts,** nucleated cells differing primarily in their color. The fourth stage is a **normoblast,** also called a "late normoblast" since the prior two stages are also referred to as "early" and "intermediate normoblasts." The nucleus of the normoblast then disintegrates and is absorbed. During this phase, the remaining endoplasmic reticulum is still evident in the cell as a network, or "reticulum." At this time, the cell is called a **reticulocyte,** the final stage before the reticulum disappears, leaving little more than a bag of hemoglobin called the erythrocyte. The mature erythrocyte then squeezes through the walls of the capillaries in the bone marrow and is borne away as part of the blood.

As erythrocytes are formed and released into the circulation, occasionally reticulocytes and, more rarely, normoblasts are also released if production is particularly rapid. Thus, the rapidity of red cell production can be estimated merely by counting the number of reticulocytes and normoblasts in the circulating blood.

Along with red blood cells, the bone marrow also produces **white blood cells** (WBCs), also called **leukocytes** (*leuko-* = white) because they lack hemoglobin and its red color. Some leukocytes, however, are formed in the lymphatic system rather than bone marrow. Leukocytes differ from erythrocytes in two major ways—they have a nucleus, and they serve mainly to defend the body from invading organisms and other substances. Leukocytes can be divided into three main types: **granulocytes, monocytes,** and **lymphocytes.** Granulocytes evolve from **myeloblasts** (*myelo-* = marrow) in the bone marrow, while lymphocytes and monocytes are formed in lymphatic tissue.

When they are stained with Romanovsky stains, granulocytes are seen to contain granules in their cytoplasm, which is the source of their name. Also called **myelocytes** because they develop from myeloblasts, granulocytes may also be further subdivided into **neutrophils, eosinophils,** and **basophils** on the basis of the color of the granules when stained. In fact, the names of these granulocytes are derived from the color of the stained granules or the chemical properties of the stains they accept; for example, eosinophils contain granules that stain orange-red and are named for the red acidic dye eosin, while basophils accept basic stains.

Neutrophils protect the body against acute invasion by bacteria and are the most numerous of the leukocytes. When bacteria cause tissue damage, the tissues release chemotactic substances, one of which is **leukotaxine** (*-taxis* = movement). These substances diffuse in all directions and create a concentration gradient. Chemotaxis, the noun form, indicates movement of cells toward areas of higher chemical concentration, and leukotaxine specifically attracts leukocytes such as neutrophils. Following the tissue injury, the chemotactic substances increase the porosity of nearby capillaries, and neutrophils adhere to the capillary walls in a process called **margination.** The neutrophils then literally squeeze through the capillary pores by **diapedesis** (*dia-* = through) into the interstitial spaces. Attracted by the chemotactic substances, neutrophils move through the tissues to the damaged area by ameboid motion. Projecting a finger-like extension called a **pseudopodium** (literally, "false foot") ahead of the main mass, the neutrophil then forces its cytoplasm to stream into the pseudopodium and move. Repeating the process over and over, the neutrophil moves to the damaged area. Because they change shapes during ameboid motion, neutrophils are also called **polymorphs** (literally meaning "many shapes") or **polymorphonucleocytes** ("nucleated cells with many shapes") and sometimes simply **polys.**

After reaching the damaged tissue, neutrophils ingest or **phagocytize** (literally, "eat the cell") foreign substances, especially bacteria, and, to a lesser extent, tissue debris. Enzymes within the neutrophils then digest bacterial proteins and other matter.

Eosinophils exhibit chemotaxis, phagocytosis, and ameboid motion as well, but they seem to respond to foreign proteins rather more than bacteria and are not effective scavengers. Basophils are also similar to neutrophils, but their function is probably related to the histamine and heparin that they contain.

Monocytes function in much the same manner as neutrophils, but they arise from the lymph nodes rather than bone marrow and do not contain granules. Monocytes initially are about the same size as neutrophils, but they move much more slowly in response to tissue damage. After they have been in the tissue for several hours, however, monocytes swell to become one of two other types of cells. The first is what are called **histiocytes** (*histio-* = tissue), which are fixed or inactive, or they may become **macrophages** (literally, "large eaters"), which are the mobile form of swollen monocyte. As macrophages, their ameboid motion increases dramatically, and they move quickly to the site of tissue damage. Macrophages are also excellent scavengers, phagocytizing many more bacterial cells and far more tissue debris than neutrophils. Monocytes, as macrophages, also contain lipases that can destroy the protective fatty shell of some bacteria. When a bacterial infection lasts more than a few days, the proportion of monocytes in the circulating blood increases until they may be even more numerous than neutrophils. Thus, neutrophils are the initial defense against bacterial invasion, but monocytes attack long-term, chronic infections. Monocytes also clean up the tissues after an infection has been eliminated.

Lymphocytes also arise from lymph tissue, but they have numerous functions. A large proportion of lymphocytes serve as part of the immune system discussed in Chapter 17. These lymphocytes, which can be "sensitized" to specific antigens, can be divided into two groups: the **thymic lymphocytes** (or simply **T-cells**) formed in the thymus and the **bursal lymphocytes** (or **B-cells**) formed in lymphoid tissue of the gastrointestinal tract and named for the "bursa of Fabricius," which is the source of these cells in birds. T-cells become sensitized to invading antigens and attack bacteria or viruses that present these antigens to the circulation. B-cells produce antibodies.

Besides these functions, lymphocytes also can become plasma cells, which produce antibodies responsible for immunity against toxins. They can also enter any tissue of the body and be converted into **fibroblasts.** Fibroblasts in turn secrete substances that become collagen fibers, elastic fibers, and other components of connective tissue. Finally, lymphocytes can enter bone marrow and become hemocytoblasts or myeloblasts.

All of these leukocytes together are produced at about the same rate as erythroblasts, but their proportion in the circulation is normally much lower. First, white blood cells are capable of leaving the circulation and entering tissues, unlike red blood cells. Secondly, with the exception of some lymphocytes, leukocytes are destroyed as they perform their defensive function and rarely exist in the circulation or tissues for longer than a few hours to a few days. Thus, the circulation usually contains about 500 erythrocytes for every leukocyte.

Platelets, also called **thrombocytes** (literally, "clot cells"), are also often considered to be white blood cells and are formed in the bone marrow. The marrow produces very large, fragile cells called **megakaryocytes.** When these are mature, they suddenly fragment into many minute parts that become the platelets. Platelets and several other factors within the blood and vessel walls are responsible for blood coagulation.

When a vessel is traumatized, the tissues at the broken edge release **thromboplastin,** a lipoprotein. Platelets also adhere to the torn edges of the vessel and each other in a process called **platelet aggregation.** The platelets then disintegrate and release **platelet factor 3,** a substance similar to thromboplastin. Thromboplastin and platelet factor 3 react with different protein factors and calcium ions to form **prothrombin activator,** which, in conjunction with calcium ions, enzymatically splits **prothrombin** into **thrombin.** Each of the coagulation factors has its own name, but they are usually referred to by an agreed-upon series of Roman numerals; e.g., factor II is prothrombin and factor VIII is **antihemophilic globulin.** Thrombin then serves as an enzyme to convert the soluble fibrinogen molecules in the circulation into insoluble **fibrin** threads. The fibrin then entraps red blood cells to form a clot, sealing the vessel. This process forms the extrinsic system of blood coagulation based on the release of **thromboplastin** and the intrinsic system based on the actions of platelet factor 3.

Different types of blood can be classified on the basis of cell membrane proteins that normally cause antibody reactions. Thus, blood may be grouped as type O, A, B, or AB. These four groups are based on the presence or absence in blood cells of the type A and type B proteins that may cause transfusion reactions. Called **agglutinogens** because they lead to agglutination (clumping) and **hemolysis** (rupture) of blood cells exposed to specific antibodies, these proteins react with agglutinins in the plasma to cause the cells to clump. Those people without a specific agglutinogen usually do have the complementary agglutinin in their plasma.

Similar to the four major blood groups, blood can be classified on the basis of **Rh factor,** also called **rhesus factor** for the rhesus monkey in which the grouping was first discovered. Rhesus factor is a group of antigens that is found on the surface of red blood cells in about 85% of all people. Those who possess the factor are called Rh positive; those whose red blood cells lack the antigens are Rh negative. When an Rh negative person is exposed to Rh positive blood, the individual will develop antibodies to the antigen; on subsequent exposures, the antigen/antibody reaction will cause agglutination.

Therapeutics

Diseases

Among the more common diseases of the hematologic system are the anemias. Derived from the prefix *a-* ("without") and the Greek word for blood (*haima,* the source of the combining form *hema-* and its derivatives), **anemia** is a relative lack of red blood cells or hemoglobin. Anemias may result from impaired production of erythrocytes or hemoglobin, premature destruction of erythrocytes, or excessive loss of blood. As a result, one or more of the quantitative measures of red blood cells such as RBC count, hemoglobin **(Hb)**, or **hematocrit (Hct)** may be below normal. RBC count is simply the number of erythrocytes in a cubic millimeter of blood. Hb is the concentration of hemoglobin in the blood, usually measured in grams per 100 ml of blood. Hct refers to the percentage of the blood consisting of red blood cells, obtained by packing the red cells with centrifugation and reported in milliliters of packed red cells per 100 ml of blood.

Acute posthemorrhagic anemia is caused by the rapid loss of a large amount of blood. Although the RBC count, hemoglobin, and hematocrit may be relatively high initially because of vasoconstriction, they usually drop within a few hours as fluid from the tissue enters the circulation and dilutes the blood. Because the change is rapid, the anemia is **normocytic** (cells are normal) and **normochromic** (normal amount of hemoglobin in the erythrocytes, resulting in normal color).

Chronic posthemorrhagic anemia, however, is **microcytic** and **hypochromic;** i.e., the RBCs are small and pale. A prolonged loss of blood causes the marrow to become hyperactive as it attempts to replace the loss rapidly. Additionally, the loss of blood causes a loss of iron since about two-thirds of the body's iron stores are in hemoglobin. The result is the release of cells that are smaller and less mature and that contain reduced amounts of hemoglobin. Chronic posthemorrhagic anemia may be caused by any prolonged excessive blood loss, including bleeding ulcers, bleeding hemorrhoids, or menometrorrhagia (excessive uterine bleeding).

Iron-deficiency anemia presents with the same cell morphology. Indeed, since chronic blood loss causes a loss of iron stores, chronic posthemorrhagic anemia actually is an iron-deficiency anemia. Whether the underlying cause is blood loss, decreased iron absorption, or inadequate dietary iron for an increased iron demand, the result is a hypochromic microcytic anemia. Symptoms of severe iron-deficiency anemia may include a craving for dirt or paint (a syndrome called **pica**) or ice **(pagophagia),** but diagnosis usually depends on a determination of plasma iron levels and the elimination of other causes.

Iron is not the only deficiency that causes anemia. Deficiency of vitamin B_{12} or folic acid can impair the production of erythrocytes, creating cells that grow slowly with many fewer divisions. The resulting cells are abnormally large **(macrocytic),** oddly shaped, and extremely fragile. **Macrocytic anemia** is often easily treated with supplementation of the deficient nutrient. One form of this condition is **pernicious anemia,** in which a deficiency of vitamin B_{12} is caused by an inability of the gastric mucosa to secrete **intrinsic factor,** a substance that facilitates B_{12} absorption. Pernicious anemia may result from atrophic gastritis, gastrectomy, or myxedema. Diagnosis may include evaluation of radioactive B_{12} absorption with and without exogenously administered intrinsic factor **(Schilling test).**

On rare occasions the bone marrow may completely stop producing erythrocytes, a condition called **aplastic anemia.** Aplastic anemia usually results from exposure of bone marrow to toxic chemicals, antineoplastic agents, or large doses of ionizing radiation, so the onset is rapid. The red blood cells already in circulation are normal (normochromic and normocytic), but the RBC count progressively diminishes since aging cells are no longer replaced. Concomitantly, leukocyte and thrombocyte production are also affected, so the patient exhibits **leukopenia** (decreased leukocyte count) and **thrombocytopenia.**

Healthy mature erythrocytes are quite flexible and shaped like a double concave disk.

Further, slightly abnormal RBCs are removed by the spleen, and more severely abnormal cells are destroyed by the liver. If the bone marrow produces erythrocytes that are abnormal, they are quickly removed by these two organs, resulting in anemia. Several such abnormalities occur. **Sickle cell anemia** occurs almost exclusively in Negroes and is characterized by sickle-shaped cells due to a homozygous inheritance trait. The sickled cells are unable to pass through capillaries, leading to thrombosis and infarction, and they are also more fragile, producing hemolysis. Similarly, **hereditary spherocytosis** (also called **chronic familial icterus**) is an inherited disease characterized by spheroidal red blood cells. These cells are hemolyzed by the spleen, which becomes enlarged. The splenomegaly results in even greater hemolysis, so the only treatment is **splenectomy,** the surgical excision of the spleen.

Polycythemia is an excess of red blood cells, and mild polycythemia is normal in those who exercise excessively or live at high altitudes. Polycythemia vera (*vera* = "true"), however, is a **myeloproliferative** (cancerous proliferation of bone marrow) disorder characterized by an increase in red blood cell mass (**erythrocytosis**) and hemoglobin concentration.

White blood cells may also increase or decrease in number. **Neutropenia** is a reduction in the number of neutrophils in the blood. It occurs in a wide variety of diseases, including certain hereditary defects, aplastic anemia, bone marrow tumors, and acute leukemias. **Granulocytopenia** is a more general term describing a reduction in the number of granulocytes (leukocytes), including neutrophils. **Agranulocytosis** applies to diminished or absent granulocyte production, essentially the same disorder. Whichever term applies, granulocytopenic conditions all result in increased susceptibility to bacterial infection and mucous membrane ulcerations, usually in relation to the degree of the deficiency.

Leukemia literally means an excess of white blood cells in the circulation, but it is an excess that is caused by cancer of the white cell–producing tissue. Leukemias are divided into myelocytic leukemias, which are cancers of the bone marrow, and lymphocytic leukemias, which are cancers of lymphoid tissues. Leukemias are discussed in Chapter 18.

Bleeding disorders also can arise from white blood cells. **Thrombocytopenia** is a reduction in the number of thrombocytes (platelets). Because platelets are necessary for coagulation, thrombocytopenia results in bleeding into the skin (**purpura**), spontaneous bruising, and prolonged bleeding after injury.

Another clotting factor frequently absent or deficient in the circulation, prothrombin, is formed by the liver and requires vitamin K as an intermediary in its production. A deficiency of vitamin K, liver disease, or a hereditary defect, therefore, can cause **hypoprothrombinemia,** resulting in increased bleeding.

Hemophilia is actually a group of diseases, each caused by a lack of a different coagulation factor. Each has slightly unique characteristics, but all involve a deficiency in the platelet-mediated clotting mechanism. The missing factors, however, are not necessary for the tissue thromboplastin mechanism for initiating blood clotting. So clotting occurs almost normally if the tissues are torn severely enough to form adequate thromboplastin. A simple rupture without much local tearing, however, causes bleeding that can last for hours.

Incompatibilities can occur with transfusions because of the four major blood groups. Since transfusion with the wrong blood type can result in agglutination and hemolysis, **cross-matching** of blood is essential. Besides typing for the correct blood group, the blood of the donor and recipient are both centrifuged to separate the plasma and the blood cells; then suspensions of cells and plasma are cross-mixed to see if agglutination occurs. If clumps of red cells are evident on microscopic examination, an antibody reaction has occurred and the bloods are mismatched.

Similar to mismatching, **erythroblastosis fetalis** is caused by an antibody reaction involving Rh factor. If an Rh positive father and Rh negative mother produce an Rh positive fetus, the Rh antigens in the fetal blood reach the maternal circulation. This causes the mother to develop Rh antibodies, which can cross the placental barrier and cause agglutination and hemolysis of the fetal blood. To offset this rapid destruction, the fetus produces red cells very quickly. Because of the speed of erythrocyte production, many early nucleated cells, including erythroblasts, are released into the circulation, giving the disease its name. Unable to match production to hemolysis, many infants with erythroblastosis fetalis are stillborn. Rare in the first Rh positive infant born to an Rh negative mother, it becomes more common with successive pregnancies. Treatment relies primarily on exchange transfusion. The condition usually can be avoided by administering anti-Rh gamma-globulin immediately after the birth to prevent the mother from becoming sensitized.

Several other common diseases and symptoms of the hematologic system are listed in Table 16.1; abbreviations are included in Table 16.2.

Diagnosis and Therapy

Both bone marrow and lymphatic tissue can be biopsied for evaluation of cell production, but the majority of diagnostic procedures applicable to the hematopoietic system take place in the laboratory. The primary tissue for evaluation is the blood itself.

The first tests usually performed are the **complete blood cell count (CBC)** and hematocrit (Hct). Hematocrit is determined by centrifuging blood in a graduated tube; the graduations allow measurement of the volume of the packed red cells as compared to the total volume. The CBC is actually a very rudimentary test, offering only a count of the total number of cells in a cubic milliliter of the blood.

Typically included with the CBC are the RBC count and hemoglobin (Hb). The RBC count tells the number of red blood cells in a cubic millimeter of blood and indicates the presence of anemia or polycythemia. Hemoglobin is essential in determining the cause of many anemias. For the RBC to remain constant, dying cells must be replaced by new cells released from the bone marrow. Reticulocytes are the immediate precursors of erythrocytes, so the **reticulocyte count** is an important gauge of marrow activity. Also included with a CBC are the red blood cell indices of **mean corpuscular volume (MCV), mean corpuscular hemoglobin (MCH),** and **mean corpuscular hemoglobin concentration (MCHC).** These measures can be derived from the RBC count, Hb, and Hct. MCV describes an anemia as microcytic, normocytic, or macrocytic. MCH and MCHC indicate whether or not the patient suffers from a hemoglobin deficiency or hypochromia. Examination of a peripheral blood smear is also essential in diagnosing many anemias since it can detect abnormal shapes and staining of corpuscles.

A CBC provides limited information; to be more meaningful, a CBC is usually completed "with differential" to differentiate variations in white cell production. The differential count separates the count for the leukocytes into the different types. Of the 7,500 white blood cells normally found in a cubic millimeter of blood, 62% are neutrophils, 30% are lymphocytes, 5% are monocytes, 2% are eosinophils, and 1% are baso-

---

Table 16.1—Common Diseases and Symptoms of the Hematologic System

Anemias:	idiopathic immune hemolytic anemia
	Fanconi syndrome
	megaloblastic anemia of infancy
	sideroblastic anemia
	thalassemia
Polycythemias:	polycythemia vera
	stress polycythemia (stress erythrocytosis)
Hemorrhagic Disorders:	allergic purpura
	disseminated intravascular coagulation (DIC)
	hereditary hemorrhagic telangiectasia
	idiopathic thrombocytopenic purpura
	Von Willebrand's disease (pseudohemophilia)

Table 16.2—Abbreviations Associated with the Hematologic System

ABMT	autologous bone marrow transplant		HBF	hepatic blood flow
ACD	anemia of chronic disease		Hct	hematocrit
AGG	agammaglobulinemia		HIT	heparin-induced thrombocytopenia
AHA	autoimmune hemolytic anemia		HTR	hemolytic transfusion reaction
AHF	antihemophilic factor		IH	indirect hemagglutination
AHG	antihemophilic globulin		ILLS	lazy leukocyte syndrome
AIHA	autoimmune hemolytic anemia		IMH	indirect microhemagglutination
ANC	absolute neutrophil count		MAHA	macroangiopathic hemolytic anemia
BM	bone marrow		MCH	mean corpuscular hemoglobin
BMA	bone marrow aspirate			
BMC	bone marrow cells		MCHC	mean corpuscular concentration
BMT	bone marrow transplant			
CBF	cerebral blood flow		MCV	mean corpuscular volume
CBFS	cerebral blood flow studies		MHA	microangiopathic hemolytic anemia
CBFV	cerebral blood flow velocity			
CBG	capillary blood glucose		MMA	monocyte monolayer assay
CDA	congenital dyserythropoietic anemia		MNC	mononuclear leukocytes
			NCF	neutrophilic chemotactic factor
CSBF	coronary sinus blood flow			
FEP	free erythrocyte protoporphyrin		NCNC	normochromic, normocytic
			PC	packed cells; platelet concentrate
HA	hemolytic anemia			
Hb	hemoglobin		PDGF	platelet-derived growth factor

PMB	polymorphonuclear basophils		**PTF**	plasma thromboplastin factor
POEMS	plasma cell dyscrasia with polyneuropathy, organomegaly, endocrinopathy, monoclonal (M)-protein, skin changes		**PV**	polycythemia vera
			RCV	red cell volume
			RE	reticuloendothelial
			RES	reticuloendothelial system
			RHE	recombinant human erythropoietin
POLY	polymorphonuclear leukocyte		**SRBC**	sickle/sheep red blood cells
PPF	plasma protein fraction		**TEC**	total eosinophil count
PRA	plasma renin angiotensin		**TCT**	thrombin clotting
PRAT	platelet radioactive antiglobulin test		**TGT**	thromboplastin generation test
PRBC	packed red blood cells		**WBC**	white blood cell/count
PRCA	pure red cell aplasia		**WC**	white count
PRV	polycythemia rubra vera			

phils. Changes in the differential can help diagnose the patient's condition. For example, neutrophils can rise to as high as 95% in severe acute infections, and monocytes can rise from 5% to as high as 40% in long-term chronic infections while the total number of white blood cells rises to 15,000 to 20,000 cells/mm^3.

When blood transfusions are needed, typing and cross-matching are mandatory. Additionally, donor blood is tested in several ways, including ABO and Rh typing, antibody screening, and tests for hepatitis B surface antigen and HIV-1 antibody.

Pronouncing Glossary

Root	Meaning	Example	Pronunciation
cyt	cell	granulocyte	GRAN u lo site
eryth-	red	erythrocyte	ee RITH ro site
hema-	blood	hemagogue	HE mah gog
hemat-		hematic	he MAT ik
hemo-		hemolysis	he MOL ee sis
hemangio-	blood vessel	hemangioma	he man gee OH mah
leuk-	white	leukemia	luk EE me ah
phleb-	vein	phlebolith	FLEB oh lith
plasma-	plasma	plasmacyte	PLAZ mah site
plasmo-		plasmocyte	PLAZ mo site
thrombo-	clot	thrombosis	throm BO sis

Glossary

agglutination—clumping together of suspended cells or particles
agglutinin—an antibody in serum that produces clumping of its antigen

agglutinogen—a substance that stimulates the production of agglutinin

agranulocytosis—a condition including decreased granulocyte count and lesions of the throat and other mucous membranes

anemia—general term for various disorders involving decrease in the number of red blood cells, hemoglobin, or packed red cells in the blood

basophil—a granular cell that stains readily with basic dyes

chemotaxis—response of cells to chemical stimuli

diapedesis—passage of blood cells through intact walls of the blood vessel

ecchymosis—a small hemorrhagic spot in the skin or mucous membrane

elinin—the part of red blood cells containing the A, B, and Rh factors

eosinophil—a type of white blood cell containing uniformly sized round granules

erythroblast—the cell from which the erythrocyte (RBC) develops

erythroblastosis—presence of erythroblasts in the circulating blood

erythrocyte—a mature red blood cell

erythropoiesis—the formation of red blood cells

erythropoietin—the hormone that stimulates red blood cell production

Fanconi syndrome—a hereditary type of anemia involving disorders of the blood, bone marrow and congenital anomalies

fibrin—a protein formed by thrombin, acts in the clotting of blood

fibrinogen—Factor I; the part of plasma that is converted to fibrin to produce coagulation of the blood

fibroblast—an immature cell found in connective tissue

granulocyte—a mature granular leukocyte

granulocytopenia—deficiency of granulocytes in the blood

hematocrit—the percentage of a blood sample composed of cells

hematology—the medical specialty pertaining to the blood and blood-forming tissues

hemocytoblast—a primitive blood cell

hemoglobin—the oxygen-carrying protein of red blood cells; laboratory test for its concentration in blood

hemolysis—destruction of red blood cells

hemolytic anemia—deficiency of red blood cells resulting from abnormal destruction in the body

hemophilia—inherited blood disorder involving a defect in coagulation

hemopoiesis—development of the blood cells

hypochromia—decrease in the percentage of hemoglobin in the red blood cells

hypoprothrombinemia—decrease in the amount of prothrombin (Factor II) in the circulating blood

leukocyte—white blood cell

leukopenia—less than normal number of white blood cells in the circulating blood

lymphocyte—white blood cell formed in lymph tissue

macrocytic—pertaining to a large erythrocyte

macrophage—one of the large mononuclear phagocytic cells

megaloblastic anemia—anemia in which there are a large number of megaloblasts, large nucleated embryonic cells

megakaryocyte—the large cell of bone marrow that produces blood platelets

monocyte—a mononuclear, phagocytic leukocyte

myelocyte—a young cell in the granulocytic series occurring normally in bone marrow

neutropenia—decrease in number of neutrophils in the blood

neutrophil—mature white blood cell in the granulocytic series

normoblast—a nucleated red blood cell, precursor of the erythrocyte

normochromia—normal color of erythrocytes

normocytic—pertaining to a red blood cell that is normal in size, shape, and color

phagocytosis—to engulf and destroy bacteria and foreign particles

plasma—the fluid or noncellular part of the circulating blood

platelet—thrombocyte; disk-shaped structure in the blood containing granules and protoplasm, but no nucleus

polycythemia—increase in the number of red cells in the blood

purpura, thrombocytopenic—disorder of extensive ecchymoses, hemorrhages from mucous membranes, anemia and decreased platelet count

reticulocyte—young red blood cell found during the process of blood rejuvenation

Romanovsky stain—laboratory procedure for blood smears involving a mixture of methylene blue and eosin

sideroblastic anemia—anemia characterized by the presence of sideroblasts, erythrocytes containing granules of ferratin

spherocytosis—presence of sphere-shaped red cells in the blood seen in familial hemolytic anemia

stromatin—an insoluble protein found in the framework of red blood cells

telangiectasia—dilation of the small blood vessels

thalassemia—an inherited disorder of hemoglobin metabolism

thrombin—an enzyme produced by the activation of prothrombin

thrombocyte—platelet

thrombocytopenia—abnormal decrease in the number of platelets in circulating blood

thromboplastin—a substance in blood and tissues that aids in coagulation

Von Willebrand's disease—a disorder characterized by bleeding from mucous membranes, prolonged bleeding time and platelet defects

CHAPTER 17

The Lymphatic/Immune System and Its Disorders

The lymphatic system forms a secondary fluid circulation system that works in conjunction with the bloodstream to maintain the proper fluid levels of tissues. As a circulatory system, the lymphatics contain a complex series of vessels throughout the body similar to the veins of the bloodstream; they also contain a pumping mechanism to move the fluid known as lymph, although the "pump" consists of several structures and mechanisms rather than a single unit like the heart. The lymphatic system, however, also serves significant immune functions. The lymph nodes located along the lymphatic vessels filter the lymph, passing it over reticuloendothelial cells, which quickly remove bacteria and particulate matter from the lymph before it is returned to the bloodstream. Lymph nodes also produce the white blood cells known as lymphocytes, which attack and destroy bacteria and other invaders in the body.

Anatomy and Physiology

The lymphatic system consists of a network of small, thin-walled vessels called **lymphatics** or **lymphoducts.** This system provides unidirectional fluid transport from the tissues of the body to the circulatory system at the **right lymph duct** or the **thoracic duct** (see Figure 17.1). The vessels of this system begin in nearly all tissue spaces with the minute dead-end structures called **initial lymphatics.** Also known as **lymphatic capillaries,** the initial lymphatics are intimately positioned between tissue cells and near the blood capillaries. Leading out of the tissue spaces and toward the center of the body, the initial lymphatics coalesce into progressively larger and larger lymphatic vessels, finally terminating in the neck at the lymph ducts. The lymphatics from the lower part of the body, the left arm, and the left side of the head come together at the thoracic duct, which empties at the junction of the left internal jugular and subclavian veins. The lymphatics from the right arm, right upper chest, and the right side of the head drain into the right lymphatic duct at the junction of the right internal jugular and subclavian veins.

The initial lymphatics are extremely permeable. Lymphatic capillary walls consist of a single layer of flat endothelial cells attached to the surrounding tissues with anchoring **ligaments,** which are thin filaments extending between surrounding cells and holding the lymphatic capillary in place. The endothelial cells slightly overlap, so the edge of one cell forms a flap over the adjacent cell, serving as a one-way valve into the initial lymphatic and increasing the vessel's porosity. The high permeability of the initial lymphatics allows interstitial fluid, particles, and protein molecules to flow into the vessel.

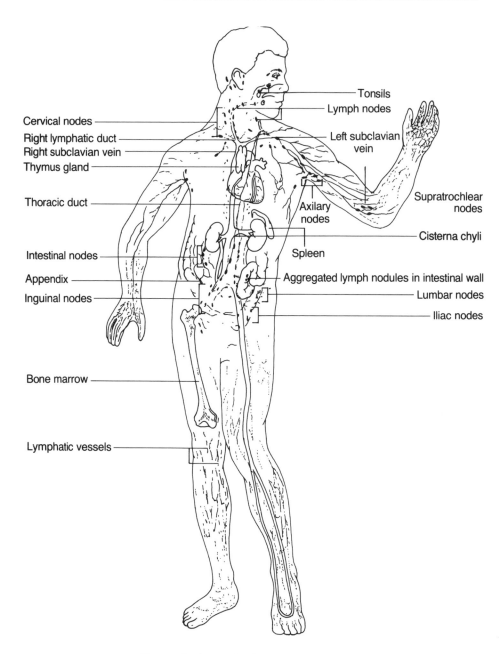

Figure 17.1——The Lymphatic System.

The fluid is essentially overflow from the interstitial spaces and has the same constituents. It is known as **lymph** from the Latin word *lympha,* meaning water. Along the course of the lymphatics, particularly where several smaller vessels join to form a larger one, the lymph passes through **lymph nodes** (also called **lymphaden**), organs whose function is to filter particles out of the lymph before it empties into the veins.

To move the lymph along its course, the system incorporates a pumping mechanism. All lymph vessels contain **lymphatic valves,** also known as **valvulae lymphatica** (singular: **valvula lymphaticum**). As a lymphatic vessel fills with lymph, it contracts in response to being stretched. The contraction forces the lymph past the lymphatic valve and into the next section of the vessel, and the valve closes from the back pressure as that new section begins to contract. Additionally, pressure is applied to the lymphatics by muscle movement, and even arterial pulsations during exercise compress the lymphatics, moving lymph along the channel. In the initial lymphatics, contraction or pressure causes the channels between overlapping endothelial cells to close, and the anchoring ligaments squeeze the lymphatic capillary as the surrounding cells move.

The single most important function of the lymphatics is to restore protein to the circulation after it leaks out of the capillaries. As protein molecules leave the circulation and enter interstitial spaces, the tissue osmotic pressure increases, drawing more fluid after the protein. Protein molecules readily enter the initial lymphatics, and the osmotic flow created by the large protein molecules increases the flow of lymph, draining the tissue. Thus, the lymphatic system picks up the large molecules that leak from the capillaries, carries them back to the central circulation, and drains the fluid, keeping the osmotic pressure of the tissue spaces below that of the blood.

Besides the protein molecules, other substances and particles must also be removed from the tissue. Large molecules such as tetanus toxin, particles that occur as debris from infectious and inflammatory processes, and cells such as bacteria cannot be absorbed by the capillaries, so they are removed by the lymphatics. As lymph passes through lymph nodes, it passes over a network of **reticuloendothelial cells,** which phagocytize foreign proteins. (Phagocytosis is discussed in Chapter 16.) Reticuloendothelial cells also contain **lipases** (enzymes that digest lipids) and other enzymes that destroy foreign cells and other substances.

The location of the lymphatics and lymph nodes plays an important role in protecting the body from microorganisms and other substances. For example, the **mesenteric lymphatics** spread through the tissue and near the blood vessels surrounding the small intestine, and the **mesocolic lymphatics** surround the large intestine. These in turn include concentrations of lymph nodes known as the **mesenteric lymph nodes** and the **mesocolic lymph nodes**. As bacteria and other particles are absorbed through the intestinal wall into surrounding tissues, they are immediately taken into the lymphatics and destroyed in the lymph nodes, preventing damage to the body. Similarly, other collections of lymph nodes protect other routes of entry into the body. As shown in Figure 17.1, the **inguinal lymph nodes** provide a defense against infections entering through the legs, the **axillary nodes** filter the lymph drained from the arms, and the **rectosacral nodes** remove gut flora entering through the rectum. Each of these lymph nodes, as are others throughout the body, is named for the area in which it is located or structures to which it is adjacent; inguinal nodes are in the inguinal notch of the groin, axillary nodes lie in the axilla (armpit), and rectosacral nodes are located near the rectum and sacrum.

Beyond filtering the lymph and phagocytizing foreign proteins and cells, the lymphatic system has two additional roles in protecting the body: producing the **lymphocytes** involved in both cellular and humoral immunity, and forming **monocytes** that scavenge the tissue debris and bacteria. Types of white blood cells (or **leukocytes,** as discussed in Chapter 16), lymphocytes, and monocytes are formed in lymphatic tissue and form important components of the body's immune system, the functional group of organs and tissues that provide immunity against a host of different agents.

Lymphocytes are chiefly formed in lymphoid tissue and can become "sensitized" to specific antigens. **Bursa-equivalent lymphocytes** (commonly called **B-lymphocytes, B-cells,** or **thymus-independent lymphocytes**) are formed primarily in lymphoid tissue of the gastrointestinal tract, although other sites also produce B-cells. Bursa-equivalent lymphocytes are named for the "bursa of Fabricius," the source of analogous cells in birds, although they are not formed in bursae in humans. When exposed to an **antigen,** B-lymphocytes become committed or **sensitized.** Antigens are primarily proteins, lipoprotein complexes, or polysaccharides and are found in toxins, bacterial cells, virus particles, or other foreign materials. They are said to be **immunogenic** ("causing immunity") since they produce an immune response. When a B-lymphocyte is sensitized, it divides many times and matures into a **plasma cell,** which produces **antibodies** that react with the specific antigen.

An antibody is an immunoglobulin molecule with a specific amino acid sequence to react with its specific antigen or closely related antigens. Antibodies are divided on the basis of their action when in contact with the antigen. **Agglutinins,** for example, cause **agglutination** or clumping of the cells with the appropriate surface antigen, and **bacteriolysins** cause bacteria to **lyse** or rupture so they are killed and their components can be removed from the body. **Opsonins** are antibodies that attach to a particulate antigen such as a bacterial cell or virion (virus particle) and make them susceptible to phagocytosis, a reaction that is essential in fighting infection by the many organisms resistant to ingestion by monocytes and neutrophils.

Opsonization is a multiphasic process. First, the antibody attaches to the antigenic determinant (chemical structure complementary to the antibody) on the bacterial surface. Then a succession of other chemicals called **complement proteins** attach to the antibody, quickly covering the surface of the bacterium with complement complex. Finally, the entire structure can be phagocytized and digested by neutrophils or monocytes.

Complement also causes the bacterial surface to become "sticky" and agglutinate (clump). Agglutination immobilizes the bacteria so they can be removed, generally by the lymphatic system. Complement complex also contains enzymes that can digest the cell wall of a bacterium, causing lysis and destroying the cell.

Each Y-shaped antibody or **immunoglobulin** is made up of two light peptide chains and two heavy chains. The arms of the Y form the **variable region,** which differs for each specific antibody; the variable region contains the **combining site (antigen-binding site)** specific for the antigens to which they attach and can be split chemically to yield the **Fab fragment (antigen-binding fragment).** There are five different kinds of heavy chains providing the classification of immunoglobulins: IgA (or gA), IgG, IgD, IgE, and IgM.

The base of the Y-shaped molecule is the **constant region,** which is fairly constant for each Ig class. Most of the constant region is found in the **Fc fragment (crystallizable fragment)** when the molecule is cleaved. After the plasma cell matures, it releases its antibodies into the circulation where they can neutralize, precipitate, opsonize, or otherwise react with antigens. Because antibodies are borne by the blood, they constitute what is called **humoral immunity,** immunity carried by the "humor" known as blood.

Thymic lymphocytes (also called **thymus-dependent lymphocytes** or **T-cells**) are so named because they are formed in the thymus, pass through it, or are influenced by it on their way to the tissue. T-lymphocytes are components of **cellular** or **cell-mediated immunity.** T-lymphocytes fall into two categories: **T-suppressor cells** inhibit the stimulation of antibody production and serve a regulatory function in immunity; **T-helper cells** (also called **CD4$^+$ cells** because of the CD4$^+$ receptor site on their surface) assist such stimulation. T-lymphocytes also can attach to and kill large antigenic cells such as cancer cells and transplant cells, so they are involved in the process of transplant rejection.

Monocytes arise from the lymph nodes, but they function much like neutrophils (as discussed in Chapter 16). Monocytes exhibit slow ameboid motion in response to the chemotactic substances released by tissue damage. After they have been in the tissue for several hours, however, monocytes swell to become either **histiocytes** (*histio-* = tissue), which are fixed or inactive, or **macrophages,** which are mobile. As macrophages, their ameboid motion increases dramatically, and they move quickly to the site of tissue damage. Macrophages are also excellent scavengers, phagocytizing bacterial cells and tissue debris. Monocytes, as macrophages, also contain lipases that can destroy the protective fatty shell of some bacteria. When a bacterial infection lasts more than a few days, the proportion of monocytes in the circulating blood increases until they may be even more numerous than neutrophils. So monocytes provide an important defense in long-term, chronic infections. Monocytes also clean up the tissues after an infection has been eliminated.

Other organs also contain significant amounts of lymphoid tissue, and their location helps protect the body from invaders. On each side of the throat is a mass of lymphoid tissue called a **palatine tonsil (tonsilla palatina** or simply **tonsil),** which acts as a source of phagocytes (phagocytic cells) to the mouth and pharynx to destroy bacteria. The spleen, located in the upper abdominal cavity, consists largely of lymphoid tissue and destroys red blood cells, serves as a reservoir of blood, and produces monocytes (known specifically as **splenocytes)** in the fetus and newborn. The thymus also produces monocytes and lymphocytes in the fetus and newborn, but the organ usually undergoes involution after early childhood.

Therapeutics

Diseases

If the lymphatic system fails to properly regulate the amount of fluid in the tissues, **edema** may result. Edema is characterized by swelling of the subcutaneous tissues caused by excess intercellular fluid. As the interstitial fluid pressure rises above the zero level, the cells spread apart, so any disorder that causes the pressure to rise will lead to edema. Heart failure, venous congestion, or arteriolar dilation will increase capillary pressure, forcing fluid into the interstitial spaces. Similarly, loss of plasma proteins through extensive burns or kidney disease decreases the osmotic pressure of the circulatory system, increasing the amount of fluid escaping to the tissue. Finally, blockage of the lymphatics decreases the drainage of the tissues, leading to edema. **Filariasis,** a South Sea Island disease in which lymph nodes become plugged with microorganisms known as filaria, can totally block nodes in certain areas. The result is the condition known as **elephantiasis,** in which one limb can expand enormously and eventually weigh as much as the rest of the body.

Much more common in the United States is an accumulation of white blood cells in the lymph nodes draining the intrapleural space, pericardial space, or other space. In such an instance, the resulting "edema" fills the space with fluid called **effusion.** If the effusion is abdominal, it is called **ascites.**

Inflammation of the lymphatic tissue also occurs because of accumulation of white blood cells and other debris in lymph nodes. **Tonsillitis** (inflammation of the tonsils), for example, is common in pharyngeal infections. **Splenitis** is an inflammation of the spleen, usually caused by **pyemia** (a septicemia with numerous abscesses or foci of infection, creating an accumulation of pus in the spleen).

Splenomegaly is enlargement of the spleen and is a symptom rather than a disease. The most common cause of splenomegaly is congestion. Many infectious processes, liver disease, and hematologic abnormalities can enlarge the spleen.

Since the lymphatic system is involved in immunity, infections are a common result of lymphatic disorders. When any part of the immune system is suppressed, as by drugs that cause leukopenia, any **lymphadenopathy** (disease of the lymph nodes), or **lymphangitis** (inflammation of the lymph vessels), the individual may become immunocompromised. Such immunosuppression may also be an intended or unavoidable result of drug therapy, as in the transplant patient who is on immunosuppressive therapy to reduce the risk of rejection or the cancer patient being treated with antineoplastic agents. These agents suppress the immune system because the immune cells are produced more rapidly than most others, making them more susceptible to the cytotoxic effects of these drugs.

In the **immunocompromised** host, normally nonpathogenic microorganisms may reproduce unabated. Further, those pathogens that are part of the normal flora but are held in check may produce serious infections. Immunocompromised patients commonly present with thrush, an oral candidiasis; vaginal yeast infections; staphylococcal infections of the skin; and numerous other infections.

Infection with **human immunodeficiency virus** (HIV) presents special problems. HIV is a retrovirus that preferentially attacks the T-helper lymphocytes, entering the host cell by attaching at the CD4$^+$ site. By reproducing within the T-lymphocytes, HIV kills the host cell and destroys the host's immune response. HIV infection may be asymptomatic, or it may progress to minor or severe immunodeficiency. The severe form is **acquired immune deficiency syndrome (AIDS),** from which fatality may result because of opportunistic infections. Among the more prominent of the HIV opportunistic infections are *Pneumocystis carinii* pneumonia, **Cytomegalovirus** pneumonia, candidiasis, toxoplasmosis, and **Herpesvirus** infections.

The objective of the immune system is to identify and remove foreign invasion. The body, however, is capable of developing antibodies and sensitized lymphocytes directed against components normally present in the individual. **Autoimmunity** (immunity to one's self) leads to a number of conditions, depending on the tissues to which the immune system reacts. For example, **systemic lupus erythematosus (SLE)** is a connective tissue disorder that presents with skin eruptions, arthralgia, leukopenia, and other symptoms. Autoimmunity is generally implicated by the presence of **hypergammaglobulinemia** (excess of gamma globulins). Other diseases with an autoimmune component include **rheumatoid arthritis** and **autoimmune thyroiditis.**

The most common disorders related to the immune system are those in which immunity itself becomes a problem for the individual, which is the case with **hypersensitivity,** an immune reaction that is exaggerated or unwanted. Often referred to simply as **allergy,** hypersensitivity reactions can occur to a wide range of **antigens.**

Hay fever is the common term associated with **pollenosis** (also spelled "pollinosis"), an allergic reaction to pollens and other airborne, naturally occurring antigens, which usually results in nasal and ocular symptoms. The **rhinitis** (literally, inflammation [*-itis*] of the nose [*rhin-*]) of hay fever occurs when the antigenic reaction occurs in the nose and nasopharynx, which is only during a specific season, depending on the blooming of the plant, use of heating systems, release of mold spores, or other event putting the antigen in the air. Thus, the symptoms are seasonal, and the disorder is called **seasonal allergic rhinitis.** When the antigenic reaction occurs in the eye, the patient develops **allergic conjunctivitis,** which is an inflammatory response in the conjunctiva of the eyelid to the **allergen.** If the antigen affecting the respiratory tract is present throughout the year, as occurs with allergy to dust, animal dander, some molds, and a variety of artificial environmental allergens, the patient may suffer from **chronic** or **perennial allergic rhinitis.**

Allergic reactions also develop outside the respiratory tract, often affecting the skin. **Contact dermatitis,** literally an inflammation (*-itis*) of the skin (*derma-*) caused by contact to an antigenic substance, is the most common skin disorder among humans and results from exposure to an enormous range of substances, including a number of drugs commonly applied to the skin. The most common symptom is **urticaria,** commonly called **hives,** although other types of skin eruptions do occur, including **vesicles, bullae, purpura, petechiae,** and **macules.**

Allergic reactions vary from the almost imperceptible to life threatening. The most severe is **anaphylaxis.** Anaphylactic reactions are systemic hypersensitivity responses to injected antigens, which can result in severe respiratory distress, unconsciousness, and death in a matter of minutes if untreated.

Several other diseases commonly affect the lymphatic and immune systems, including those listed in Table 17.1; abbreviations are listed in Table 17.2.

Diagnosis and Therapy

The most common diagnostic technique employed to evaluate the immune system is laboratory examination of the blood to determine the **complete blood count (CBC)** with **differential.** The differential establishes the percentage of each of the leukocytes in the blood, as described in Chapter 16. Advances made during the last fifteen years in response to the worldwide AIDS crisis have added several laboratory tests that are useful in evaluating immune status, including a T-lymphocyte count and the ratio of T-helpers to T-suppressors, both of which indicate cell-mediated immune function.

Immune reactions play a vital role in a number of diagnostic tests. Several infections, including HIV, hepatitis B, and **Cytomegalovirus (CMV),** are identified by detecting antibodies in the blood. The **complement fixation (CF)** test is used in the diagnosis of viral diseases by detecting specific antibodies in the patient's serum. The presence of antibodies is assumed to be indicative of infection, and **antibody titer** (concentration) indicates degree of response or whether the infection is active. Antibodies are detected with **immunofluorescence, enzyme-linked immunosorbent assay (ELISA),** agglutination tests, and **iontophoresis.** Without the immune response, there would be no antibodies to detect.

Immune activity is also demonstrated with a direct skin test of antigenic extracts. Used to diagnose **type I (immediate** or **IgE-mediated) hypersensitivity** reactions, direct skin tests involve application of extracts with a scratch or needle prick to break the skin.

Table 17.1—Common Disorders Involving the Lymphatic/Immune System

Hypersensitivity:	allergic conjunctivitis
	angioedema
	anaphylaxis
	asthma
	drug allergy
	eczema
	hay fever (pollinosis)
	perennial allergic rhinitis
	serum sickness
	urticaria (hives)
Immunodeficiencies:	chronic granulomatous disease
	DiGeorge syndrome (thymic hyperplasia)
	selective IgA deficiency
Autoimmunity:	pernicious anemia
	photosensitivity

Table 17.2—Abbreviations Associated with the Lymphatic/Immune System

ABL	allograft bound lymphocytes	**FEL**	familial erythrophagocytic lymphohistiocytosis
AHO	autoimmune hemolytic disease	**GIC**	general immunocompetence
AIDS	acquired immunodeficiency syndrome	**GLNH**	giant lymph node hyperplasia
AILD	angioimmunoblastic lymphadenopathy	**HIV**	human immunodeficiency virus
ALG	antilymphocyte globulin	**IAHA**	immune adherence hemagglutination
ARC	AIDS-related complex	**IMIG**	intramuscular immunoglobulin
ARV	AIDS-related virus	**IMN**	internal mammary (lymph) node
CDLE	chronic discoid lupus erythematosus	**IVIG**	intravenous immunoglobulin
CFIDS	chronic fatigue and immune dysfunction system	**LAF**	lymphocyte activating factor
		LAG	lymphangiogram
CIAED	collagen-induced autoimmune ear disease	**LAN**	lymphadenopathy
		LCT	lymphocytotoxicity
CIC	circulating immune complexes	**LED**	lupus erythematosus disseminatus
CIDS	cellular immunodeficiency syndrome	**LN**	lymph nodes
		LND	lymph node dissection
CMI	cell-mediated immunity	**LTT**	lymphocyte transformation test
CTL	cytotoxic T-lymphocytes		
DILE	drug-induced lupus erythematosus	**LYG**	lymphomatoid granulomatosis
DLE	discoid lupus erythematosus	**MALT**	mucosa-associated lymphoid tissue
ELISA	enzyme-linked immunosorbent assay	**MCA**	monoclonal antibodies
EMG	essential monoclonal gammopathy	**MCLNS**	mucocutaneous lymph node syndrome

MGUS	monoclonal gammopathies of undetermined significance	**PLN**	pelvic/popliteal lymph node
MIDD	monoclonal immunoglobulin deposition	**RPLND**	retroperitoneal lymphadenectomy
MLC	mixed lymphocyte culture	**SCID**	severe combined immunodeficiency syndrome
MLNS	mucocutaneous lymph node syndrome		
		SLE	systemic lupus erythematosus
PBL	peripheral blood lymphocyte		
PBMC	peripheral blood mononuclear cell	**TANI**	total axial node irradiation
		TLC	total lymphocyte count
PBMNC	peripheral blood mononuclear cell	**TLI**	total lymphocyte irradiation
		TNI	total nodal irradiation
PGL	persistent generalized lymphadenopathy	**VIG**	vaccina immune globulin
		WDL	well-differentiated lymphocyte

Antigens may also be injected intradermally. Development of a **wheal-and-flare** reaction shows a positive response and the presence of IgE-sensitized basophils and mast cells, which release histamine and other immunologically active substances.

Type IV (cell-mediated or **delayed) hypersensitivity** reactions are most frequently diagnosed with **patch tests.** To identify an antigen causing a dermatitis, suspected antigens are applied to the skin under an occlusive patch and left for 48 hours. Burning, itching, erythema, induration, and vesicle formation all indicate a positive reaction. The sites must be reinspected after 72 hours since the reaction may not be apparent when the patch is first removed.

Loss of immune function can also be detected with these same skin tests. The severely immunocompromised person may develop **anergy,** lack of response to antigens, even if the antibodies are present, because of suppressed cell-mediated response. Skin testing to detect anergy is used in evaluating immunosuppression in transplant recipients, AIDS patients, and others.

The inverse procedures are also used. **Monoclonal antibodies**, antibodies specific to one antigen, are produced by fusing mouse lymphoma cells and human lymphocytes. Those monoclonal antibodies can be used *in vitro* to agglutinate antigens in body fluids to detect the presence of certain foreign proteins and other chemicals or *in vivo* to transport other agents to antigenic tissue. The technique is currently used in drug testing as well as in the diagnosis and treatment of disease such as tumors.

The lymphatic system can be visualized by injecting radiopaque dyes into the lymphoducts and then taking roentgenograms of the individual. Roentgenographic visualization of the lymphoducts and lymph nodes is called **lymphography.** If the vessels are primarily visualized, the procedure is referred to as **lymphangiography. Lymphadenography** is visualization of the lymph nodes.

When the same procedures are used to image the spleen, it is called **splenography** and results in a **splenogram.**

Pronouncing Glossary

Root	Meaning	Example	Pronunciation
lieno-	spleen	lienopathy	leen AH path ee
lymph-	lymph	lymphadenopathy	LIMPF add in OP a thee
splen-	spleen	splenomegaly	splen o MEG ah lee

Glossary

agglutinin—an antibody that causes clumping of bacterial cells

agglutination—formation of suspended cells into clumps or masses

ascites—accumulation of serous fluid in the abdominal cavity

autoimmunity—condition of having an immune response against the body's own tissues

bacteriolysin—antibody that causes dissolution of bacterial cells

complement—protein found in normal serum that combines with a specific antibody to destroy bacteria

cytomegalovirus—a group of viruses having an affinity for the salivary glands, causing development of characteristic inclusions in the cell cytoplasm or nucleus

edema—abnormal accumulation of fluid in intercellular spaces of the body

filariasis—presence of parasitic worms in the body fluids or tissues, found in tropical and subtropical regions

histiocyte—a macrophage found in connective tissue

humoral immunity—acquired nonsusceptibility to disease primarily associated with circulating antibodies

immunity—resistance to disease

immunocompromised—deficiency in the immunologic mechanism due to disease, irradiation, or drugs

immunogenic—referring to the property of a substance to provoke an immune response

immunoglobulin—protein with antibody activity found in body tissues and fluids, classified in amounts present in normal serum as IgA, IgD, IgE, IgG, or IgM

iontophoresis—introduction of ions of a medication into the body by means of electric current

lymph—transparent, opalescent fluid in the lymphatic vessels that is collected from all body tissues and returned to the blood through the lymphatic system

lymph duct—channel for conducting lymph

lymph node—accumulation or masses of lymphoid cells along the course of lymphatic vessels

lymphadenopathy—disease of the lymph nodes

lymphangitis—inflammation of the lymph vessels

lymphatics—collective term for lymph nodes and lymph vessels

lymphocyte—a white blood cell formed in lymph tissue

macrophage—large mononuclear phagocytic cells that interact with lymphocytes to promote antibody production

monocyte—a large mononuclear white blood cell normally found in lymph nodes, bone marrow, and some connective tissue

phagocytic—referring to any cell that ingests microorganisms or other foreign particles

plasma cell—derived from lymphocytes and active in the formation of antibodies

reticuloendothelial—referring to the system of cells in different organs all primarily concerned with macrophagocytosis

spleen—the large vascular lymphatic organ that stores red corpuscles

splenitis—inflammation of the spleen

splenomegaly—enlargement of the spleen

thrush—infection of the oral mucous membranes with *Candida albicans*

thymus—the lymphoid organ in which T-lymphocytes are produced, necessary in early life for normal development of immunological function

tonsil—any collection of lymphoid tissue

tonsillitis—inflammation of a tonsil

valvula lymphaticum—one of the valves occurring at close intervals along the walls of lymph vessels

CHAPTER 18

Oncology

Oncology (*onco* = tumor, mass; *-ology* = study of) is the term that denotes the branch of medicine devoted to the study of tumors. Physicians specializing in this area of practice are **oncologists** or **hematologists** (those who treat disorders of the blood).

The term **cancer** denotes abnormal growth of cells that spread beyond the original site. These cancer cells differ from normal cells in that they lack the controlling device to stop reproducing after the typical number of cell divisions. Many of these cells die before becoming harmful. Those that survive, however, are strong, and they grow and spread so rapidly that they consume all available nutrients, essentially killing the normal cells by starvation. This abnormal growth of new tissue is called a **neoplasm** (*neo* = new; *plasma* = form). Neoplasms are classified as either **benign** or **malignant**. A **tumor** is the correct term for any abnormal mass or swelling.

Pathology

Benign neoplasms do not spread beyond the original site. Although they sometimes become malignant, detection and removal are usually not difficult and no complications result. A malignant tumor, in contrast, is cancerous; it has the ability to spread to other locations in the body by a process called metastasis (Figure 18.1). Malignant neoplasms grow rapidly in an uncontrollable and unorganized manner and are recognized by their many chromosomal changes as well as other changes, in the cells and tissues.

The three primary types of malignant neoplasms are usually classified by the type of body tissue from which they originate. **Carcinomas** (from the Greek for "cancer") arise in epithelial tissues that form the skin and linings of inner organs. These are the most common types of cancer, usually spread by the lymphatic system. Examples of carcinoma would be malignant melanoma of the skin, as well as neoplasms of the lungs, breasts, intestines, stomach, uterus, and mouth. **Sarcomas** (derived from the Greek term for "fleshy growth") originate in connective tissue and may be found anywhere in the body. They usually spread in the bloodstream. Osteosarcoma or osteogenic sarcoma of the bone, myeloma of the bone marrow (*myel-* = marrow, as well as spinal cord), and neoplasms of joint and cartilage are all examples of sarcomas. **Mixed tissue neoplasms** arise from tissue that can differentiate into either connective or epithelial tissue and therefore are composed of several types of cells. Table 18.1 lists a number of both benign and malignant neoplasms. Note that, except for the leukemias (blood disorders), all terms end with the suffix *-oma*, denoting tumor.

Cancers are caused most often by agents called **carcinogens** (literally, "cancer maker"), which disrupt the **homeostasis** ("same state," or tendency to stability) of

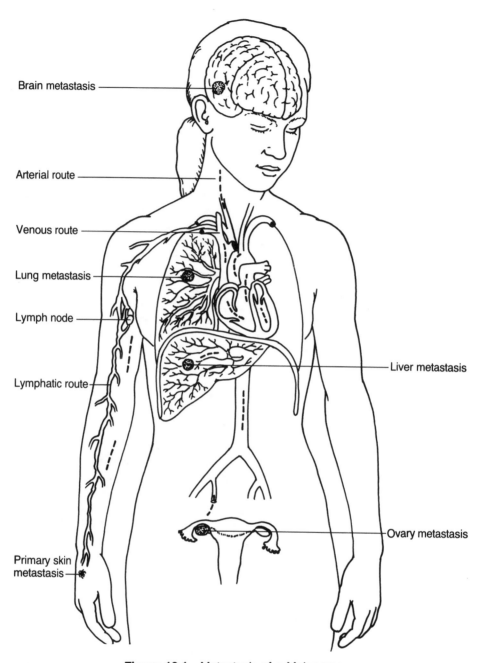

Figure 18.1—Metastasis of a Melanoma.
Cancer spreads when malignant cells break away from the primary neoplasm and
enter the circulatory system through the lymphatic vessels or the blood vessels.
Melanoma frequently spreads to the brain, lungs, liver, and ovaries.

Table 18.1—Terms Relating to Types of Neoplasms

adenocarcinoma	lipoma
adenoma	liposarcoma
adenosarcoma (Wilms' tumor)	lymphangioma
angioma	lymphangiosarcoma
angiosarcoma	lymphomas:
astrocytoma	Burkitt's lymphoma
basal cell carcinoma	diffuse histiocytic lymphoma
carcinoma	(DHL)
cholangiocarcinoma	diffuse lymphocytic lymphoma
chondroma	lymphogranuloma (Hodgkin's dis-
chondrosarcoma	ease)
choriocarcinoma	medulloblastoma
epithelioma	melanoma
fibroma	myeloma
fibrosarcoma	myoma
glioblastoma	neuroblastoma
glioma	neurolymphoma
hemangioendothelioma	oat cell carcinoma
hemangioma	osteoma
hepatoblastoma	retinoblastoma
hepatocarcinoma	rhabdomyosarcoma
hepatoma (hepatocellular carci-	sarcomas:
noma)	Ewing's sarcoma
hypernephroma (renal cell carci-	osteogenic sarcoma (osteosarcoma)
noma)	seminoma
insulinoma	small cell lung cancer
leiomyosarcoma	squamous cell carcinoma
leukemias:	teratoma
acute lymphocytic/lymphoblastic	
leukemia (ALL)	
acute myelocytic leukemia (AML)	
acute nonlymphocytic leukemia	
(ANLL)	
chronic lymphocytic leukemia	
(CLL)	
chronic myelogenous leukemia	
(CML)	

normal cells. The three main types of carcinogens are chemicals, radiation, and viruses. The chemicals include arsenic, asbestos, benzene, benzidine, hydrocarbons (tobacco smoke), synthetic estrogens, and vinyl chloride. Types of radiation are ultraviolet rays, X rays, and radioactive substances. Diet has also been associated with cancer, especially of the colon. A newer development in the study of cancer includes the discovery of **oncogenes,** or ''cancer genes,'' which are present and active in all cells only during the

Table 18.2—Staging Classification for Tumors (TNM)

T:	Primary tumor (T)	N:	Regional lymph nodes (N)
T_0:	No evidence of tumor	N_0:	No metastasis to regional lymph nodes
T_1:	Mass less than 3 cm in diameter, no evidence of invasion	N_1:	Metastasis to regional lymph nodes
T_2:	Mass greater than 3 cm in diameter, no evidence of invasion	N_{2-4}:	Metastasis to distant lymph nodes
T_3:	Mass greater than 3 cm in diameter, invasion into adjacent tissue	N_x:	Lymph nodes not assessed
		M:	Distant Metastasis (M)
T_4:	Tumor of any size with direct extension to chest wall or skin	M_0:	No distant metastasis
		M_{1-3}:	Evident metastasis
T_x:	Tumor not assessed		

early stages of development. Reactivation of these genes by an abnormal process causes the growth of cancerous cells through several mechanisms.

Symptoms

A number of general symptoms are associated with the oncologic disorders. **Anemia** is present in over half of patients with disseminated cancer and may be the first symptom of malignant disease. **Hemorrhage** occurs as a result of tumor invasion of blood vessels, causing intravascular coagulation and thrombocytopenia. **Fever** occurs in many patients with cancer, usually due to infections. Malnutrition, or the **cachexia** of malignancy, is often the most debilitating aspect, resulting from a combination of anorexia, loss of adipose tissue and protein stores, and abnormal glucose tolerance effects. Other manifestations may include neurological disorders, effusions, obstruction of the superior vena cava, hypercalcemia, and psychological effects. Most patients experience pain.

Diagnosis

Cancer is more likely to occur in areas of the body where cell division is frequent and rapid, such as in the lining of the digestive and respiratory tracts. Cancers in males are most often found in the lungs, prostate, colon, and rectum. In females, cancer occurs most frequently in the breasts, colon, rectum, uterus, and lungs.

A number of diagnostic procedures are utilized to determine if a symptom is cancer related. These usually include physical examination, chest X ray, blood chemistry studies and biopsies in addition to specific testing. **X rays, computerized tomography** (CT), **nuclear scanning techniques,** and **magnetic resonance imaging** (MRI) are used in radiographic diagnosis and later to assess response and toxicity of therapy. These parameters are also used to stage the disease and grade the tumor. Staging by **TNM** (tumor, lymph node status, metastasis) classifies tumor aggressiveness, spread, sites of metastases, and prognosis (see Table 18.2). Positron-emission tomography (**PET** scan) measures glucose-fluorodeoxyglucose (FDG) metabolism to monitor tumor growth. Structural changes can be detected by MRI or CT. PET is used to distinguish new growth from necrotic tissue after therapy.

Most recent research indicates that cancer is closely related to lifestyle. Preventive measures are effective in identifying risk factors and detecting early warning signs.

Treatment

The human body's immune system contains **T-cells** that continuously monitor the body for cancer cells and destroy most of them before they can multiply and spread. This internal mechanism sometimes fails, and external treatments are therefore necessary. Conventional treatment is primarily in the form of surgery, radiation therapy, and drug therapy, often referred to as **chemotherapy.**

Surgery is very effective for removal of benign tumors and is used as the primary treatment in most early cancers. Surgery may also be performed solely for staging purposes; for example, laparotomy (incision into the abdominal cavity) is useful in evaluating lymphomas. Malignant neoplasms cannot be entirely removed if the cells of the neoplasm have spread, so the degree of spreading can profoundly affect the extent or even advisability of surgical excision. Because of the chance of spreading, adjacent tissue and lymph nodes are usually included in a surgical procedure to remove a malignant neoplasm. Use of the laser has improved this approach. Tumors of the breast, colon, rectum, stomach, lung, thyroid, uterus, and prostate are primarily treated by surgery. Terms commonly associated with surgical treatment include excisions with the suffix-*ectomy* denoting removal (e.g., mastectomy = breast, hysterectomy = uterus); **cryosurgery,** freezing and removal of malignant tissue; **electrocauterization**, destruction of malignant tissue by burning; **fulgeration,** destruction of tissue by using a high-frequency current to generate electric sparks; and **exenteration,** removal of the tumor, organ, and surrounding tissue in that area of the body.

Radiation therapy involves the use of X rays or rays from radioactive substances **(cobalt, radium)** to destroy cancer cells in a specific location. Doses of radiation are expressed in units called **rads.** Equipment such as the **cyclotron, supervoltage X-ray** machine, and **linear accelerator** allow for deeper penetration and less harm to healthy tissue than with previous approaches. This form of treatment is used most often on cancer of the bladder, cervix, skin, testes, and parts of the head and neck as well as on lymphomas. **Fractionation** refers to the process of giving radiation in small repetitive doses. Tumors may be referred to as **radiocurable** (complete eradication), **radiosensitive** (destruction of tumor cells without significant damage to surrounding tissues), or **radioresistant** (requiring large amounts of radiation that may damage surrounding cells). **Radiosensitizers** are drugs that increase the sensitivity of tumors to the effects of radiation.

Radiation implant treatment—placing a small amount of radioactive material either directly into a cancer cell or in the affected area of the body—allows for use of higher doses. It also has the benefit of sparing most of the surrounding healthy tissue. **Bone marrow transplantation** (BMT) is another treatment approach that allows for delivery of higher doses of chemotherapy and/or radiation. The two primary types are **allogenic** (bone marrow from donor) and **autologous** (patient's own bone marrow). Peripheral blood stem cells (PBSCs) are also used in this procedure.

Palliative radiation has several applications in the treatment of metastatic cancer. Acute toxic effects of radiation are nausea, vomiting, fatigue, erosion of the gastrointestinal mucosa, bone marrow suppression, weight loss, and possible skin reactions. Chronic toxicity is associated with fibrous dysplasia and sterility. Radiation is known to be carcinogenic, particularly when used in combination with drug treatment.

Chemotherapy has become increasingly effective in treating cancer, especially **leukemia** and **lymphoma.** It is used in advanced stages of many cancers, often as an adjunct to surgery and/or radiation therapy. A number of metastatic cancers are now considered curable by chemotherapeutic regimens. The approximately fifty drugs that have been used to destroy or retard the growth of cancer cells are categorized as

- alkylating agents, which prevent cell division by disrupting DNA
- alkaloids
- antimetabolites, agents that impair cell metabolism
- antitumor antibiotics that disrupt synthesis of RNA
- endocrine or hormonal agents
- immunologic stimulants

These drugs are classed as **antineoplastics** and are often referred to as **cytotoxic** agents since their use in cancer treatment is to destroy the abnormal cells. Hormonal therapy is employed to treat tumors that arise from hormonally mediated tissues such as the breast, prostate, and endometrium. Chemotherapeutic regimens of multiple agents are often used and are commonly referred to by abbreviations listed in Table 18.3 A number of adverse effects on various parts of the body are associated with the use of these antineoplastic drugs. Some of the terms frequently associated with these adverse effects are listed in Table 18.4

Pain management is also a significant component of the treatment of cancer patients since chronic pain occurs in approximately one-third of patients with metastatic disease, especially when the bones or nerves are involved. Selection of **analgesics** is based on consideration of the severity of pain.

An area of increasing interest and activity in cancer treatment involves the use of **monoclonal antibodies** (see Figure 18.2). The term *monoclonal* is comprised of the prefix *mono-*, denoting one and the adjective *clonal,* which refers to a clone, a cell identical to the one from which it was formed. Monoclonal antibodies are produced by a process involving injection of cancerous tissue from a patient into a laboratory mouse. The resultant antibody-producing lymphocytes are then mixed with malignant white blood cells from another mouse. These produce a hybrid cell called a **hybridoma** that begins to divide repeatedly and form **clones.** The clone cells are tested for the desired antibody to obtain those suitable for use in treatment. This method permits production of large amounts of antibodies to the specific type of cancer. They have been useful in treating colorectal cancer, leukemias, melanoma, breast cancer, and others. If cytotoxic drugs are attached to the antibodies, the agents can be administered to a patient with little or no adverse effect on normal tissue; the antibodies attach directly to the cancer cells, isolating the cytotoxic drug to the site where it is needed. Other uses for monoclonal antibodies in oncology include diagnosis of tumors by detecting antigen in serum, tumor localization by using labelled antibodies, monitoring therapeutic and intrinsic agents by detection in serum, and monitoring immune and hematopoietic (blood cell formation) status of cancer patients by assay of number and proportions of different cell types.

Some forms of cancer are genetically transmitted because of inherited or acquired abnormalities in the suppression of genes that control growth and differentiation. **Cyto-**

Table 18.3—Abbreviations Associated with Chemotherapeutic Regimens

Abbreviation	Drugs	Location/Disorder
ABVD	Adriamycin, bleomycin, vinblastine, dacarbazine	Hodgkin's
ACE	Adriamycin, cyclophosphamide, etoposide	lung
BEP	bleomycin, etoposide, cisplatin	testicular
CAE	cyclophosphamide, etoposide, Adriamycin	lung
CAF	cyclophosphamide, Adriamycin, fluorouracil	breast
CHOP	cyclophosphamide, hydroxydaunorubicin,	non-Hodgkin's
	Oncovin, prednisone	lymphoma
CMF	cyclophosphamide, methotrexate, fluorouracil	breast
CMFVP	cyclophosphamide, methotrexate, fluorouracil, vincristine, prednisone	breast
CP	cyclophosphamide, cisplatin	ovarian
DDP	cisplatin	pancreas, lung, head, neck
EAP	etoposide, A(doxorubicin), cisplatin	gastric
EVA	etoposide, vinblastine, Adriamycin	non-Hodgkin's lymphoma
5-FU	fluorouracil	colorectal, gastric, esophagus
FAM	fluorouracil, Adriamycin, mitomycin	gastric, pancreatic
FCBM	fluorouracil, cisplatin, bleomycin, mitomycin	esophagus
H-CAP	hexamethylmelamine, cyclophosphamide, Adriamycin, cisplatin	ovary
HEXA-CAF	hexamethylmelamine	ovary
M-BACOD	melphalan, bleomycin, Adriamycin, cyclophosphamide, O(vincristine), dexamethasone	non-Hodgkin's lymphoma
MP+IFN	melphalan, interferon, prednisone	multiple myeloma
M-VAC	methotrexate, vinblastine, Adriamycin, cisplatin	bladder
MACOP-B	mitomycin, Adriamycin, cyclophosphamide, Oncovin, prednisone, bleomycin	non-Hodgkin's lymphoma
MOPP	mechlorethamine, Oncovin, prednisone, procarbazine	Hodgkin's
MP	melphalan, prednisone	multiple myeloma
MVP	mitomycin, vincristine, cisplatin	lung
PACE	cisplatin, Adriamycin, cyclophosphamide, etoposide	lung
PVB	cisplatin, vinblastine, bleomycin	testicular
VAD	vinblastine, Adriamycin, dexamethasone	multiple myeloma
VIP	vinblastine, ifosfamide, cisplatin	testicular

Table 18.4—Terms Associated with Antineoplastic Adverse Effects

Bone marrow:	anemia leukopenia myelosuppression neutropenia thrombocytopenia	CNS:	ataxia autonomic neuropathy encephalopathy neurotoxicity palsy paresthesia
Heart:	cardiomyopathy congestive heart failure dysrhythmia		somnolence
		Reproductive:	sterility teratogenic effects
Lung:	dyspnea fibrosis infiltrates pneumonitis rales tachypnea	Skin:	alopecia extravasation hyperpigmentation local reactions nail changes
Kidney/ bladder:	hematuria hemorrhagic cystitis nephrotoxicity tubular necrosis/ degeneration	Gastrointestinal:	esophagitis lower bowel distur- bances mucositis nausea & vomiting stomatitis
Liver:	hepatotoxicity		xerostomia
Hematologic:	cytopenia	Other:	erythema (local tissue necrosis) hypersensitivity reac- tions vesication

genics is a relatively recent term that reflects the use of genetic information to help classify patients as to risks of treatment failure and to assist in determining treatment regimens.

A number of terms are used in relation to treatment. **S phase** (DNA synthesis phase), **M phase** (mitosis), G_1 (Gap 1—periods of RNA and protein synthesis), G_2 (Gap 2), and G_0 (resting phase) refer to stages of the cell cycle. **Recruitment, growth fraction, synchronization, irradiation, induction therapy, consolidation therapy,** and **maintenance therapy** are terms often encountered in discussion of cancer treatment. Recruitment indicates the use of agents with an effect on cells in the cell cycle and in the Go or resting phase. Growth fraction is that portion of cancer cells that are actively dividing, often the cells that are the direct target of the treatment. Synchronization refers to the use of two anticancer drugs in sequence to achieve maximum efficacy. Induction therapy is the use of drug treatment during periods of remission; consolidation therapy is a period of intensive therapy after complete remission; and maintenance therapy (also known as con-

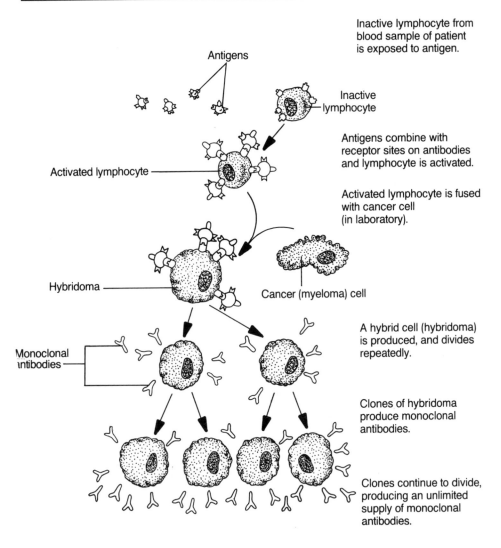

Antigens

Inactive lymphocyte from blood sample of patient is exposed to antigen.

Inactive lymphocyte

Activated lymphocyte

Antigens combine with receptor sites on antibodies and lymphocyte is activated.

Activated lymphocyte is fused with cancer cell (in laboratory).

Hybridoma

Cancer (myeloma) cell

A hybrid cell (hybridoma) is produced, and divides repeatedly.

Monoclonal antibodies

Clones of hybridoma produce monoclonal antibodies.

Clones continue to divide, producing an unlimited supply of monoclonal antibodies.

Figure 18.2—Monoclonal Antibodies.
The mechanism for the production of monoclonal antibodies.

tinuation therapy) is an empiric approach to balance the risk of treatment or relapse with the eradication of remaining cancer cells. **Eradication, palliation,** and **remission** refer to the effects or goals of treatment.

Alternative treatments utilize physiological and psychological therapies to strengthen the immune system. **Antineoplastin** therapy is based on the theory that the body has a parallel biochemical defense system (BDS) that is independent of the immune system and can help reprogram defective cancer cells to begin normal functions. These polypeptides are given in synthetic form in treatment of lymphoma, leukemia, and several other types of cancers. **Botanical** medications utilized successfully include shiitake and maitake mushrooms (to stimulate immune function), shark cartilage (an anti-angiogenic that inhibits blood supply in tumors), shark liver oil (to generate antibody response), and hydrazine sulfate (to treat cachexia). Nutritional and vitamin therapies, emotional and sociological support, visualization, and biopsychosocial programs (e.g., Block's) are also utilized, as is traditional Chinese medicine in the form of acupuncture, herbs, meditation, and exercise therapies.

Specific Oncologic Disorders

Blood

The **leukemias** are neoplastic disorders of the blood-forming cells of the bone marrow that result in the growth and accumulation of immature and defective blood cells in the marrow and bloodstream. The term *leukemia,* like most neoplastic disorders, is less intimidating if analyzed by its word parts: *leuk-,* meaning "white," plus the suffix *-emia,* meaning "blood," to denote a disorder of the white blood cells. **Leukocytes** (*leuk-* again, plus *cyt,* meaning cell) are the cells usually involved; however, there are several different forms of the disease. Leukemias are classed as acute or chronic, referring to the survival time. Acute leukemias are generally divided into **acute lymphocytic** (lymph cell) **leukemia (ALL)** and **acute nonlymphocytic leukemia (ANLL).** The latter group can also affect other cell lines and be further described as **myelocytic** (*myel* = bone marrow; *cyt* = cell), **monocytic** (*mono* = one), **promyelocytic** or **erythrocytic** (*erythr* = red).

Both immunologic and biochemical markers are used to identify subtypes of leukemia cells. **Immunologic** refers to the surface immunoglobulin (**SIg**) located on the cell membrane of malignant leukocytes or to their cytoplastic immunoglobulins (**CIg**). These markers change with cell differentiation and can be used to determine the degree and type of cell involved. **Biochemical** markers refer to altered concentration of enzymes such as terminal deoxynucleotidyltransferase (**TdT**), which may be found in various forms of leukemia. Other diagnostic parameters include possible **myeloperoxidase** and **Sudan black stain** in ANLL and possible periodic acid-Schiff (**PAS**) reaction in ALL. In most cases, the cause of leukemia cannot be determined. Studies are being done on isolation of the human T-cell lymphotropic virus (**HTLV**) from human lymphomas.

The primary approach to treatment of acute leukemias is combination drug therapy. **Bone marrow transplantation** is becoming increasingly utilized for treatment of both ALL and ANLL. The procedure requires total body irradiation, often with high-dose drug therapy to destroy residual leukemia cells and produce irreversible bone marrow suppression. The bone marrow for transplant is obtained from a human lymphocyte antigen (HLA)-matched donor (**allogenetic**), an identical twin (**syngenetic**), or from the patient in remission (autologous). Complications include failure to engraft, infection from immunosuppression, and graft-versus-host disease (**GVHD**). Plasma cell disorders (PCD) involve production of excessive amounts of an immunoglobulin, such as in multiple myeloma.

Lymph

Lymphomas (*lymph,* referring to the lymphatic system, plus the suffix *-oma,* tumor) are malignant disorders that originate in lymphoreticular cells and spread through lymphatics or the bloodstream to other lymph nodes and organ systems. Malignant lymphomas are classified as either **Hodgkin's disease** or one of several non-Hodgkin's lymphomas **(NHLs).**

The etiology of malignant lymphoma is uncertain; however, there seems to be an association with the Epstein-Barr virus **(EBV).** Patients with primary immunodeficiency disease, acquired immunodeficiency syndrome (AIDS), and those on immunosuppressive therapy are at risk of developing lymphoma. Terms associated with the pathology include **Reed-Sternberg (R-S) cells; Rye classification** (histology); **Rappaport system** (categorization of morphology, cell type, differentiation); and large-cell, small-cell **lymphoblastic.**

Lymphadenopathy (*aden-,* gland, plus **pathy,** disease) is a symptom present in the majority of patients. Treatment primarily involves radiation therapy and the use of chemotherapeutic agents. Other terms associated with diagnosis and treatment of lymphomas include **lymphography** and **splenectomy** (surgical removal of the spleen).

Breast

Carcinoma of the breast originates in the epithelial tissues that are the ductal or lobular components. The tumors are characterized as **infiltrating** (invasive) or **noninfiltrating** (noninvasive). Staging classification for breast cancer is by the **TNM** method, with specific application for this type of neoplasm.

Diagnosis is encouraged by breast self-examination **(BSE). Mammography** is used to locate tumors and to distinguish between benign and malignant masses, although it does not provide definitive diagnosis by itself. Liquid crystal **thermography** is a procedure that detects masses based on their heat-producing ability. **Ultrasound** is also being used increasingly as a noninvasive procedure to distinguish solid masses from cystic masses. **Immunologic** tests are used to identify antigens that are specifically associated with breast cancer.

Surgical treatment options for excision of breast cancer include **mastectomy (radical, extensive radical, modified radical, simple [total], or subcutaneous),** and **lumpectomy (tylectomy). Oophorectomy** (removal of the ovaries) is another surgical procedure sometimes used to reduce the level of endogenous ovarian hormones and temporarily regress hormone-dependent tumors. **Adrenalectomy** and **hypophysectomy** (excision of the adrenal and pituitary glands, respectively) are also utilized to decrease hormone secretions. Radiation therapy has been used for all types of breast cancer as primary, adjuvant, and palliative treatment. A number of chemotherapeutic agents are used successfully in treatment, particularly in multidrug regimens. Hormonal manipulation has also been a significant addition to treatment options. Use is determined by the presence of **estrogen receptor protein (ERP)** in the tumor tissue.

Lung

Lung cancers are classed as **small cell carcinoma** (SCLC) or the non-small cell carcinomas (NSCLC), which include **squamous cell (epidermoid) carcinoma, adenocarcinoma,** and **large cell carcinoma.** Staging by **TNM** is designated after use of chest X-ray, fiberoptic **bronchoscopy,** computed tomography, and routine laboratory tests to identify any metastases. In early stages of NSCLC, surgery is the treatment of choice. Radiation is used as an adjunct and for nonsurgical candidates. Combination chemotherapy regimens are also being used increasingly for NSCLC and as the standard treatment for both limited and extensive SCLC.

Gastrointestinal

The most common types of neoplasms found in the gastrointestinal tract are **squamous cell carcinoma** of the esophagus, **adenocarcinoma** of the stomach, and colorectal adenocarcinoma. Terms associated with diagnosis include **dysphagia,** stool **guaiac,** carcinoembryonic antigen (CEA) assay, biopsy/brush **cytology, proctoscopy, endoscopy, colonoscopy,** barium enema, and **sigmoidoscopy.** Surgery is the primary approach to treatment for all types of gastrointestinal neoplasms and may involve procedures such as esophagectomy, gastrectomy, or hemicolectomy. Radiation and chemotherapy are used as adjunctive treatment, particularly for metastatic involvement, although results are not encouraging. Early detection has been the primary factor in decreasing mortality from these neoplasms.

One of the most common sites for both primary and metastatic tumors is the liver. Primary tumors of the benign type include **cavernous hemangioma** (*hem-,* meaning "blood"; *angi-,* meaning "vessel"; plus *-oma,* "tumor"), **focal nodular hyperplasia,** hepatic cell **adenoma** (*aden-,* "gland"), and infantile **hemangioendothelioma** (*endothel-,* arising from linings of the blood vessel). The most prevalent malignant tumor of the liver is hepatocellular (*hepato-,* "liver") carcinoma (**HCC**). In children it is a hepatoblastoma. Others occurring less frequently are intrahepatic **cholangiocarcinoma, angiosarcoma,** epithelioid **hemangioendothelioma,** and undifferentiated **sarcoma.**

HCC is associated with exposure to the hepatitis B virus; many cases have preexisting cirrhosis. Terms encountered in diagnosis include **hepatomegaly, alpha-fetoprotein (AFP)** level, **arteriography,** radionuclide **liver-spleen scanning, ultrasound,** computer **tomography,** and **magnetic resonance imaging.** Surgical resection, liver transplantation, radiotherapy, and hepatic arterial chemotherapy are methods of treatment. More recent treatment approaches include embolization and **chemoembolization,** which involve radiographic placement of a catheter into the hepatic artery and injection of a substance to occlude blood flow in the tumor capillaries and produce ischemia of tumor tissue.

Reproductive Organs

Carcinoma of the **prostate** is a commonly diagnosed neoplasm in elderly males. It is a slow-growing tumor; early detection has had significant impact on survival rates. Diagnosis is established by rectal examination, closed needle biopsy of nodules, serum prostatic acid phosphate (**PAP**) and serum prostate-specific antigen (**PSA**) measurements, radionuclide bone scan, pelvic computed tomography, and excretory urogram.

Treatment of early stage disease is started with external beam irradiation and lymph node dissection, followed by radical **prostatectomy** (surgical removal of the prostate gland). Disseminated carcinoma treatment involves hormonal manipulation to decrease the effect of androgens on cancer cell growth. This involves use of estrogens, antiandrogens, other hormonally active agents, and LH-RH antagonists, as well as surgical excision of the testes (**orchiectomy, orchidectomy, orchectomy**). Chemotherapy is used as an adjuvant and when response to hormone therapy fails.

Carcinoma of the cervix is a commonly occurring oncologic disorder in females. The Papanicolaou (Pap) smear as a diagnostic tool has allowed for reduction of the incidence of invasive cervical cancer and for diagnosis at earlier stages. **Adenocarcinoma** of the endometrium is the most frequently occurring neoplasm of the uterus, seen primarily in older females. Metastasis occurs most commonly in nearby areas or in the lung. **Carcinoma of the ovary** has a less favorable prognosis since early detection is difficult and recurrence rates after surgery are high.

Skin

Skin cancer is an increasingly diagnosed neoplasm. **Squamous cell carcinoma** is the most common type and tends to be quite invasive and to develop metastasis in the greater degrees of undifferentiation. **Basal cell carcinomas** present as nodular ulcerative, pigmented, sclerosing, or superficial. Topical chemotherapy can be utilized in treating these types of tumors. Malignant **melanomas** (*melan-*, black), tumor of the pigment-producing cells, can disseminate widely, with metastasis via the blood or lymphatics.

Other

Neoplasms arising in the brain and other parts of the nervous system are mostly **gliomas** or **glioblastomas** (Greek *glio-*, connective tissue of the central nervous system, plus *blast-*, denoting a formative cell). **Meningiomas** are benign neoplasms arising in the arachnoid region of the brain.

Neoplasms seen in the pediatric population in addition to the acute leukemias include **rhabdomyosarcoma** (a soft tissue sarcoma), **Ewing's sarcoma** (a highly malignant sarcoma of bone), **medulloblastoma** (primary brain tumor), **neuroblastoma** (often seen in the spinal cord), osteogenic sarcoma or **osteosarcoma** (malignant bone tumor), and **Wilms' tumor** (an abdominal malignant solid tumor).

Abbreviations associated with oncological disorders are listed in Table 18.5.

Table 18.5—Abbreviations Associated with Oncologic Disorders

ABMT	autologous bone marrow transplantation	**APL**	acute promyelocytic leukemia
		BCC	basal cell carcinoma
ACC	adenoid cystic carcinomas	**CA**	carcinoma
AGL	acute granulocytic leukemia	**CALGB**	Cancer and Leukemia Group B
ALL	acute lymphocytic leukemia		
ALM	acral lentiginous melanoma	**CALLA**	common acute lymphoblastic leukemia antigen
AmegL	acute megokaryoblastic leukemia		
		CCG	Children's Cancer Group
AML	acute myelogenous leukemia	**CDC**	Cancer Detection Center
AMMOL	acute myelomonoblastic leukemia	**CEA**	carcinoembryonic antigen
		CF	cancer-free
AMOL	acute monoblastic leukemia	**CFS**	cancer family syndrome
ANC	absolute neutrophil count	**CGL**	chronic granulocytic leukemia
ANLL	acute nonlymphoblastic leukemia	**CIS**	carcinoma *in situ*
		CLL	chronic lymphocytic leukemia

CML	chronic myelogenous leukemia		**NPDL**	nodular poorly differentiated lymphocyte
CMM	cutaneous malignant melanoma		**NSCLC**	non-small cell lung cancer
CMV	cytomegalovirus		**NWTS**	National Wilms' Tumor Study
COG	Central Oncology Group		**OPM**	occult primary malignancy
CRC	colorectal cancer		**PLL**	prolymphocytic leukemia
CTNM	clinical-diagnostic staging of cancer		**POG**	Pediatric Oncology Group
DHL	diffuse histiocytic lymphoma		**POS**	parosteal osteosarcoma
DPDL	diffuse poorly differentiated lymphocytic lymphoma		**RBB**	right breast biopsy
			RCC	renal cell carcinoma
DWDL	diffuse well differentiated lymphocytic lymphoma		**RTx**	radiation therapy
			SCBC	small cell bronchogenic carcinoma
FNH	febrile nonhemolytic reaction		**SCC**	squamous cell
GVHD	graft versus host disease		**SCLC**	small cell lung cancer
HCC	hepatocellular carcinoma		**SqCCa**	squamous cell carcinoma
HCL	hair cell leukemia		**SSM**	superficial spreading melanoma
HD	Hodgkin's disease			
HDC	high-dose chemotherapy		**STNM**	surgical-evaluative staging of cancer
HTL	human thymic leukemia			
HTLC	human T-cell leukemia virus		**SWOG**	Southwest Oncology Group
IORT	intraoperative radiation therapy		**TAA**	tumor-associated antigen (antibodies)
IT	intrathecal		**TANI**	total axial node irradiation
LCLC	large cell lung carcinoma		**TCA**	terminal cancer
LBB	left breast biopsy		**TCCB**	transitional cell carcinoma of bladder
LSA	lymphosarcoma			
MFH	malignant fibrous histiocytoma		**TCMH**	tumor-direct cell-mediated hypersensitivity
MM	multiple myeloma		**TDF**	tumor dose fractionation
MTI	malignant teratoma interminate		**TLI**	total lymphoid irradiation
			TLS	tumor lysis syndrome
MTU	malignant teratoma undifferentiated		**TNI**	total nodal irradiation
			TNF	tumor necrosis factor
NCI	National Cancer Institute		**WDLL**	well-differentiated lymphocyte lymphoma
NHL	non-Hodgkin's lymphoma; nodular histiocytic lymphoma		**XRT**	radiotherapy

Pronouncing Glossary

Root	Meaning	Example	Pronunciation
blast-	bud, germ	neuroblastoma	nur oh BLAST oh mah
carcin-	cancer	carcinomatosis	car sin OH MAH to sis
chemo-	chemistry	chemotherapy	KEY mo ther a pee
neo-	new, strange	neoplasm	NEE oh plas ehm
onco-	mass, swelling	oncocyte	ON koh site

Glossary

adenocarcinoma—a malignant neoplasm of epithelial cells

adenoma—a benign tumor of epithelial tissue

angioma—a swelling or tumor caused by proliferation

angiosarcoma—a malignant neoplasm occurring most often in the breast and skin, believed to originate from endothelial cells of blood vessels

antibody—an immune or protective protein that reacts specifically with an antigen

antigen—any substance capable of inducing a specific immune response

antineoplastic—referring to an agent used to destroy or retard the growth of cancer cells

astrocytoma—a relatively well differentiated glioma

basal cell carcinoma—a slow-growing, locally invasive neoplasm derived from the epidermis or hair follicles

benign—referring to a tumor that is not malignant and does not spread to distant sites in the body

cancer—any malignant tumor

carcinogen—any substance that causes cancer

carcinoma—any malignant new growth that arises in epithelium

chemoembolization—radiographic placement of a catheter into an artery with injection of a substance to occlude blood flow in the tumor capillaries and produce ischemia of tumor tissue

chemotherapy—the prevention or treatment of disease with use of chemical agents

cholangiocarcinoma—an adenocarcinoma, primarily in intrahepatic bile ducts

chondroma—a benign neoplasm derived from cells that form cartilage

chondrosarcoma—a malignant neoplasm derived from cartilage cells

clone—genetically identical cells or organisms derived from a single source by asexual reproduction

cobalt—a metallic element used in radiation therapy

cytogenetics—the branch of genetics dealing with cells

cytotoxic—referring to an agent that damages or destroys specific cells, used to treat various types of cancer

epithelioma—a carcinoma of the skin derived from squamous, basal, or adnexal cells

erythrocytic—pertaining to a red blood cell

fibroma—a benign neoplasm derived from fibrous connective tissue

fibrosarcoma—a malignant neoplasm derived from fibrous connective tissue

glioblastoma—Grade IV astrocytoma; a glioma consisting chiefly of cells that are precursors of astrocytes

glioma—any neoplasm derived from one of the various types of cells that form the interstitial tissue of the brain, spinal cord, pineal gland, posterior pituitary gland, and retina

hemangioendothelioma—a neoplasm derived from blood vessels

hemangioma—a congenital abnormality with a proliferation of vascular endothelium resembling neoplastic tissue

hematologist—specialist in blood and blood forming tissues and the disorders associated with them

hepatoblastoma—a malignant neoplasm occurring primarily in children, primarily in the liver

hepatocarcinoma—malignant hepatoma

hepatoma—hepatocellular or liver cell carcinoma

homeostasis—the physiological process by which the internal systems of the body are maintained at equilibrium, despite variations in the external condition

hybridoma—a culture of hybrid cells produced by fusion of lymphocyte tissue cells, used in the production of monoclonal antibodies

hypernephroma—renal cell carcinoma

immune—resistance to disease because of sensitization from previous contact

immunoglobulin—structurally related proteins that act as antibodies

insulinoma—an islet cell adenoma that secretes insulin

irradiation—the diagnostic or therapeutic application of electromagnetic radiation to a particular structure

leiomyoma—a benign neoplasm derived from smooth muscle

leiomyosarcoma—a malignant neoplasm derived from smooth muscle

leukemia—leukocytic sarcoma; progressive proliferation of abnormal leukocytes found in hemopoietic tissues

leukopenia—a decrease in the number of white blood cells in the blood

lipoma—a benign neoplasm of adipose tissue

liposarcoma—a malignant neoplasm usually occurring deep in intermuscular or periarticular areas

lymphadenopathy—any disease of the lymph glands

lymphangioma—nodule or mass of lymphatic vessels or channels, usually in the neck or axilla

lymphangiosarcoma—malignant neoplasm derived from vascular tissue

lymphoblast—a young immature lymph cell

lymphocyte—white blood cells formed in lymphoid tissue

lymphography—technique of injecting radio-opaque material into the lymphatic system to obtain X-ray photographs of the vessels and nodes

lymphoma—malignant neoplasm of lymph or reticuloendothelial tissues

lymphotropic—referring to nourishment of the tissues by lymph in parts without blood vessels

malignant—describing a tumor that invades and destroys the tissue in which it originates and can spread to other sites in the body via the bloodstream and lymphatic system

mammography—radiography of the breast

medulloblastoma—a glioma consisting of neoplastic cells, usually in the spinal cord, brainstem, or cerebellum

melanoma—malignant neoplasm derived from melanin-forming cells in the skin

metastasis—the distant spread of malignant tumor from its site of origin

mitosis—a type of cell division in which a single cell produces two genetically identical daughter cells

monoclonal—derived from a single cell, having identical molecules

monocytic—referring to a type of white blood cell formed in the bone marrow

myelocytic—describing an immature form of granulocyte occurring normally in bone marrow

myeloma—a malignant tumor from cells normally found in the bone marrow

myelosuppression—decrease in blood cell production by the bone marrow

myoma—a benign neoplasm of muscular tissue

neoplasm—new and abnormal growth; any benign or malignant tumor

neuroblastoma—malignant neoplasm with nerve cells of embryonic type

oncogene—a viral gene that can cause cancer

oncologist—a specialist in the study and treatment of tumors

osteoma—benign, slow-growing mass of bone, usually arising from the skull or mandible

osteosarcoma—osteogenic sarcoma; most common and malignant of bone tumors

palliation—providing temporary relief from symptoms of disease, not a cure

promyelocytic—describing one of the series of cells that gives rise to the granulocytes

radium—a metallic element used in radiotherapy for the treatment of cancer

rads—units that express a dose of radiation

remission—a lessening in the severity or progression of symptoms during the course of an illness

retinoblastoma—a malignant neoplasm composed of primitive retinal cells

rhabdomyosarcoma—a malignant neoplasm derived from skeletal muscle

sarcoma—a connective tissue neoplasm, usually highly malignant

seminoma—a malignant testicular neoplasm

T-cell—a type of long-lived lymphocyte responsible for cell-mediated sensitivity

teratoma—a neoplasm composed of multiple tissues not normally found in the organ in which it arises

thermography—a technique for measuring and recording the heat produced by different parts of the body

thrombocytopenia—decrease in number of platelets in the blood

tomography—a diagnostic technique of using X rays or ultrasound waves to produce an image of structures at a particular depth within the body

tumor—any abnormal growth of tissue

tylectomy—lumpectomy; surgical removal of a tumor from the breast

CHAPTER 19

Trauma and Poisoning

Many of the physical disorders that plague mankind cannot be classified according to the body system affected. Some affect several systems at once; others are not specific to any system at all. Trauma, for example, ranks high among the causes of morbidity and mortality, and traumatic injury can affect any portion of the body. Similarly, poisoning is a major cause of death that can, depending on the poisonous agent, affect all types of cells through a wide range of mechanisms.

Trauma

Trauma, the same word in English as in Latin and Greek, refers to any injury or wound, whether physical or psychic. The terms describing the results of psychic trauma are discussed in Chapter 14, so the psychic manifestations of trauma are not discussed here. However, **psychic trauma** implies a sudden traumatic event, a useful analogy for trauma due to physical insult. A traumatic event is important since physical trauma is the result of a relatively sudden external force or agent. Traumatic disorders include the effects of the kinetic forces that cause fractures, lacerations, contusions, and abrasions, and they also include reactions to other forms of energy—sunlight, heat, cold, radiation, and electric shock.

Kinetic trauma can take many forms, to which any emergency room personnel can attest. Trauma to the skeletal system can result in **fractures** and **dislocations,** as discussed in Chapter 7. A fracture is a broken bone, and the way in which the bone breaks gives the injury its specific name. A **greenstick** fracture, for example, occurs when a long bone is bent to the point of breaking one side while the other side only bends, much like the partial break occurring in a thin tree branch that is bent; if a long bone is twisted, it may break in a **spiral** or **torsion** fracture; a **transverse** fracture is a break directly across a bone's axis; if the bone is splintered or crushed, the fracture is **comminuted;** and an **impacted** fracture results when one fragment of the bone is driven into another fragment. The location of a fracture can also determine its name. For example, a **Colles'** fracture occurs in the wrist at the lower end of the radius when the radial end is displaced posteriorly, a common fracture among patients who have fallen and attempted to ''catch'' themselves on their hands. A **reverse Colles'** fracture (also called **Smith's** fracture) is in the same place but with an anterior displacement. Even the involvement of other tissues may determine the nomenclature, as with a **compound** fracture, an open fracture in which the bone is exposed.

To allow a fracture to heal properly, the break is **reduced** (the fragments of bone

281

returned to the proper position). After reduction, the bones are supported in the proper position with a cast, splint, or bandage to allow recalcification.

Unlike bone, soft tissue tears rather than fractures. When the skin and underlying tissue is pulled excessively, it tears in an irregular, mangled wound known as a **laceration,** from the Latin word meaning "to tear." Rubbing the tissue on a coarse surface, however, causes an **abrasion,** denuding the surface of skin or mucous membrane. Application of a blunt trauma to soft tissue results in a **contusion,** a bruise caused by compressing the tissue and rupturing or injuring capillaries.

A violent jar or shock is known as a **concussion.** Unlike blunt trauma, concussion is a more generalized force. The resulting injury, which is also known as a concussion, may affect any part of the body. Concussion of the brain causes loss of consciousness because of the impact to the brain. In a mild brain concussion, there is temporary loss of consciousness with possible impairment of higher functions, such as retrograde amnesia and emotional lability. Severe concussion produces prolonged unconsciousness with impairment of brainstem function such as pupillary dilation, vasomotor activity, or temporary loss of respiratory reflex. Concussion of the brain, which is functional, may be differentiated from contusion, which is organic.

Concussion may be caused by a blow to the head, causing a generalized trauma to the brain, but it may also result from any other generalized force. For example, **hydraulic concussion** is an abdominal injury resulting from a violent underwater explosion, and **air concussion** may result from the increased air pressure in the vicinity of a blast.

The forces causing physical trauma may be less obvious than those causing fractures, contusions, concussions, lacerations, or abrasions. Sunlight, for example, can have profound effects on the body. Chronic effects of excessive exposure to sunlight include such problems as **actinic keratoses** (precancerous keratotic lesions) and wrinkling. Acute exposure, of course, can cause the familiar **sunburn;** the initial symptoms of erythema and pain may lead to swelling and blisters with more prolonged exposure. If large parts of the body are affected, sunburn can produce constitutional symptoms such as fever, chills, weakness, and shock.

The systemic effects of sunburn may be due to **heat hyperpyrexia (heatstroke)** or **heat prostration.** Heat causes the dilation of cutaneous blood vessels, and failure to adjust to this dilation can lead to the exhaustion and circulatory collapse of heat prostration. Cooling the body provides a rapid response. Heat hyperpyrexia, however, is a disturbance of the heat regulatory mechanism, and it is characterized by high fever and collapse, sometimes leading to convulsions, coma, and death. Immediate treatment to reduce body temperature is essential. Untreated, heat prostration progresses to heat hyperpyrexia.

Extremely high temperatures also cause burns, although the term **burn** technically applies to tissue injury from **electrical** or **chemical** insult as well as **thermal** injuries. Burns can be classified as **superficial,** in which regeneration occurs rapidly from uninjured epidermal elements, or **deep** burns, which destroy the epidermis and much of the dermis. Electrical burns result from heat generated at the point of skin contact with the conductor, the area of highest electrical resistance, which can reach temperatures up to 5000° Celsius. Because of the intense heat, tissue damage is often more severe and widespread than at first apparent. Chemical burns result from exposure to irritating chemicals of various types and may slowly extend for several hours. **Inhalation** burns usually are caused by inhalation of the products of incomplete combustion, which are irritants, rather than by heat. Usually, only steam inhalation causes actual thermal damage to the respiratory tract.

Burns are also classified into three categories by the degree of tissue damage. **First degree** burns damage only the outer layer of the epidermis and result in erythema, increased warmth, tenderness, and pain. **Second degree** burns extend the damage through the epidermis and to the dermis, but not enough to interfere with tissue regeneration. **Vesicles** (blisters) are the hallmark of second degree burns. **Third degree** burns, also called **full-thickness** burns, destroy both the epidermis and dermis. Because of nerve damage, pain is usually acute initially with a full-thickness burn but quickly disappears. The appearance of areas of third degree burn will vary, depending on the cause of the burn. For example, steam may cause pale tissue while flames may char it.

Estimation of the area of a burn is often performed using the **"rule of nines,"** which divides the body into areas each corresponding to a multiple of 9% of the **body surface area (BSA).** Treatment of all burns involves strict **asepsis** (freedom from infection; *a* = without, *sepsis* = infection) and care of the wound, relief of pain, control of infection, correction of attendant anemia, maintenance of nutrition, and prevention or relief of shock. Treatment of shock always takes precedence since the fluid and protein loss through burned surfaces can be enormous. Local treatment of the wound may be **open** (exposed to the air) or **closed** (covered), depending on the type of wound and area burned.

Excessively low temperatures also cause injury. **Frostnip** leaves firm, white, cold areas on the face, ears, or extremities after exposure to cold. If it is not promptly treated, frostnip may cause peeling or blistering similar to sunburn. In **frostbite,** which is more severe than frostnip, the injured area is hard, white, and numb; as the area is warmed, it becomes blotchy-red, swollen, and painful. Severe frostbite can lead to gangrene. Cold exposure also can lead to a decrease in core body temperature, which is called **hypothermia** or **severe exposure** and which requires emergency treatment to slowly warm the patient and support respiration and circulation.

Ionizing radiation is another possible traumatizing source of energy, although more radiation reactions occur from prolonged exposure than from acute exposure. The somatic and genetic effects of radiation—whether in the form of X rays, neutrons, protons, or alpha, beta, or gamma rays—are determined by the total dose and the dose rate. Radiation dose is measured in terms of the **rad** (radiation absorbed dose), the energy actually absorbed by tissues, which is a function of both time of exposure and amount of radiation. The **roentgen (R)** is the international unit of x- or gamma-radiation in the air. Low doses over prolonged periods of time can cause genetic effects; high doses are usually of concern because they cause immediate somatic effects. Acute radiation syndromes include the **cerebral syndrome,** which is produced by very high total body doses and is always fatal; **gastrointestinal syndrome,** producing intractable nausea and diarrhea at lower doses; and **hematopoietic syndrome,** with atrophy of the lymph nodes, spleen, and bone marrow.

Electric shock also causes trauma, including burns at the site of current entry into the body, cardiac arrest from electrical stimulation of cardiac pathways, respiratory paralysis, and even fractures caused by rapid contraction of skeletal muscles.

Also included in the general category of trauma is **asphyxiation.** Derived from the Greek for "a stopping of the pulse," the term **asphyxia** describes a condition caused by a lack of oxygen in the respired air. Asphyxiation can result from near-drowning, in which **hypoxemia** may be caused by aspiration of fluid or respiratory paralysis. Aspiration of water causes loss of surfactant in the lungs, **atelectasis** (collapse of the lung), and shunting of blood in the pulmonary circulation, leading to hypoxemia. Aspiration of fresh water also can cause profound electrolyte imbalances and hemolysis.

Among the more frequent severe problems associated with trauma are bleeding, **shock** (inadequate tissue perfusion), **respiratory arrest,** and **cardiac arrest,** all of which are often interrelated in their etiology. For example, consider a single hypothetical accident victim with a severe bleeding injury and no other trauma. Bleeding by such a victim can quickly cause severe blood loss, resulting in decreased perfusion of tissues. Psychic trauma associated with pain, anxiety, and fright from the accident may cause rapid vasodilation, further exacerbating the hypoperfusion through **primary (neurogenic)** shock. When the hypoperfusion is sufficient to threaten inadequate oxygenation of tissues, blood is shunted to vital organs to the detriment of other tissue. Severe or sudden hypovolemia from the bleeding can result in **secondary** shock and can cause **cardiac arrest,** which in turn causes **respiratory arrest.** Because of this interactive cascade of events, emergency procedures in cases of trauma usually focus first on **cardiopulmonary resuscitation (CPR,** the physical maintenance of circulation and respiration) and control of bleeding.

Poisoning

Aside from the large number of specific poisons, the terminology associated with poisoning is fairly limited. A **poison** is a substance that causes damage to structure or disturbance of function by its chemical action when it is ingested, inhaled, or absorbed or when injected into or produced within the body in small amounts. Although this definition is quite complex, it includes some distinct criteria. First, only a small amount of a poison is required to cause damage, distinguishing poisons from other harmful chemicals. Second, the damage is caused by a chemical action, distinguishing poisons from infectious agents and antigenic substances. Finally, poisons can enter the body by any route of administration or can even be toxic substances produced within the body. Poisoning, also called **intoxation** or **intoxication** (from the Latin *in-,* meaning "intensive," and the Greek *toxikon,* meaning poison), is the morbid condition produced by a poison.

The term **toxin** comes from the Latin word for poison. Although a toxin in its simplest sense is any poison, in medical usage the word *toxin* is almost always applied specifically to toxic proteins produced by some higher plants and animals.

Most other medical terms specific to poisoning apply to the treatment of patients who have been poisoned. The first therapeutic measure in dealing with ingested poisons is often chemical or physical induction of **emesis** (vomiting) to empty the stomach of the toxic substance. **Emetics,** medications that induce vomiting, such as syrup of ipecac, usually evacuate the stomach within 15–30 minutes and are much more effective than physically induced vomiting. When emesis is contraindicated, **gastric lavage** (the French word for "washing") is employed to wash the contents from the stomach. Gastric lavage is performed through a large-bore tube such as an **Ewald** tube, which is passed through the mouth to the stomach; further, the tube may be **cuffed** (i.e., incorporate a cuff or protrusion to protect the trachea) to prevent aspiration of lavage products.

Absorption of poisons from the GI tract may also be reduced by administering an **adsorbent** such as activated charcoal to adsorb the toxin and either remove it with lavage

Table 19.1—Abbreviations Associated with Trauma and Poisoning

AA	auto accident	**FAS**	fetal alcohol syndrome
ADAU	adolescent drug abuse unit	**GSW**	gunshot wound
ADDU	alcohol and drug dependency unit	**GWA**	gunshot wound of the abdomen
ADR	adverse drug reaction	**GWT**	gunshot wound of the throat
AKA	alcoholic ketoacidosis	**HI**	head injury
BSB	body surface burned	**HIR**	head injury routine
CC	cerebral concussion	**MSW**	multiple stab wounds
CHI	closed head injury	**MVA**	motor vehicle accident
DAWN	Drug Abuse Warning Network	**OD**	overdose
DIE	die in emergency department	**SIW**	self-inflicted wound
DOA	dead on arrival	**STU**	shock trauma unit
DOI	date of injury	**SWT**	stab wound of the throat
EBI	estimated blood loss	**TBSA**	total burn surface area

or allow it to pass through the gut without absorption into the body. Adsorbents are often administered in conjunction with saline **cathartics,** most frequently sorbitol although magnesium sulfate (Epsom salt) was used more commonly in the past. Saline laxatives decrease the GI transit time, so they may be administered with an adsorbent to reduce the amount of time the poison is available for absorption.

Once a poison has been absorbed, the only alternatives are to remove it from the body or render it less harmful. Removal from the body can involve accelerating the normal elimination by pathways (e.g., alkalinization of the urine), either **hemodialysis** or **peritoneal lavage** to remove the poison from the blood, or **chelation** of the substance to increase its excretion and decrease its toxicity.

Therapy for poisoning by a specific agent may include the use of an **antidote** (literally, "to give against"). An antidote counteracts a specific poison, either inactivating it, facilitating its elimination, or blocking its activity. Activated charcoal was formerly administered in combination with magnesium oxide and tannic acid in what was called the **"universal antidote";** the usefulness of the combination, however, is questionable and it is seldom used any longer.

Most of the other terms associated with the treatment of poisonings refer to specific toxins and reactions to them, antidotes, and chelating agents. A good medical dictionary can help the pharmacist apply these specialized terms. Abbreviations commonly associated with trauma and poisoning are listed in Table 19.1.

Glossary

abrasion—a wound scraped or rubbed in tissue, denuding the surface of skin or mucous membrane

actinic keratoses—precancerous keratotic lesions

air concussion—injury resulting from a sudden, severe increase in air pressure, such as is experienced in the vicinity of a blast

antidote—a substance that counteracts a specific poison

asphyxiation—a condition caused by a lack of oxygen in the respired air

atelectasis—collapse of the lung in the adult; failure of the lung to properly expand in the neonate

Colles' fracture—fracture of the lower end of the radius in which the radial end is displaced posteriorly

comminuted fracture—a fracture in which the bone is splintered or crushed

compound fracture—an open fracture in which the bone is exposed

concussion—a violent jar or shock causing injury

concussion of the brain—the injury resulting from a violent jarring of the brain

contusion—a bruise

dislocation—disarticulation; injury to a joint causing misalignment of the bones

emesis—vomiting

emetic—chemical agent that induces vomiting

exposure injury—hypothermia

first degree burn—thermal injury causing damage only to the outer layer of the epidermis

fracture—broken bone

frostnip—injury of the face, ears, or extremities caused by exposure to low temperatures and leaving firm, white, cold areas

frostbite—injury of the face, ears, or extremities caused by exposure to low temperatures and leaving hard, white, numb tissue; as the area is warmed, it becomes blotchy-red, swollen, and painful

gastric lavage—removal of the stomach contents by washing through a tube inserted through the mouth to the stomach

hypothermia—decrease in core body temperature sufficient to impair the body's ability to control internal temperature

full-thickness burn—third degree burn

greenstick fracture—a bone that is bent to the point of breaking on one side while the opposite side remains intact

heat prostration—failure to adjust to the vasodilation of blood vessels in response to heat

heat hyperpyrexia—a disturbance of the heat regulatory mechanism characterized by high fever and collapse, sometimes leading to convulsions, coma, and death

heatstroke—heat hyperpyrexia

hydraulic concussion—an abdominal injury resulting from a violent underwater explosion

impacted fracture—fracture occurring when one fragment of the bone is driven into another fragment

intoxation—intoxication

intoxication—morbid condition produced by a poison

laceration—an irregular, mangled wound caused by tearing the tissue

neurogenic shock—primary shock

poison—any substance that causes damage to structure or disturbance of function by its chemical action when it is ingested, inhaled, or absorbed or when injected into or produced within the body in small amounts

primary shock—decreased tissue perfusion caused by rapid vasodilation associated with pain, anxiety, and fright

psychic trauma—a shocking event causing prolonged emotional injury, particularly to the subconscious

rad—acronym for "radiation absorbed dose," a unit of exposure to ionizing radiation

reduce—align properly; especially fragments of bone returned to the proper position after a fracture

roentgen—a unit or x-or gamma-radiation in the air; identified by the symbol *R*

reverse Colles' fracture—fracture of the lower end of the radius in which the radial end is displaced anteriorly

second degree burn—thermal injury in which the damage extends through the epidermis and to the dermis, but insufficient to interfere with tissue regeneration

secondary shock—shock in response to severe or sudden hypovolemia

shock—inadequate tissue perfusion to sustain life

spiral fracture—a fracture caused by twisting a long bone

sunburn—acute injury of the skin caused by excessive exposure to ultraviolet light

third degree burn—thermal injury that destroys both the epidermis and dermis

torsion fracture—a spiral fracture

toxin—a poison, specifically applied to certain proteins produced by some higher plants and animals that are toxic to other organisms

transverse fracture—a fracture directly across the axis of the bone

trauma—any injury or wound, whether physical or psychic

universal antidote—a mixture of 2 parts activated charcoal, 1 part magnesium oxide, and 1 part tannic acid, given as 15 ml in a glass of warm water, to be followed by emesis or gastric lavage

vesicle—blister

CHAPTER 20

Nutritional Disorders/Alternative Medicine

A number of disease states can be classified under the heading of nutritional disorders, but all relate to the body's supply of or need for one or more nutrients and usually arise from either altered consumption or absorption. Some are usually unintentionally induced, such as the variety of conditions resulting from either an excess **(hypervitaminosis)** or a deficiency **(hypovitaminosis)** of the vitamins. Others such as malnutrition are often either economic in origin or arise from an inappropriate diet for other reasons. And some are often considered to be psychological disorders—anorexia nervosa, bulimia, and obesity—although they have been presented in this section since their effects are manifested on the nutritional status of the body.

Vitamin Deficiency/Excess

Vitamins are organic compounds necessary for regulation of metabolism. The original term of ''vitamine'' was a combination of *vita* meaning life and *amine* for what was thought to be the chemical structure of these compounds. The final *e* was omitted from the spelling after it was discovered that not all vitamins are amines.

Vitamins A, D, E, and K are classified as **fat-soluble** because of their lipophilic (Greek *lipos,* meaning ''fat,'' plus *phil-,* meaning ''craving for'') nature. They must be emulsified by bile salts in the gastrointestinal tract before absorption into the bloodstream and can then be stored in the body's fat tissue for periods of time. Conversely, vitamin C and the B vitamins are **water-soluble;** they are easily absorbed, are degraded by heat, and must be constantly replenished in the body. Table 20.1 lists the vitamins and their chemical names.

Toxicity of the fat-soluble vitamins may be caused by diminished urinary excretion of normal body stores, as well as ingestion of excess amounts. Acute vitamin A toxicity can occur after a single large dose. The chronic toxicity of **hypervitaminosis A** results in pruritus (itching), dry scaly skin, changes in nail and hair texture, bone pain, increased cerebrospinal fluid pressure, and hypercalcemia. Prolonged use of vitamin A, even in therapeutic doses, can cause fatigue, nausea, vomiting, dizziness, irritability, cheilosis (inflammation at the corners of the mouth), and generalized skin desquamation (shedding).

Tolerance to vitamin D is variable. Hypervitaminosis D may cause **hypercalciuria** (increased calcium levels in the urine,-*uria*) or **hypercalcemia** (-*emia,* blood) with symptoms of weakness, anorexia, vomiting, diarrhea, excessive thirst (polydipsia), excessive

Table 20.1—The Vitamins

Vitamins	Chemical Name
A	carotene, retinol
B_1	thiamine
B_2	riboflavin
B_3	niacin, nicotinic acid
B_5	pantothenic acid
B_6	pyridoxine
B_{12}	cyanocobalamin
Biotin	
C	ascorbic acid
D_2	calciferol, ergocalciferol
D_3	cholecalciferol
AT_{10}	dihydrotachysterol
E	tocopherols
Folic acid	folacin, pteroylglutamic acid
Inositol	
K	phylloquinone

urination (polyuria), mental changes and proteinuria. Because of vitamin D's role in calcium utilization, deposits of calcium salts in soft tissue may result if the condition is prolonged. Chronic overdosage of vitamin D can lead to irreversible renal failure.

The other fat-soluble vitamins are less likely to cause a hypervitaminosis. **Vitamin E** excess is not associated with severe toxic effects. Gastrointestinal disturbances are the most common complaint with large doses. Low birth weight infants are at risk of greater morbidity and mortality if given IV dosages of the vitamin. **Vitamin K** is relatively nontoxic, although adverse effects have been noted in premature infants and following rapid IV administration.

Toxicity from the water-soluble vitamins is not a common clinical problem since these compounds are more readily excreted from the body. They can, however, be toxic when large amounts are ingested for long periods. **Sensory neuropathy** (disease of the nerves) has been reported with vitamin B_6 excess. Flushing, burning, and tingling around the neck, face, and hands are associated with high vitamin B_3 intake. Kidney stones (nephrolithiasis) are listed as an effect of vitamin C excess.

Deficiency of **vitamin A** is usually due to malabsorption syndromes or malnutrition. It is related to impaired resistance to infection and produces a number of symptoms: night blindness (nyctalopia), extreme dryness of the conjunctiva (xerophthalmia), development of a horny layer of skin (keratinization), growth failure (from imbalance in the ratio of osteoblasts and osteoclasts), fetal malformations, and diminished corticosteroid production. **Vitamin D deficiency** can be caused by malabsorption syndromes as well as by renal disease, hypoparathyroidism, short bowel syndrome, and long-term anticonvulsant use. Deprivation of sunshine or ultraviolet (U/V) light causes deficiency of vitamin D that is necessary for active absorption of calcium into the blood. The deficiency produces inadequate mineralization in bones and teeth, resulting in the condition known as **rickets** in children and **osteomalacia** in adults. **Vitamin E deficiency** is seen in severe malabsorption and in premature infants. It has been associated with increased rate of onset of Alzheimer's disease. Results are seen in a neurologic syndrome of ataxia (incoordination), muscle weakness, nystagmus (oscillation of the eyeballs), and loss of sensation. **Vitamin K deficiency** is associated with antibiotic use, concurrent use of large amounts of vitamins A and E, and advanced liver damage. Newborn infants require vitamin K supplementation until development of the intestinal tract's ability to synthesize the vitamin.

Water-soluble vitamins can be deficient as the result of stress from injury or surgery, hyperthyroidism, diarrhea, or fever. Clinical symptoms include anorexia (loss of appetite), weight loss, headache, insomnia, apathy or irritability. Specific clinical syndromes occur in severe deficiency states.

The most common cause of **thiamine (B$_1$) deficiency** in this and other developed countries is alcoholism. The condition is also seen in the clinical setting with use of peritoneal or hemodialysis. The two primary syndromes of the deficiency affect the cardiovascular system (**wet beriberi**) and the nervous system (**dry beriberi, Wernicke-Korsakoff** syndrome). Cardiovascular symptoms involve peripheral vasodilation, myocardial failure, and sodium-water retention leading to edema. Peripheral neuropathy (nerve disorder), Wernicke's encephalopathy (cerebral beriberi), and Korsakoff syndrome with amnesic psychosis are nervous system manifestations.

Niacin (B$_3$) deficiency caused by alcoholism or protein-calorie malnutrition produces a state known as **pellagra** with skin eruptions, dermatitis, dementia, and diarrhea. Deficiency of vitamin B$_{12}$ is manifested as pernicious anemia or as an uncomplicated deficiency, such as seen in vegetarian diets. **Pyridoxine (B$_6$)** deficiency is seldom caused by dietary restrictions except in association with alcoholism. Drug-induced deficiency is more common with use of hydralazine, penicillamine, isoniazid, or cycloserine. Symptoms include peripheral sensory neuropathy with ataxia, numbness, skin lesions on the face, glossitis (inflammation of the tongue), stomatitis (inflammation of the mucous membrane of the mouth), and anemia.

Ascorbic acid (C) deficiency results in impaired synthesis of collagen, the major protein of the white fibers of connective tissue, bone, and cartilage. Symptoms include joint pain, anemia, delayed wound healing, and increased risk of infection. The severe form of deficiency is **scurvy** with hemorrhages in the skin, gum inflammation with loosening of the teeth, muscle weakness, and joint pain. The disorder is no longer common in the general population. It is seen in areas of urban poverty, during the first year of life when infant formulas are not supplemented with vitamin C, and occasionally in middle age to elderly males because of poor diet. Symptoms of deficiency occur after discontinuation of large doses of vitamin C; therefore, dosages should be tapered.

Treatment of the hypervitaminoses would primarily be directed toward removal of continued dietary intake. Dietary supplementation is the basis for correcting deficiency disorders.

Body Element Disorders

Water, electrolyte, and element deficiencies are generally categorized as those involving either metabolic acidosis (loss of alkali) or alkalosis (acid defect). Specific acid-base disorders more closely related to nutrition are included in Table 20.2. Potassium deficiency or **hypokalemia** (*hypo* = less,*-emia* = blood) usually occurs from vomiting or diarrhea. A deficiency of calcium (**hypocalcemia**) is sometimes equated with the term

---

Table 20.2—Terms Associated with Parenteral Nutrition

Anabolic	Ideal body weight (IBW)
Basal energy expenditure (BEE)	Lipogenesis
Bolus	Micronutrients
Central venous catheter	Osmolality
Essential fatty acid deficiency (EFAD)	Polymeric
Fat emulsion	Resting energy expenditure (REE)
Hyperglycemic, hyperosmolar, nonketotic	Substrate
dehydration (HHND)	Total daily energy requirement (TDE)
Hyperosmolarity	Trace minerals
Hypertonic	

---

tetany, muscular spasms with systemic effects. Other element deficiency disorders include **hypophosphatemia,** anemia (iron deficiency), and goiter (iodine deficiency).

Accumulation of sodium in the body occurs primarily in the extracellular fluid (ECF). **Hypernatremia** can result from various causes and produce hypertonic dehydration. **Hyperkalemia,** or excess potassium, can arise from excess ingestion or infusion of potassium salts or in conditions such as acute renal failure or adrenal insufficiency.

Malnutrition

The term *malnutrition* means disordered nutrition. **Protein energy malnutrition (PEM)** can manifest as semistarvation, general inanition, hunger, or underfeeding.

Two types of primary malnutrition are **marasmus** (from the Greek word meaning "withering") and **kwashiorkor,** usually seen in children. Marasmus occurs after a long period of inadequate caloric and protein intake. The body lowers its metabolic rate to preserve proteins in the tissues and fat becomes the major energy substrate. Individuals with this form of malnutrition would be described as **cachectic,** showing a lack of nutrition and wasting. The word *cachexia* is derived from the Greek *kakos,* meaning "bad," and *hexis,* a habit of body. Kwashiorkor, on the other hand, develops rapidly when protein intake is deficient, although caloric intake is adequate. Visceral protein stores become depleted when they are consumed to provide for caloric metabolism and storage. Individuals with this disorder are often obese and appear to be well nourished or appear with the pot belly appearance seen in starving children. Many disorders can combine aspects of both of these with changes in protein and energy deficiency accompanied by depletion of vitamins, minerals, and electrolytes.

Secondary malnutrition occurs when an adequate diet is available but the patient is still undernourished. Undernourishment develops due to inadequate intake, malabsorption, inadequate utilization of nutrients, increased requirements, increased losses, or drug-nutrient interactions. Malnutrition occurs in hospitalized patients when a marginal nutritional state is compromised by effects of disease, injury, and/or surgery.

Diagnosis of malnutrition is based on an extensive history to determine possible primary causes; alcoholism, poverty, a diet high in foods with a low nutrient-density, and/or solitary life style are among the etiologic factors. Chronic disease states, gastrointestinal difficulty, or prolonged fever are indicators of secondary malnutrition. Patient appearance is likely to reflect listlessness; pallor; drawn face; swelling (edema); and dry, cracked skin hanging in folds with possible dermatitis (inflammation of the skin) and pigmentation changes. **Emaciation** is evidenced by protrusion of bones in areas of normal fat deposit, such as buttocks, thighs, or the back. Growth is retarded in children. **Anthropometric** measurements of triceps skin fold **(TSF)** and midarm muscle circumference **(AMC)** reflect deficiencies in subcutaneous fat stores and lean body mass. Laboratory indices of nutritional status and metabolic expenditure include serum albumin and transferrin levels and urea nitrogen excretion. Laboratory test abnormalities associated with starvation include decreases in urinary excretion of 17-hydroxysteroids/ketosteroids, decreased metabolic cortisol clearance, and decreased thyroid hormone levels, all in conjunction with normal or increased plasma cortisol concentration. Achlorhydria, absence of hydrochloric acid from gastric juice, is frequent.

When normal dietary intake is not possible, aggressive nutritional support is indicated and may take the form of **enteral** (*enter-*, intestine) **nutrition (EN)** or **total parenteral nutrition (TPN).** Nutritional support may be needed when surgery is performed or in conditions such as coma, gastrointestinal disorders (obstruction, fistulas, inflammatory bowel disease), psychiatric disorders (anorexia nervosa), increased nutritional demands (trauma, sepsis), and other advanced or chronic disease states. In general, EN is indicated when gastrointestinal function is intact and such nutrition is not contraindicated. Enteral nutrition is usually administered via a naso-gastric (NG) tube from the nose *(naso-)* into the stomach *(gastric)* or a naso-duodenal (ND) or naso-jejunal (N-J) tube into the indicated portion of the intestine.

For long-term nutritional support and in patients at risk of choking, a gastrostomy tube (G-tube) or jejunostomy tube can be used. These terms refer to feeding tubes inserted through the abdominal wall into the stomach or jejunum, named for the procedure by which they are inserted (*gastrostomy* means ''establishment of a new opening into the stomach''). TPN is utilized when adequate nutrition cannot be provided by the enteral route and requires placement of a catheter into a peripheral vein or through the subclavian vein (located beneath the clavicle or collarbone) into the vena cava.

Determination of the required composition of nutritional solutions is a complex and individualized process based on specific needs of individual patients. Adequate sources of the basic categories of protein, fats, carbohydrates, electrolytes, vitamins, minerals, and water are necessary to maintain energy balance and tissue synthesis. The nutritional standard that specifies the amount and type of nutrients required to maintain health is the **recommended dietary allowance (RDA),** formerly referred to as the minimum daily requirement (MDR). These units, used as legal standard for labeling nutritional products, are grouped by age, weight, and sex requirements. A number of terms are encountered in relation to nutritional support. Those listed in Table 20.2 are frequently encountered by pharmacists who consult about, prepare, or deliver TPN solutions.

Other Nutritional Disorders

Anorexia nervosa (*an* = without; *-orexis* = a longing) is a disorder seen primarily in adolescent females who produce a state of voluntary starvation. The condition is associated with psychological dysfunction; however, the mechanisms have not been defined. These individuals are emaciated but deny that they are hungry, fatigued, or even thin. Common symptoms include amenorrhea (absence of menstruation), lanugo (fetal hair), episodes of bulimia, vomiting, periods of overactivity, and slow heartbeat (bradycardia). Criteria for diagnosis of the disorder are onset prior to age 25; weight loss of at least 25 percent of original body weight; distorted attitude toward food that is not influenced by hunger, reassurance, or admonitions; no known causative medical illness; and no other known psychological disorder. Except for correction of weight loss and malnutrition, there is no specific therapy for anorexia nervosa, although early identification and removal of the patient from the environment are the most significant aspects of supportive treatment. Antidepressant drugs are useful in some patients. Parenteral nutrition may be indicated in cases of extreme starvation.

Bulimia, also called **bulimia nervosa** or **gorge-purge syndrome,** is a disorder most often found in young females who gorge on food several times weekly, ingesting as many as 40,000 calories. These episodes are followed by self-induced vomiting and/or abuse of laxatives or diuretics. Dehydration and metabolic imbalances may result. Other complications can include impaired liver and kidney function, dry skin, frequent infections, and muscle spasms. The disorder is believed to be a psychological response to stress. Treatment includes behavior modification and psychotherapy along with nutritional guidance. Medical treatment is directed to the specific consequences.

Food intolerance can be defined as a reproducible adverse reaction to a specific food or food ingredient. Food aversion does not occur if the food is given in disguised form. **Food allergies** involve a hypersensitivity reaction, associated with elevated serum IgE, circulating immune complexes and eosinophilia.

Food poisoning involves gastrointestinal symptoms after consumption of foods or drink, usually due to salmonella or an enterotoxin. Foods, water or milk can also be carriers for the enteric (intestinal) fevers—typhoid or paratyphoid—caused by *Salmonella* organisms. Bacillary dysentery *(Shigella)* and cholera *(Vibrio cholerae)* are other bacterial diseases spread through food or drinking water. Amebic dysentery, caused by the protozoan *Entamoeba histolytica,* is transmitted by water or uncooked foods contaminated with human feces. The term *traveler's diarrhea* refers to the gastrointestinal disorder that occurs from strains of enterobacteria to which immunities have not been developed.

Obesity

The regulation of eating behavior is located in the hypothalamic area of the brain, which may be influenced by psychological, social, and genetic factors. Several terms are associated with this function. **Adipostat** or set point is a theoretical level of fat tissue to which the body adjusts and which it tries to maintain; the term employs the same suffix as "thermostat." **Adiposis** is simply the level of adipose tissue (connective tissue packed with fat cells) in the body. The **satiety center** is the center in the brain controlling the perception of satisfaction or fullness from food. **Thermogenesis** refers to the creation of heat, specifically the physiologic process of heat production in the body.

When an individual exceeds 20–25 percent of the recommended body weight, the condition is known as **obesity** or **adiposity.** In most cases, this is due to exogenous intake of calories rather than hormonal imbalance. Secondary causes of obesity include hypothyroidism, Cushing's disease, insulinoma, and hypothalamic disorders.

Obesity occurs with the combination of excessive food (caloric) intake and inadequate expenditure of energy (calories) by exercise. Assessment of obesity is most easily done by using height and weight ranges; however, this method has some disadvantages. More precise measurements are based on body density or isotropic dilution methods; however, these are too complicated for routine clinical use. **Anthropometry** assesses the degree of adiposity by measurement of skin fold thickness, usually in the triceps and subscapular areas and relating these figures to height, weight, and age.

Treatment of primary obesity falls into the major areas of (a) caloric restriction, (b) behavior modification (**BMOD**), (c) exercise, (d) drugs, and (e) surgery. Caloric restriction involves a very low calorie diet (**VLCD**) designed to produce rapid initial weight loss. A variety of nutritional counseling programs are available for maintenance purposes. Behavior modification includes techniques such as biofeedback, counseling, and support groups such as Weight Watchers, Overeaters Anonymous (OA), and Take Off Pounds Sensibly (TOPS). Drugs include the anorexiants (*an* = without; *-orexia* = appetite), usually referred to as appetite suppressants, or the newer intestinal-acting (fat absorption) type. Surgical procedures are designed to alter the normal digestive route. For example, **gastroplication,** also called **gastroptyxis** or **gastrorrhaphy,** involves suturing a longitudinal fold to reduce the size of the stomach. This procedure is commonly referred to as a "stomach staple." **Jejunoileal shunt, gastric bypass,** and **gastroplasty** are other terms that may be encountered in association with treatment of obesity.

Common disorders and abbreviations relating to nutrition are summarized in Tables 20.3 and 20.4, respectively.

Table 20.3—Common Nutritional Disorders

Anorexia nervosa	
Bulimia	
Malnutrition:	primary, secondary
Obesity	
Vitamin deficiency:	Beriberi
	Osteomalacia
	Rickets
	Wernicke-Korsakoff syndrome
Vitamin toxicity:	hypervitaminosis
Bacterial:	Cholera
	Dysentery
	Food poisoning
Acid-base disorders:	Bicarbonate ingestion
	Gastrointestinal loss of acid
	Gastrointestinal loss of base
	Milk-alkali syndrome
	Phosphorus deficiency (hypophosphatemia)
	Phosphorus excess (hyperphosphatemia)
	Potassium deficiency (hypokalemia)
	Potassium excess (hyperkalemia)
	Sodium deficiency (hyponatremia)
	Sodium excess (hypernatremia)
Ammonium chloride ingestion	
Methyl alcohol intoxication	

Table 20.4—Abbreviations Associated with Nutritional Disorders

AMC	arm muscle circumference	**MDR**	minimum daily requirement
BEE	basal energy expenditure	**NG**	nasogastric (tube)
BMI	body mass index	**NPU**	net protein utilization
BMOD	behavior modification	**OA**	Overeaters Anonymous
BMR	basal metabolic rate	**PEM**	protein energy malnutrition
CDS	chronic dieting syndrome	**PER**	protein efficiency ratio
ECF	extracellular fluid	**RDA**	recommended dietary
EFA	essential fatty acids		allowance
EFAD	essential fatty acid deficiency	**REE**	resting energy expenditure
EN	enteral nutrition	**TDE**	total daily energy requirement
HDL	high density lipoproteins	**TOPS**	Take Off Pounds Sensibly
HHND	hyperglycemic, hyperosmolar,	**TPN**	total parenteral nutrition
	nonketotic dehydration	**TSF**	triceps skin fold
IBW	ideal body weight	**VLCD**	very low calorie diet
LDL	low density lipoproteins	**VLDL**	very low density lipoproteins
MCT	medium chain triglycerides		

Alternative Medicine

Although nutritional deficiencies are relatively uncommon in the United States, the typical pharmacy still sells scores or even hundreds of different vitamin and mineral preparations. Most communities support one or more retailers whose entire market is little more than selling nutritional supplements for medical purposes, and traditional medicine might maintain that such sales do not satisfy any real medical need in most developed countries. Yet sales are often brisk; the reason is that such sales are usually not because patients are treating actual deficiencies but are using nutritional supplements to accomplish a variety of medical purposes that may be outside the scope of traditional medicine.

Nutrition has long been an important part of traditional medical practice, but in more recent years it has taken on a new image as something that can provide healing beyond the concepts of deficiency and excess. Nutritional supplements are now part of the entire alternative medical market, an arena of which pharmacists and other health practitioners should be aware. Traditional medicine in western cultures includes primarily **allopathic** medicine, **osteopathic** medicine (as it is practiced today), their related technologies, and pharmaceuticals. **Alternative medicine** is the term frequently applied to a variety of increasingly common approaches to the management of mental and physical disorders that do not always follow the standard scientific method. The distinguishing difference between traditional and alternative medicine seems to be that most of the alternative approaches are based on a specific theory of healing or a philosophy of health rather than arising from a more strictly scientific, empiric approach. In short, each method has an underlying philosophy or theory that often relies of theoretical ''forces'' and ''balances'' rather than on biochemistry and physiology.

One feature often attributed to alternative medicine is that it is **holistic,** meaning that the mind and body are viewed as a living, integrated system and that they continually interact. Although not excluded by traditional medicine, this holistic approach of whole body medicine sometimes combines many different Eastern and Western medical specialties such as those described below.

Osteopathy (*osteo* = bone; *pathy* = disease) is a branch of medicine focusing on the shape and position of the skeletal structure as a means of improving health and aiding in the body's inherent healing ability. It focuses more on health of the arteries and flow of blood and lymphatics than does chiropractic medicine. **Osteopaths** or Doctors of Osteopathy **(DO)** can provide comprehensive medical and surgical care.

Chiropractic medicine is primarily oriented toward adjusting the spinal vertebra to eliminate any subluxation (an incomplete dislocation) that can cause impingement and pressure or irritation of the surrounding nerves. The distorted nerve messages can damage surrounding muscle or other tissues. Some practitioners **(chiropractors)** utilize a method they term **contact reflex analysis (CRA)** to incorporate physical therapy, nutrition, and acupressure/acupuncture in treating emotional, mental, and chemical factors that can produce tension in the spinal system and soft tissues. It has been used successfully in treatment of such disorders as carpal tunnel syndrome (CTS) and reflex sympathetic dystrophy (RSD).

Chinese medicine encompasses terms such as the forces of **yin** (cold, rest, passivity, darkness, inwardness, decrease) and **yang** (heat, activity, stimulation, light, outwardness, increase) emanating from the **Tai,** an integrated whole present in everything. The balance of yin and yang is manifest in the flow of an energy called **chi** (life force), which flows through the body in meridians. All treatment is directed toward bringing harmony/balance between deficiency (yin) and excess (yang). Foods, herbs, and other therapeutic techniques are used, including such things as **moxibustion** (heat applied to acupuncture points), massage to increase or decrease the chi flow, acupuncture, or acupressure.

Acupuncture is used for anesthesia, in addition to rebalancing a chi disturbance. In the procedure, needles are inserted just below the epidermis and serve as antennas to stimulate body tissue at locations along the **meridians,** the lines connecting different anatomical sites. More recent uses in this country include treatment of alcoholism and opiate addiction and to induce smoking cessation. **Acupressure** utilizes fingers and thumbs rather than needles to press chi points on the body's surface. It serves to relieve muscle tension, thereby promoting blood flow throughout the body. It has been used successfully to treat mental tension and stress, eyestrain, headaches, menstrual cramps, and joint inflammation.

Kinesiology is a diagnostic approach using individual muscle functions to provide information about overall health. Analysis of posture and gait and testing of muscle strength and mobility contribute to treatment regimens for a given illness. **Rolfing** is a deep massage technique that uses manipulation of the connective tissue to restore the body's natural alignment.

Hydrotherapy involves use of the physical properties of water to facilitate healing. These are buoyancy (to facilitate movement), temperature (to promote relaxation and decrease pain), viscosity (to provide resistance), and hydrostatic or circumferential pressure (to enhance blood circulation).

Nutrition is an aspect of health that is becoming increasingly associated with both maintenance of good health and affecting diseases such as cardiovascular disorders, cancer, diabetes, arteriosclerosis, and cerebrovascular accidents.

Traditions of **botanical medicines,** also called herbal medicines or **phytopharma-ceuticals** (*phyto-* meaning "plants") can be found in all cultures, designated by a variety of terms, some indigenous to a specific group, others more commonly recognized. Botanical medicines are available in the forms listed in Table 20.5. Patients may be taking a variety of these substances in conjunction with prescription medication. Some of the most widely used are listed in Table 20.6.

Table 20.5—Availability of Botanical Medicines	
Encapsulated	Fresh plant
Extracts:	Infusion
freeze-dried	Plaster
solid	Poultice
standardized	Tea
Fomentation	Tincture

Homeopathic medicine or **homeopathy,** from the Greek words *homoios* ("like") and *pathos* ("suffering" or "sickness"), differs from the general medical viewpoint in considering the symptoms to be part of the curative process rather than as a manifestation of the disease itself. In this practice, a homeopathic substance is matched with the patient's symptoms and given in small amounts. The substance may contain chemicals, minerals, plant extracts, preparations of diluted animal and insect venoms, disease-causing germs, or standard drugs. These contribute to the body's defensive reaction in trying to eliminate the underlying disease. **Potentization** is an essential concept, and the extremely low concentration of active ingredient is a primary difference between homeopathy and use of herbal preparations.

Hypnosis is utilized in both traditional and alternative medicine to induce a positive mental state of healing. The Office of Alternative Medicine (**OAM**) at the National Institutes of Health (NIH) has reported usefulness of hypnosis in providing more rapid healing and less pain. It has been successful in adjunctive treatment for weight loss, smoking cessation, phobias, eating disorders, and mental disorders.

Biofeedback is a training technique that enables an individual to obtain some control over autonomic body functions. Patients are connected to machines that monitor skin temperature, blood pressure, perspiration, and electrical responses. Using this information, the patient can then determine the physiological effects of consciously willing for changes to take place. The technique has been most successful with treatment of insomnia, menstrual cramping, asthma, irritable bowel syndrome, migraine headaches, and other pain associated with muscle tightness.

Table 20.6—Commonly Used Botanical Medicines	
Blue-green algae	Ginkgo
Aloe vera	Ginseng
Bitter melon	Goldenseal
Chamomile	Green tea
Chinese skullcap	Hawthorn berry
Cranberries	Licorice
Dandelion	Maitake mushrooms
Dong quai	Milk thistle
Echinacea	Mistletoe
Garlic	Pokeweed
Ginger	Shitaake mushrooms

Table 20.7—Abbreviations Relating to Alternative Medicine

AHMA	American Holistic Medicine Association	BMOD	behavior modification
AHP	Association for Humanistic Psychology	CRA	contact reflex analysis
		DC	Doctor of Chiropractic
AMTA	American Massage Therapy Association	DO	Doctor of Osteopathy
		OAM	Office of Alternative Medicine
		TM	transcendental meditation

Yoga focuses on altering an individual's state of mind and using mind power to generate healing within the body. Various positions, known as asanas, along with concentration on breathing serve to maintain suppleness of the spine and exercise all of the major muscle groups, thereby strengthening organs due to increased respiration and blood flow. Breathing is central, as it is the vehicle for the **prana** or vital life force to enter the body. Yoga is often recommended by a variety of medical practitioners for remedial and preventive measures for the spine and as a stress-reduction technique. Massage, hypnosis, music therapy, and meditation/visualization techniques such as transcendental meditation (**TM**) are other forms of relaxation and concentration approaches to induce a positive mental state of healing.

Naturopathic medicine or **naturopathy** can be defined as the use of nontoxic healing methods derived from Greek, Oriental, and European medical tradition. In this approach, the body's striving for health is assumed as the focus of healing and when possible, nontoxic, noninvasive treatments are utilized. Many practitioners called **naturopaths** do utilize drugs or surgery in crisis situations and are licensed to do so in most states.

Ayurvedic medicine, from the Sanskrit meaning ''the science of life and longevity,'' is based on the premise that health is a state of balance among the body's physical, emotional, and spiritual systems. Treatment regimens can include yoga, diet, herbal preparations, dietary and sleep pattern revisions, massage, sound and **aromatherapy** (treatment with scents), and/or meditation.

Other treatment approaches that may be viewed as types of alternative medicine include **gemmotherapy, auto-sanguis dilution therapy, neural therapy, Anthroposophic medicine,** and **immunotherapy.**

Abbreviations associated with the area of alternative medicine are listed in Table 20.7.

Pronouncing Glossary

Root	Meaning	Example	Pronunciation
metron-	measure	anthropometric	an thro po MET rek
orexia-	appetite	anorexia	an oh REX ee ah
phyto-	plant	phytotoxin	FI to TOK sin
troph-	nourishment	hypertrophy	hi PURR tro fee

Glossary

acupuncture—ancient Oriental therapy utilizing puncture with fine, long needles

adiposity—obesity

allopathy—treatment of disease by producing a second condition that is incompatible with the first

anabolic—promoting tissue growth by increasing the metabolic processes involved in protein synthesis

anorexia—loss of appetite; aversion to food

anorexiant—a drug, process, or event that leads to an aversion to food

anthropometry—the comparative measurements of various parts of the human body

Anthroposophic medicine—focus on management (herbal and homeopathic support) of acute limited inflammatory diseases in childhood as an alternative to vaccinations

auto-sanguis dilution therapy—form of homeopathy utilizing patient's own blood and homeopathic remedies to detoxify and stimulate the immune system

beriberi—a condition of polyneuritis and other disorders resulting from thiamine deficiency

biofeedback—technique based on the learning principle of association when information indicates that a specific thought or action produces a desired response

bolus—a soft mass of chewed food or a pharmaceutical preparation that is ready to be swallowed

cachexia—a state of general poor health and malnutrition during the course of a chronic disease or emotional disturbance

chiropractic—science that utilizes the recuperative powers of the body and the relationship between the musculoskeletal structures and functions of the body

dysentery—frequent watery stools, often with blood and mucous, characterized by pain, fever, dehydration, and tenesmus

emaciation—a wasted state of the body with extreme loss of flesh

enteral—of or relating to the intestinal tract

exogenous—originating or produced outside the organism

fomentation—application of warmth and moisture in the treatment of disease

gastric bypass—surgical formation of an anastomosis to the jejunum and closure of the distal portion of the stomach, used for treatment of morbid obesity

gastroplasty—surgical reconstruction of the stomach or lower esophagus utilizing the stomach wall

gastrostomy—establishment of an artificial opening into the stomach

gemmotherapy—plant-based homeopathy used in treatment of acne, asthma, headaches, eczema, hypertension and prostate dysfunction

hydrotherapy—use of water by external application, either for pressure effects or for application of physical energy to the tissues

hyperosmolarity—elevated osmolality of serum or plasma

hypertonic—describing a solution that has a greater osmotic pressure than another solution, usually greater than normal for a body fluid

hypnosis—an artificially induced trancelike state in which the subject is highly susceptible to suggestions

immunotherapy—stimulation and support of the immune system through specialized vaccines, diet, and individually tailored supplement programs and psychological counseling

jejunostomy—establishment of a permanent opening through the wall of the abdomen into the jejunum

kinesiology—the science or study of movement and the active and passive structures involved

lipogenesis—the process of conversion to fat in the body

malabsorption—impaired gastrointestinal absorption

micronutrients—those vitamins and minerals that the body requires in only small quantities

naturopathic medicine—naturopathy; a system of therapeutics depending primarily on natural or nonmedicinal forces

neural therapy—injection of anesthetics into scars or nerve ganglia for pain relief

nutrient—food or nourishment

osmolality—concentration of a solution expressed as per kilograms of solvent

osteomalacia—gradual softening of the bones

pellagra—a nutritional disease due to a deficiency of niacin, manifested by skin, gastrointestinal, and psychic disturbances

polymeric—having the properties of a polymer, a substance of high molecular weight

potentiation—concept used in chemotherapy of a degree of synergism that is greater than additive

potentization—successive geometric dilution of an active ingredient using a specialized mixing technique to produce less concentrated but more potent homeopathic medications

rickets—condition due to vitamin D deficiency with associated skeletal deformities and other disorders

scurvy—a disease due to a deficiency of vitamin C, marked by anemia, ulceration of the gums, and hemorrhages into the skin

substrate—the specific substance on which an enzyme acts

thermogenesis—the production of heat in the body

APPENDIX A

Medical Abbreviations

A	alive; ambulatory; apical; artery; assessment
A₂	aortic second sound
AA	amino acid; achievement age; active assistance; arm ankle (pulse ratio); authorized absence; auto accident; Alcoholics Anonymous
AAA	abdominal aortic aneurysmectomy/aneurysm
AAC	antibiotic agent-associated colitis
AAFP	American Academy of Family Physicians
AAL	anterior axillary line
AAMA	American Association of Medical Assistants
AAN	analgesic-associated nephropathy; analgesic abuse nephropathy; attending's admission notes
AAO × 3	awake and oriented to time, place and person
AAP	assessment adjustment pass; American Academy of Pediatrics
AAPA	American Academy of Physician Assistants
AAPC	antibiotic acquired pseudomembranous colitis
AAROM	active assistive range of motion
AAS	atlanto axis subluxation
AAV	adeno-associated virus
AAVV	accumulated alveolar ventilatory volume
Ab	abortion; antibody
A & B	apnea and bradycardia
ABC	airway, breathing, circulation; absolute band counts; artificial beta cells
ABCDE	botulism toxoid pentavalent
Abd	abdomen; abdominal
ABDCT	atrial bolus dynamic computer tomography
ABE	acute bacterial endocarditis
ABG	arterial blood gases
ABI	atherothrombotic brain infarction
ABL	allograft bound lymphocytes
ABLB	alternate binaural loudness balance
ABMT	autologous bone marrow transplantation
ABN	abnormality
Abnor.	abnormal
ABR	absolute bed rest; auditory brain (evoked) responses
ABS	at bedside; admitting blood sugar; absorption
ABT	aminopyrine breath test
ABW	actual body weight
ABx	antibiotics
AC	acute; before meals; acromio-clavicular; air conduction; air conditioned; assist control; abdominal circumference; anchored catheter

A/C	anterior chamber (of the eye)
ACA	anterior cerebral artery; acrodermatitis chronicum atrophicans; acute or chronic alcoholism
ACB	antibody-coated bacteria
AC & BC	air and bone conduction
ACBE	air contrast barium enema
ACC	accommodation; adenoid cystic carcinomas; administrative control center
ACD	anterior chest diameter; anterior chamber diameter; anemia of chronic disease; absolute cardiac duliness
ACEI	angiotensin-converting enzyme inhibitor
ACH	adrenal cortical hormone
ACI	aftercare instructions
ACL	anterior cruciate ligament
ACLS	advanced cardiac life support
ACPP-PF	acid phosphatase prostatic fluid
ACT	automated coagulation time; allergen challenge test
Act Ex	active exercise
ACOA	adult children of alcoholics
ACS	American Cancer Society; American College of Surgeons
ACTH	adrenocorticotropic hormone
ACTSEB	anterior chamber tube shunt encircling band
ACV	atrial/carotid/ventricular
A & D	admission and discharge
AD	Alzheimer's disease; right ear; accident dispensary
ADA	American Diabetes Association; American Dental Association
ADAU	adolescent drug abuse unit
ADCC	antibody-dependent cellular cytotoxicity
ADD	attention deficit disorder; adduction
ADDU	alcohol and drug dependence unit
ADEM	acute disseminating encephalomyelitis
ADH	antidiuretic hormone
ADHD	attention deficit hyperactivity disorder
ADL	activities of daily living
ad lib	as desired; at liberty
ADM	admission
adol	adolescent
ADPKD	autosomal dominant polycystic kidney
ADR	adverse drug reaction; acute dystonic reaction
ADP	adenosine diphosphate
ADS	anonymous donor's sperm; anatomical dead space
ADT	anticipate discharge tomorrow
ADX	adrenalectomy
AE	above elbow; air entry
AEC	at earliest convenience
AED	automated external defibrillator
AEG	air encephalogram
AER	acoustic evoked response; auditory evoked response
Aer. M	aerosol mask
Aer. T	aerosol tent
AES	anti-embolic stocking
AF	atrial fibrillation; acid-fast; amniotic fluid; anterior fontanel
AFB	acid-fast bacilli; aorto-femoral bypass

AFC	air filled cushions
A.fib	atrial fibrillation
AFO	ankle-foot orthosis
AFP	alpha-fetoprotein
AFV	amniotic fluid volume
AFVSS	afebrile, vital signs stable
A/G	albumin to globulin ratio
Ag	antigen
AG	anti-gravity; anion gap
AGA	acute gonococcal arthritis; appropriate for gestational age
AGD	agar gel diffusion
AGE	angle of greatest extension
AGF	angle of greatest flexion
AGG	agammaglobulinemia
aggl.	agglutination
AGL	acute granulocytic leukemia
AGN	acute glomerulonephritis
AGNB	aerobic gram-negative bacilli
AGPT	agar-gel precipitation test
AGS	adrenogenital syndrome
AH	airway hyperresponsiveness
AHA	autoimmune hemolytic anemia; American Heart/Hospital Association
AHC	acute hemorrhagic conjunctivitis; acute hemorrhagic cystitis
AHD	autoimmune hemolytic disease
AHF	antihemophilic factor
AHG	antihemophilic globulin
AHM	ambulatory Holter monitoring
AHT	autoantibodies to human thyroglobulin
AI	aortic insufficiency; artificial insemination; allergy index
A & I	Allergy and Immunology department
AI-Ab	anti-insulin antibody
AICA	anterior inferior communicating artery; anterior inferior cerebellar artery
AICD	automatic implantable cardioverter/defibrillator
AID	artificial insemination donor; automatic implantable defibrillator
AIDS	acquired immune deficiency syndrome
AIE	acute inclusion body encephalitis
AIF	aortic-iliac-femoral
AIH	artificial insemination with husband's sperm
AIHA	autoimmune hemolytic anemia
AILD	angioimmunoblastic lymphadenopathy
AIMS	abnormal involuntary movement scale; arthritis impact measure scale
AIN	acute interstitial nephritis
AINS	anti-inflammatory nonsteroidal
AION	anterior ischemic optic neuropathy
AIP	acute intermittent porphyria
AIR	accelerate idioventricular rhythm
AIVR	accelerated idioventricular rhythm
AJ	ankle jerk
AK	above knee
AKA	above knee amputation; alcoholic ketoacidosis; all known allergies
ALAT	alanine transaminase (alanine aminotransferase; SGPT)
Alb	albumin

ALC	acute lethal catatonia; alcohol
ALC R	alcohol rub
ALD	alcoholic liver disease; adrenoleukodystrophy
ALDOST	adosterone
ALFT	abnormal liver function tests
ALG	antilymphocyte globulin
alk	alkaline
ALK-P	alkaline phosphatase
ALL	acute lymphocytic leukemia
ALM	acral lentiginous melanoma
ALMI	anterolateral myocardial infarction
ALP	alkaline phosphatase
ALS	amyotrophic lateral sclerosis; acute lateral sclerosis; advanced life support
ALT	alanine aminotransferase (SGPT); Argon laser trabeculoplasty
ALWMI	anterolateral wall myocardial infarct
AM	myopic astigmatism; amalgam; morning
AMA	against medical advice; antimitochondrial antibody; American Medical Association
AMAP	as much as possible
A-MAT	amorphous material
Amb	ambulate; ambulatory
AMC	arm muscle circumference
AMD	age-related macular degeneration
AMegL	acute megokaryoblastic leukemia
AMG	acoustic myography
AMI	acute myocardial infarction
AML	acute myelogenous leukemia
AMM	agnogenic myeloid metaplasia
AMMOL	acute myelomonoblastic leukemia
amnio	amniocentesis
AMOL	acute monoblastic leukemia
AMP	amputation; ampule
A-M pr	Austin-Moore prosthesis
AMR	alternating motor rates
AMS	acute mountain sickness; amylase
AMV	assisted mechanical ventilation
AMSIT	A—appearance; M—mood; S—sensorium; I—intelligence; T—thought process (portion of the mental status examination)
amt	amount
AMY	amylase
ANA	antinuclear antibody; American Nurses/Neurologic Association
ANAD	anorexia nervosa and associated disorders
ANC	absolute neutrophil count
AND	anterior nasal discharge
anes	anesthesia
ANF	antinuclear factor; atrial natriuretic factor
ANG	angiogram
ANLL	acute nonlymphoblastic leukemia
ANOVA	analysis of variance
ANP	atrial natriuretic peptide
ANS	autonomic nervous system; answer
ant	anterior

ante	before
A & O	alert and oriented
AOA	American Optometric Association
AOAP	as often as possible
AOB	alcohol on breath
ao-il	aorta-iliac
AOC	area of concern
AODM	adult onset diabetes mellitus
AOM	acute otitis media
AOP	aortic pressure
A&O × 3	awake and oriented to person, place, and time
A&O × 4	awake and oriented to person, place, time and date
AOSD	adult onset Still's disease
A & P	auscultation and percussion; anterior and posterior; assessment and plans
AP	anterior-posterior; antepartum; apical pulse; abdominal-peritoneal; appendicitis
$A_2 > P_2$	second aortic sound greater than second pulmonic sound
APB	atrial premature beat; abductor pollicis brevis
APC	atrial premature contraction
APCD	adult polycystic disease
APD	automated peritoneal dialysis; atrial premature depolarization
APE	acute psychotic episode
APKD	adult onset polycystic kidney disease
APL	acute promyelocytic leukemia; abductor pollicis longus; accelerated painless labor; chorionic gonadotropin
appr	approximate
appt	appointment
APR	abdominoperineal resection
APTT	activated partial thromboplastin time
AQ	achievement quotient
aq	water
aq dist	distilled water
AR	aortic regurgitation
A & R	advised and released
A-R	apical-radial (pulse)
ARB	any reliable brand
ARC	AIDS-related complex; anomalous retinal correspondence
ARD	adult respiratory distress; acute respiratory disease; antibiotic removal device
ARDMS	American Registry of Diagnostic Medical Sonographers
ARDS	adult respiratory distress syndrome
ARF	acute renal failure; acute rheumatic fever; acute respiratory failure
ARLD	alcohol-related liver disease
ARM	artificial rupture of membranes
ARMD	age-related macular degeneration
AROM	active range of motion; artificial rupture of membranes
ARS	antirabies serum
ART	arterial; automated reagin test (for syphilis)
ARV	AIDS-related virus
AS	aortic stenosis; arteriosclerosis; anal sphincter; left ear; activated sleep; ankylosing spondylitis
ASA I	healthy patient with localized pathological process
ASA II	patient with mild to moderate systemic disease
ASA III	patient with severe systemic disease limiting activity but not incapacitating

ASA IV	patient with incapacitating systemic disease
ASA V	moribund patient not expected to live (American Society of Anesthesiologist classifications)
ASAA	acquired severe aplastic anemia
ASAP	as soon as possible
ASAT	aspartate transaminase (aspartate aminotransferase) (SGOT)
ASB	anesthesia standby; asymptomatic bacteriuria
ASC	altered state of consciousness; ambulatory surgery center
ASCP	American Society of Clinical Pathologists
ASCVD	arteriosclerotic cardiovascular disease
ASD	atrial septal defect
ASE	acute stress erosion
ASH	asymmetric septal hypertrophy
ASHD	arteriosclerotic heart disease
ASIS	anterior superior iliac spine
ASL	airway surface liquid
AsM	myopic astigmatism
ASMI	anteroseptal myocardial infarction
ASO	antistreptolysin-O titer; arteriosclerosis obliterans
ASOT	antistreptolysin-O titer
ASP	acute suppurative parotitis
ASS	anterior superior supine
AST	aspartic acid transaminase; astigmatism
ASTZ	antistreptozyme test
ASU	acute stroke unit
ASVD	arteriosclerotic vessel disease
AT	applanation tonometry; atraumatic; antithrombin
ATB	antibiotic
ATC	around the clock
ATD	autoimmune thyroid disease; antithyroid drug
AtFib	atrial fibrillation
ATG	antithymocyte globulin
ATgA	antithyroglobulin antibodies
ATHR	angina threshold heart rate
ATL	Achilles tendon lengthening; atypical lymphocytes; adult T-call leukemia
ATLS	advanced trauma life support
ATN	acute tubular necrosis
ATNC	atraumatic normocephalic
aTNM	autopsy staging of cancer
ATNR	asymmetrical tonic neck reflux
ATPS	ambient temperature and pressure; saturated with water vapor
ATR	Achilles tendon reflex; atrial
ATT	arginine tolerance test
AU	allergenic units; both ears
AUC	area under the curve
AV	arteriovenous; atrioventricular; auditory-visual
AVA	arteriovenous anastomosis
AVD	apparent volume of distribution
AVF	arteriovenous fistula
AVH	acute viral hepatitis
AVM	atriovenous malformation
AVN	atrioventricular node; arteriovenous nicking; avascular necrosis

AVR	aortic valve replacement
AVS	atriovenous shunt
AVSS	afebrile, vital signs stable
AVT	atypical ventricular tachycardia
A&W	alive and well
A waves	atrial contraction waves
AWI	anterior wall infarct
AWOL	absent without leave
ax	axillary
A-Z test	Aschheim-Zondek test; diagnostic test for pregnancy
B	bacillus; bands; bloody; black; both; buccal
Ba	barium
BA	backache; bile acid; blood alcohol; Bourns assist
BAC	blood alcohol content; buccoaxiocervical
BAD	bipolar affective disorder
BaE	barium enema
BAE	bronchial artery embolization
BAEP	brain stem auditory evoked potential
BAER	brain stem auditory evoked response
BAL	blood alcohol level; bronchoalveolar lavage
BAO	basal acid output
BAP	blood agar plate
baso.	basophil
BAVP	balloon aortic valvuloplasty
BB	bed bath; bowel or bladder; breakthrough bleeding; blood bank; blow bottle
BBA	born before arrival
BBB	bundle branch block; blood brain barrier
BBBB	bilateral bundle branch block
BBD	benign breast disease; biparietal diameter
BBM	banked breast milk
BBS	bilateral breath sounds
BBT	basal body temperature
BBVM	brush border vesicle membrane
BC	birth control; blood culture; bone conduction; Bourn control; bed and chair
BCA	balloon catheter angioplasty; basal cell atypia; brachiocephalic artery
BCAA	branched-chain amino acids
BCC	basal cell carcinoma
BCD	basal cell dysplasia
BCE	basal cell epithelioma
B cell	large lymphocyte
BCG	bacillus Calmette-Guérin vaccine
BCL	basic cycle length
BCP	birth control pills
BCS	battered child syndrome; Budd-Chiari syndrome
BD	birth defect; brain dead; bronchial drainage
BDAE	Boston Diagnostic Aphasia Examination
BDI SF	Beck's Depression Index—Short Form
BDR	background diabetic retinopathy
BE	barium enema; below elbow; bacterial endocarditis; base excess; bread equivalent
BEAM	brain electrical activity mapping
BEC	bacterial endocarditis

BEE	basal energy expenditure
BEI	butanol-extractable iodine
BEP	brainstem evoked potentials
BF	black female
BFO	balance forearm orthosis
BFP	biologic false positive
BFT	bentonite flocculation test
BFUE	erythroid burst-forming unit
BG	blood glucose
BGC	basal ganglion calcification
BGM	blood glucose monitoring
BHI	biosynthetic human insulin
BHN	bridging hepatic necrosis
BHR	bronchial hyperresponsiveness
BHS	beta-hemolytic streptococci
BI	bladder irritation; bowel impaction; bioelectric impedance
BIB	brought in by
BID	twice daily
BIG 6	analysis of 6 serum components
BIH	bilateral inguinal hernia; benign intracranial hypertension
bil	bilateral
BILAT SLC	bilateral short leg cast
BILAT SXO	bilateral salpingo-oophorectomy
bili	bilirubin
BILI-C	conjugated bilirubin
BIMA	bilateral internal mammary arteries
BIW	twice a week
BJ	bone and joint
BJE	bones, joints, and examination
BJM	bones, joints, and muscles
BJ protein	Bence-Jones protein
BK	below knee
BKA	below knee amputation
Bkg	background
BLB	Boothby-Lovelace-Bulbulian (oxygen mask)
bl cult	blood culture
BLE	both lower extremities
BLESS	bath, laxative, enema, shampoo, and shower
BLOBS	bladder obstruction
BLS	basic life support
B.L. unit	Bessey-Lowry unit
BM	basal metabolism; black male; bone marrow; bowel movement; breast milk
BMA	bone marrow aspirate
BMC	bone marrow cells
BMI	body mass index
BMJ	bones, muscles, joints
BMR	basal metabolic rate
BMT	bone marrow transplant; bilateral myringotomy tubes
BMTU	bone marrow transplant unit
BNO	bladder neck obstruction
BNR	bladder neck retraction
BO	body odor; bowel obstruction; behavior objective

BOA	born on arrival; born out of asepsis
BOM	bilateral otitis media
BOO	bladder outlet obstruction
BOT	base of tongue
BOW	bag of water
BP	blood pressure; bed pan; British Pharmacopeia
BPD	biparietal diameter; bronchopulmonary dysplasia
BPF	bronchopleural fistula
BPG	bypass graft
BPH	benign prostatic hypertrophy
BPM	breaths per minute; beats per minute
BPPV	benign paroxysmal positional vertigo
BPRS	Brief Psychiatric Rate Scale
BPSD	bronchopulmonary segmental drainage
BPV	benign paroxysmal vertigo
Bq	becquerel
BR	bathroom; bedrest; Benzing retrograde
BRAO	branch retinal artery occlusion
BRATT	bananas, rice, applesauce, tea, and toast
BRB	blood-retinal barrier
BRBPR	bright red blood per rectum
BRJ	brachial radialis jerk
BRM	biological response modifiers
BRP	bathroom privileges
BS	blood sugar; bowel sounds; breath sounds; bedside; before sleep
B & S	Bartholin and Skene (glands)
BSA	body surface area
BSB	body surface burned
BSC	bedside commode
BSE	breast self-examination; bovine spongiform encephalopathy
BSER	brainstem evoked responses
BSGA	beta Streptococcus group A
BSO	bilateral salpingo-oophorectomy
BSOM	bilateral serous otitis media
BSPM	body surface potential mapping
BSS	balanced salt solution; black silk sutures
BSU	Bartholin, Skene's, urethra
BT	bladder tumor; brain tumor; breast tumor; blood transfusion; bedtime; bituberous
BTB	breakthrough bleeding
BTFS	breast tumor frozen section
BTL	bilateral tubal ligation
BTPS	body temperature pressure saturated
BTR	bladder tumor recheck
BU	Bodansky unit
BUE	both upper extremities
BUN	blood urea nitrogen
BUR	backup rate (ventilator)
BUS	Bartholin, urethral and Skene's glands
BVL	bilateral vas ligation
BW	birth weight; body weight; body water
BWCS	bagged white cell study
BWFI	bacteriostatic water for injection

BWS	battered woman syndrome
Bx	biopsy
C	carbohydrate; Celsius; hundred; cyanosis; clubbing
C1	first cervical vertebra
C1 to C9	precursor molecules of the complement system
C-II	controlled substance, class 2
CA	cardiac arrest; carcinoma; carotid artery; chronologic age; coronary artery
C & A	Clinitest and Acetest
CAA	crystalline amino acids
CAB	coronary artery bypass
CABG	coronary artery bypass graft
CaBI	calcium bone index
CABS	coronary artery bypass surgery
CACI	computer-assisted continuous infusion
CAD	coronary artery disease
CAE	cellulose acetate electrophoresis
CAFT	Clinitron® air fluidized therapy
CAH	chronic active hepatitis; chronic aggressive hepatitis; congenital adrenal hyperplasia
CAL	calories; callus; chronic airflow limitation
CALD	chronic active liver disease
CALGB	Cancer and Leukemia Group B
CALLA	common acute lymphoblastic leukemia antigen
cAMP	cyclic adenosine monophosphate
CAN	cord around neck
CAO	chronic airway obstruction
CAP	capsule; compound action potentials
CAPD	chronic/continuous ambulatory peritoneal dialysis
CAR	cardiac ambulation routine
CARB	carbohydrate
CAS	carotid artery stenosis
CAT	computed axial tomography; children's apperception test; cataract
cath	catheter; catheterization
CAVB	complete atrioventricular block
CAVC	common atrioventricular canal
CAVH	continuous arteriovenous hemofiltration
CB	code blue; chronic bronchitis; cesarean birth; chair and bed
C & B	crown and bridge
CBA	chronic bronchitis and asthma
CBC	complete blood count
CBD	common bile duct; closed bladder drainage; cannabidiol
CBF	cerebral blood flow
CBFS	cerebral blood flow studies
CBFV	cerebral blood flow velocity
CBG	capillary blood glucose
CBI	continuous bladder irrigation
CBN	chronic benign neutropenia
CBR	complete bedrest; chronic bedrest; carotid bodies resected
CBS	chronic brain syndrome
CC	chief complaint; cubic centimeter; critical condition; creatinine clearance; cerebral concussion; chronic complainer; clean catch (urine); cord compression

CCA	common carotid artery
CCAP	capsule cartilage articular preservation
CC & C	colony count and culture
CCE	clubbing, cyanosis, and edema
CCF	compound comminuted fracture; crystal-induced chemostatic factor
CCG	Children's Cancer Group
CCHD	cyanotic congenital heart disease
CCI	chronic coronary insufficiency
CCMSU	clean catch midstream urine
CCNS	cell cycle nonspecific
C-collar	cervical collar
CCPD	continuous cycling/cyclical peritoneal dialysis
CCR	continuous complete remission
CCRU	critical care recovery unit
CCS	cell cycle specific; Cooperative Care Suite
CCT	congenitally corrected transposition
CCTGA	congenitally corrected transposition of the great arteries
CCTV	closed circuit television
CCU	coronary care unit
CCUP	colpocystourethropexy
CCX	complications
CD	Crohn's disease; cesarean delivery; continuous drainage
C/D	cup to disc ratio
C & D	cytoscopy and dilatation; curettage and desiccation
CDA	congenital dyserythropoietic anemia
CDAI	Crohn's Disease Activity Index
CDB	cough, deep breathe
CDC	Cancer Detection Center; Centers for Disease Control; calculated day of confinement
CDE	common duct exploration
CDH	congenital dysplasia of the hip; chronic daily headache
CDLE	chronic discoid lupus erythematosus
CDS	chronic dieting syndrome
cdyn	dynamic compliance
CE	cardiac enlargement; contrast echocardiology; central episiotomy; continuing education
CEA	carotid endarterectomy; carcinoembryonic antigen
CECT	contrast enhancement computed tomography
CEI	continuous extravascular infusion
CEP	congenital erythropoietic porphyria; countercurrent electrophoresis
CEPH	cephalic
CEPH Floc	cephalin flocculation
CE & R	central episiotomy and repair
CERA	cortical evoked response audiometry
CERV	cervical
CES	cognitive environmental stimulation
CF	cystic fibrosis; Caucasian female; complement fixation; cardiac failure; cancer-free; count fingers; Christmas factor; contractile force
CFA	common femoral artery; complete Freund's adjuvant
CFIDS	chronic fatigue and immune dysfunction syndrome
CFM	close fitting mask
CFP	cystic fibrosis protein

CFS	cancer family syndrome; chronic fatigue syndrome
CFT	complement fixation test
CF test	complement fixation test
CFU	colony forming units
CFU-S	colony forming unit—spleen
CG	cholecystogram
CGB	chronic gastrointestinal bleeding
CGD	chronic granulomatous disease
CGI	Clinical Global Impression (scale)
CGL	chronic granulocytic leukemia; with correction/with glasses
CGN	chronic glomerulonephritis
CGTT	cortisol glucose tolerance test
CH	child; chronic; chest; chief; crown-heel; convalescent hospital; cluster headache
CHAI	continuous hepatic artery infusion
CHB	complete heart block
CHD	congenital heart disease; childhood diseases
CHF	congestive heart failure; Crimean hemorrhagic fever
CHFV	combined high frequency of ventilation
CHI	closed head injury
CHO	carbohydrate
chol	cholesterol
chr	chronic
CHRS	congenital hereditary retinoschisis
CHS	Chédiak-Higashi syndrome
CHU	closed head unit
CI	cardiac index; cesium implant; complete iridectomy
Ci	curie(s)
CIA	chronic idiopathic anhidrosis
CIAED	collagen-induced autoimmune ear disease
CIB	cytomegalic inclusion bodies
CIBD	chronic inflammatory bowel disease
CIC	circulating immune complexes
CICE	combined intracapsular cataract extraction
CICU	cardiac intensive care unit
CID	cytomegalic inclusion disease
CIDP	chronic inflammatory demyelinating polyradineuropathy
CIDS	continuous insulin delivery system; cellular immunodeficiency syndrome
CIE	counterimmunoelectrophoresis; crossed immunoelectrophoresis
CIN	chronic interstitial nephritis; cervical intraepithelial neoplasia
Circ	circumcision; circumference; circulation
CIS	carcinoma *in situ*
CIU	chronic idiopathic urticaria
CJD	Creutzfeldt-Jakob disease
Ck	check; creatinine kinase
CK-MB	a creatine kinase isoenzyme
cl	cloudy
CL	critical list
CLA	community living arrangements
clav	clavicle
CLBBB	complete left bundle branch block
CLC	cork leather and celastic (orthotic)
CLD	chronic lung disease

CLF	cholesterol-lecithin flocculation
CLH	chronic lobular hepatitis
CLL	chronic lymphocytic leukemia
CLLE	columnar-lined lower esophagus
cl liq	clear liquid
CLO	cod liver oil; close
CL & P	cleft lip and palate
ClH	hepatic clearance
CLT	chronic lymphocytic thyroiditis
Cl VOID	clean voided specimen
clysis	hypodermoclysis
cm	centimeter
CM	Caucasian male; costal margin; continuous murmur; contrast media; centimeter; cochlear microphonics; culture media; common migraine
CMA	certified medical assistant
CMBBT	cervical mucous basal body temperature
CMC	chronic mucocutaneous moniliasis
CME	continuing medical education; cystoid macular edema
CMG	cystometrogram
CMHC	Community Mental Health Center
CMHN	Community Mental Health Nurse
CMI	cell-mediated immunity; Cornell Medical Index
CMJ	carpometacarpal joint
CMK	congenital multicystic kidney
CML	cell-mediated lympholysis; chronic myelogenous leukemia
CMM	cutaneous malignant melanoma
CMRNG	chromosomally resistant Neisseria gonorrhoeae
CMRO$_2$	cerebral metabolic rate for oxygen
CMS	circulation motion sensation
CMSUA	clean midstream urinalysis
CMT	chiropractic manipulative treatment
CMV	cytomegalovirus; cool mist vaporizer; controlled mechanical ventilation
CN	cranial nerve
CNA	chart not available
CNH	central neurogenic hyperpnea
CNP	continuous negative pressure ventilation
CNS	central nervous system; clinical nurse specialist
C/O	complains of; complaints; under care of
CO	cardiac output; carbon monoxide
Co	cobalt
CO$_2$	carbon dioxide
CoA	coarctation of the aorta
COAD	chronic obstructive airway disease; chronic obstructive arterial disease
COAG	chronic open angle glaucoma
COC	combination oral contraceptive
COD	cause of death
COEPS	cortically originating extrapyramidal symptoms
COG	cognitive function tests; Central Oncology Group
COH	carbohydrate
Coke	Coca-Cola
Collyr	eye wash
col/ml	colonies per milliliter

COLD	chronic obstructive lung disease
COLD A	cold agglutinin titer
COMP	complications; compound
conc	concentrated
CONG	congenital
COPD	chronic obstructive pulmonary disease
COPE	chronic obstructive pulmonary emphysema
cor	coronary
CORF	comprehensive outpatient rehabilitation facility
COT	content of thought
COTX	cast off to X ray
COU	cardiac observation unit
CP	cerebral palsy; cleft palate; creatine phosphokinase; chest pain; chronic pain; chondromalacia patella
C & P	cystoscopy and pyelography
CPA	costophrenic angle; cardiopulmonary arrest; cerebellar pontile angle
CPAF	chlorpropamide-alcohol flush
CPAP	continuous positive airway pressure
CPB	cardiopulmonary bypass
CPBA	competitive protein-binding assay
CPC	clinicopathologic conference; cerebral palsy clinic
CPCR	cardiopulmonary-cerebral resuscitation
CPD	chorioretinopathy and pituitary dysfunction; cephalopelvic disproportion; chronic peritoneal dialysis
CPDD	calcium pyrophosphate deposition disease
CPE	chronic pulmonary emphysema; cardiogenic pulmonary edema
CPGN	chronic progressive glomerulonephritis
CPH	chronic persistent hepatitis
CPI	constitutionally psychopathia inferior
CPID	chronic pelvic inflammatory disease
CPK	creatinine phosphokinase
CPKD	childhood polycystic kidney disease
CPM	central pontine myelinolysis; continuous passive motion; continue present management; counts per minute
CPmax	peak serum concentration
CPmin	trough serum concentration
CPN	chronic pyelonephritis
CPP	cerebral perfusion pressure
CPPB	continuous positive pressure breathing
CPPV	continuous positive pressure ventilation
CPR ·	cardiopulmonary resuscitation
CPS	complex partial seizures
CPT	chest physiotherapy
CPTH	chronic posttraumatic headache
Cr	creatinine
CR	cardiorespiratory; controlled release; cardiac rehabilitation; colon resection; closed reduction; complete remission
CRA	central retinal artery
CRAO	central retinal artery occlusion
CRBBB	complete right bundle branch block
CRC	colorectal cancer
CrCl	creatinine clearance

CRD	chronic renal disease
CREST	calcinosis, Raynaud's phenomenon, esophageal dysmotility, sclerodactyly and telangiectasia
CRF	chronic renal failure; corticotropin-releasing factor
CRI	chronic renal insufficiency
CRIE	crossed radioimmuno-electrophoresis
crit	hematocrit
CRL	crown rump length
CRO	cathode ray oscilloscope
CRP	C-reactive protein
CRPF	chloroquine-resistant plasmodium falciparum
CRST	calcification, Raynaud's phenomenon, scleroderma, and telangiectasia
CRT	copper reduction test; cathode ray tube; central reaction time; cadaver renal transplant
CrTr	crutch training
CRTX	cast removed take X ray
CRUMBS	continuous remove, unobtrusive monitoring of biobehavioral systems
CRVO	central retinal vein occlusion
CS	coronary sclerosis; central supply; clinical stage; conjunctiva-sclera; consciousness; cat scratch
C & S	culture and sensitivity
C/S	cesarean section; culture and sensitivity
CSBF	coronary sinus blood flow
CSC	cornea, sclera, conjunctiva
CS & CC	culture, sensitivity, and colony count
CSD	cat scratch disease
CSE	cross section echocardiography
C sect	cesarean section
CSF	cerebrospinal fluid; colony-stimulating factor
C-Sh	chair shower
CSH	carotid sinus hypersensitivity
CSICU	cardiac surgery intensive care unit
CSH	continuous subcutaneous insulin infusion
CS IV	clinical stage 4
CSLU	chronic status leg ulcer
CSM	circulation, sensation, movement; cerebrospinal meningitis
CSOM	chronic serous otitis media
CSP	cellulose sodium phosphate
CSR	Cheyne-Stokes respiration; central supply room; corrective septorhinoplasty
CST	convulsive shock therapy; contraction stress test; cosyntropin stimulation test; certified surgical technologist
CSU	cardiac surveillance unit; cardiovascular surgery unit
CT	computed tomography; circulation time; coagulation time; clotting time; corneal thickness; cervical traction; Coomb's test; cardiothoracic; coated tablet
Cta	catamenia (menses)
CTA	clear to auscultation
CTB	ceased to breathe
CT & DB	cough, turn, and deep breathe
CTD	chest tube drainage; cumulative trauma disorder
CTF	Colorado tick fever
CTL	cytotoxic T lymphocytes
CT/MPR	computed tomography with multiplanar reconstructions

cTNM	clinical-diagnostic staging of cancer
CTP	comprehensive treatment plan
CTR	carpal tunnel release
CTS	carpal tunnel syndrome
CTSP	called to see patient
CTW	central terminal of Wilson
CTXN	contraception
CTZ	chemoreceptor trigger zone
Cu	copper
CU	cause unknown
CUC	chronic ulcerative colitis
CUD	cause undetermined
CUG	cystourethrogram
CUS	chronic undifferentiated schizophrenia
CUSA	Cavitron® ultrasonic aspirator
CV	cardiovascular; cell/closing volume
CVA	cerebrovascular accident; costovertebral angle
CVAT	costovertebral angle tenderness
CVC	central venous catheter
CVD	collagen vascular disease
CVI	cerebrovascular insufficiency; continuous venous infusion
CVID	common variable immune deficiency
CVO	central vein occlusion; conjugate diameter of pelvic inlet
CVP	central venous pressure
CVRI	coronary vascular resistance index
CVS	clean voided specimen; cardiovascular system; chorionic villus sampling
CVUG	cysto-void urethrogram
C/W	consistent with; crutch walking
CWE	cottonwool exudates
CWMS	color, warmth, movement sensation
CWP	coal worker's pneumoconiosis
CWS	cotton wool spots
Cx	cervix; culture; cancel
CxMT	cervical motion tenderness
CXR	chest X ray
CYSTO	cystoscopy; cystogram
CZI	crystalline zinc insulin
D	diarrhea; day; divorced; distal; dead; right; diopter
D1,D2	dorsal vertebra #1, #2
DA	direct admission
DAD	drug administration device
DAF	decay-accelerating factor
DAI	diffuse axonal injury
DAH	disordered action of the heart
DAL	drug analysis laboratory
DANA	drug-induced antinuclear antibodies
DAPT	draw-a-person test
DAT	direct agglutination test; diet as tolerated; dementia of the Alzheimer type
DAW	dispense as written
DAWN	Drug Abuse Warning Network
dB	decibel

DB	date of birth
DB & C	deep breathing and coughing
DBE	deep breathing exercise
DBIL	direct bilirubin
DBP	diastolic blood pressure
DBS	diminished breath sounds
D & C	dilation and curettage
DC, d/c	discontinue; discharge; decrease; diagonal conjugate; Doctor of Chiropractic
DCH	delayed cutaneous hypersensitivity
DCO	diffusing capacity of carbon monoxide
DCR	delayed cutaneous reaction
DCSA	double contrast shoulder arthrography
DCT	direct (antiglobulin) Coombs test; deep chest therapy
DCTM	delay computer tomographic myelography
DD	differential diagnosis; down drain; dependent drainage; dry dressing; Duchenne's dystrophy
D & D	diarrhea and dehydration
DDD	degenerative disc disease; dense deposit (renal) disease
DDS	dialysis disequilibrium syndrome; Doctor of Dental Surgery
DDST	Denver Development Screening Test
DDx	differential diagnosis
D & E	dilation and evacuation
DEC	decrease
decub	decubitus
DEF	decayed, extracted, or filled
degen	degenerative
del	delivery, delivered
DEP ST SEG	depressed ST segment
DER	disulfiram-ethanol reaction
DES	disequilibrium syndrome; diffuse esophageal spasm
DEV	duck embryo vaccine; deviation
DEVR	dominant exudative vitreoretinopathy
dex.	dexter (right)
DEXA	dual energy X-ray absorptiometry
DF	decayed and filled
DFD	defined formula diets
DFE	distal femoral epiphysis
DFMC	daily fetal movement count
DFR	diabetic floor routine
DFU	dead fetus in uterus
DGI	disseminated gonococcal infection
DGM	ductal glandular mastectomy
DH	developmental history; diaphragmatic hernia; delayed hypersensitivity
DHBV	duck hepatitis B virus
DHF	dengue hemorrhagic fever
DHHS	Department of Health and Human Services
DHL	diffuse histiocytic lymphoma
DHS	duration of hospital stay
DI	diabetes insipidus; detrusor instability
diag	diagnosis
Diath SW	diathermy short wave
DIC	Drug Information Center; disseminated intravascular coagulation

DIE	die in emergency department
DIFF	differential blood count
DIJOA	dominantly inherited juvenile optic atrophy
dil	dilute
DILD	diffuse infiltrative lung disease
DILE	drug-induced lupus erythematosus
dim	diminish
DIMOAD	diabetes insipidus, diabetes mellitus, optic atrophy, and deafness
DIP	distal interphalangeal; desquamative interstitial pneumonia; drip infusion pyelogram
dis	dislocation
DIS	Diagnostic Interview Schedule questionnaire
disch	discharge
DISH	diffuse idiopathic skeletal hyperostosis
dist	distilled
DIV	double inlet ventricle
DIVA	digital intravenous angiography
DJD	degenerative joint disease
DK	diabetic ketoacidosis; dark
DKA	diabetic ketoacidosis
dl	deciliter
DL	danger list; deciliter; direct laryngoscopy; diagnostic laparoscopy
DLE	discoid lupus erythematosus
DLIS	digitalis-like immunoreactive substance
DLMP	date of last menstrual period
DLNMP	date of last normal menstrual period
DM	diabetes mellitus; diastolic murmur; dermatomyositis
DMARD	disease-modifying antirheumatic drug
DMD	Duchenne's muscular dystrophy
DME	durable medical equipment
DMF	decayed, missing, or filled
DMKA	diabetes mellitus ketoacidosis
DMOOC	diabetes mellitus out of control
DMX	diathermy, massage, and exercise
DN	down
DNI	do not intubate
DNKA	did not keep appointment
DNP	do not publish
DNR	do not resuscitate/report
DNS	do not show; deviated nasal septum; dysplastic nevus syndrome
DO	right eye; Doctor of Osteopathy
DOA	dead on arrival; date of admission
DOA-DRA	dead on arrival, despite resuscitative attempts
DOB	date of birth; doctor's order book
DOC	drug of choice; died of other causes
DOE	dyspnea on exertion
DOI	date of injury
DOLV	double outlet left ventricle
DORV	double outlet right ventricle
DORx	date of treatment
DOT	Doppler ophthalmic test; died on table
DP	dorsalis pedis (pulse); diastolic pressure

DPC	discharge planning coordinator; delayed primary closure
DPDL	diffuse poorly differentiated lymphocytic lymphoma
DPM	disintegrations per minute; Doctor of Podiatric Medicine
DPN	diabetic peripheral neuropathy
DPT	diphtheria, pertussis, tetanus
DPV	delayed pressure urticaria
DR	delivery room; diabetic retinopathy
DREZ	dorsal root entry zone
DRG	diagnosis-related groups
DRSG	dressing
DS	discharge summary; Down's syndrome; double strength; disoriented; dextrose stick
DSA	digital subtraction angiography
DSAP	disseminated superficial actinic porokeratosis
DSD	dry sterile dressing; discharge summary dictated
dsg	dressing
DSI	deep shock insulin
DSIAR	double-stapled ileoanal reservoir
DSM	drink skim milk; Diagnostic & Statistical Manual
DSS	dengue shock syndrome
DST	dexamethasone suppression test; donor specific transfusion
DT	delirium tremens; discharge tomorrow
DTD #30	dispense 30 such doses
DTH	delayed-type hypersensitivity
DTR	deep tendon reflexes
DTs	delirium tremens
DTS	donor specific transfusion
DTT	diphtheria tetanus toxoid
DTV	due to void
DTX	detoxification
DU	duodenal ulcer; duroxide uptake; diabetic urine; diagnosis undetermined
DUB	dysfunctional uterine bleeding
DUE	drug use evaluation
DUI	driving under the influence
DUR	drug utilization review
DVD	dissociated vertical deviation
DVIU	direct vision internal urethrotomy
DVR	double valve replacement
DVT	deep vein thrombosis
DW	dextrose in water; distilled water; deionized water
DWDL	diffuse, well-differentiated lymphocytic lymphoma
Dx	diagnosis
Dz	disease; dozen
E	edema
4E	4 plus edema
E>A	say EEE, comes out as A,A,A upon auscultation of lung, showing consolidation
EAA	electrothermal atomic absorption
EAC	external auditory canal
EAHF	eczema, allergy, hay fever
EAM	external auditory meatus
EAR	early asthmatic response

EAST	external rotation, abduction stress test
EAT	ectopic atrial tachycardia
EB	epidermolysis bullosa
EBL	estimated blood loss
EBV	Epstein-Barr virus
EC	enteric coated; eyes closed; extracellular
ECBD	exploration of common bile duct
ECC	emergency cardiac care docervical curettage
ECCE	extracapsular cataract extraction
ECD	endocardial cushion defect
ECEMG	evoked compound electromyography
ECF	extracellular fluid; extended care facility; eosinophilic chemotactic factor
ECG	electrocardiogram
ECHO	echocardiogram
ECL	extent of cerebral lesion; extracapillary lesions
ECM	erythema chronicum migrans
ECMO	extracorporeal membrane oxygenation
ECN	extended care nursery
ECR	emergency chemical restraint
ECRL	extensor carpi radialis longus
ECT	electroconvulsive therapy; enhanced computer tomography; emission computed tomography
ECU	extensor carpi ulnaris
ECW	extracellular water
ED	emergency department; epidural
ED50	median effective dose
EDC	estimated date of confinement; estimated date of conception; end diastolic counts; digitorum communis
EDD	expected date of delivery
EDF	extension, derotation, flexion
EDM	early diastolic murmur
EDS	Ehlers-Danlos syndrome
EDV	end-diastolic volume
EE	equine encephalitis; end to end
EEE	Eastern equine encephalomyelitis; edema, erythema, and exudate
EEG	electroencephalogram
EENT	eyes, ears, nose, throat
EF	extended-field (radiotherapy); endurance factor; ejection fraction
EFAD	essential fatty acid deficiency
EFE	endocardial fibroelastosis
EFM	external fetal monitoring
EFW	estimated fetal weight
EGA	estimated gestational age
EGBUS	external genitalia, Bartholin, urethral, Skene's glands
EGD	esophagogastroduodenoscopy
EGF	epidermal growth factor
EGTA	esophageal gastric tube airway
EH	essential hypertension; enlarged heart; extramedullary hematopoiesis
EHB	elevate head of bed
EHF	epidemic hemorrhagic fever
E & I	endocrine and infertility
EIA	exercise-induced asthma; enzyme immunoassay

EIAB	extracranial-intracranial arterial bypass
EIB	exercise-induced bronchospasm
EID	electronic infusion device
EIF	eukaryotic initiation factor
EIS	endoscopic injection scleropathy
EJ	external jugular; elbow jerk
EKC	epidemic keratoconjunctivitis
EKG	electrocardiogram
EKY	electrokymogram
E-L	external lids
ELF	elective low forceps
ELH	endolymphatic hydrops
ELISA	enzyme-linked immunosorbent assay
elix	elixir
ELOP	estimated length of program
ELP	electrophoresis
EM	electron microscope; ejection murmur; erythema multiforme
EMB	endomyocardial biopsy
EMC	encephalomyocarditis
EMD	electromechanical dissociation
EMF	erythrocyte maturation factor; evaporated milk formula; electromotive force
EMG	electromyography; essential monoclonal gammopathy
EMIC	emergency maternity and infant care
E-MICR	electron microscopy
EMIT	enzyme multiplied immunoassay technique
EMR	emergency mechanical restraint; empty, measure and record; educable mentally retarded
EMS	emergency medical services/systems
EMT	emergency medical technician
EMV	eye, motor, verbal
EMW	electromagnetic waves
ENA	extractable nuclear antigen
ENDO	endotracheal
ENG	electronystagmography
ENL	erythema nodosum leprosum
ENP	extractable nucleoprotein
ENT	ears, nose, throat
EO	eyes open
EOA	examine, opinion, and advice; esophageal obturator airway
EOG	electro-oculogram; Ethrane®, oxygen, and gas
EOM	extraocular movement; extraocular muscles
EOMI	extraocular muscles intact
EORA	elderly onset rheumatoid arthritis
eos	eosinophil
EP	endogenous pyrogen; electrophysiologic
EPA	eicosapentaenoic acid
EPB	extensor pollicis brevis
EPIS	episiotomy
epith	epithelial
EPL	extensor pollicis longus
EPM	electronic pacemaker
EPO	recombinant human erythropoietin

EPP	erythropoietic protoporphyria
EPR	electrophrenic respiration; emergency physical restraint
EPS	electrophysiologic study; extrapyramidal syndrome/symptoms
EPT®	early pregnancy test
EPTS	existed prior to service
ER	emergency room; estrogen receptor; external rotation
ERA	evoked response audiometry; estrogen receptor assay
ERCP	endoscopic retrograde cholangiopancreatography
ERFC	erythrocyte rosette forming cells
ERG	electroretinogram
ERL	effective refractory length
ERP	estrogen receptor protein; endoscopic retrograde pancreatography
ERPF	effective renal plasma flow
ERPS	event-related potentials
ERT	estrogen replacement therapy
ERV	expiratory reserve volume
ESAP	evoked sensory (nerve) action potentiation
ESC	end systolic counts
ESM	ejection systolic murmur
ESP	end systolic pressure
ESR	erythrocyte sedimentation rate; electric skin resistance
ESRD	end-stage renal disease
ess	essential
EST	electroshock therapy
ESWL	extracorporeal shockwave lithotripsy
ET	endotracheal; esotropia; eustachian tube; ejection time; exercise treadmill
et	and
et al	and others
ETF	eustachian tubal function
ETO	estimated time of ovulation
ETS	environmental tobacco smoke
ETT	endotracheal tube; exercise tolerance test
EU	excretory urography
EUA	examine under anesthesia
EUS	endoscopic ultrasonography
EVAC	evacuation
eval	evaluate
EWB	estrogen withdrawal bleeding
EWSCLs	extended-wear soft contact lenses
exam	examination
EXP	exploration; experienced
exp lap	exploratory laparotomy
ext	extract; external
ext rot	external rotation
EX U	excretory urogram
F	Fahrenheit; female; flow; facial; firm; French
F1	offspring from first generation
F2	offspring from second generation
FA	folic acid; femoral artery
FAAP	family assessment adjustment pass
FAC	fractional area concentration

FACH	forceps to after-coming head
FACS	Fellow of the American College of Surgeons
FAD	Family Assessment Device
FAI	functional assessment inventory
FALL	fallopian
FAM	family
FANA	fluorescent antinuclear antibody
FAP	fibrillating action potential; familial amyloid polyneuropathy; familial adenomatous polyposis
FAS	fetal alcohol syndrome
FAST	functional assessment staging (of Alzheimer's disease); fluoro-allegro sorbent test; fetal acoustical stimulation test
FAT	fluorescent antibody test
FB	fasting blood sugar; foreign body; finger breadth
FBG	fasting blood glucose
FBM	fetal breathing movements
FBN	fibronectin
FBP	fetal biophysical profile
FBS	fasting blood sugar; fetal bovine serum
FBU	fingers below umbilicus
FBW	fasting blood work
FC	Foley catheter; finger counting; fever, chills
F+C	flare and cells
F & C	foam and condom
F cath	Foley catheter
FCC	follicular center cells; familial colonic cancer; fracture compound comminuted
FCDB	fibrocystic disease of the breast
FCH	familial combined hyperlipidemia
FCMC	family-centered maternity care
FCMD	Fukuyama's congenital muscular dystrophy
FCMN	family-centered maternity nursing
FCP	flow cytometric platelet crossmatching
FCR	flexor carpi radialis
FCRB	flexor carpi radialis brevis
FCSNVD	fever, chills, sweating, nausea, vomiting, diarrhea
FCU	flexor carpi ulnaris
FD	focal distance; familial dysautonomia
F & D	fixed and dilated
FDA	fronto-dextra anterior
FDIU	fetal death in utero
FDP	fibrin-degradation products; flexor digitorum profundus
FDS	flexor digitorum superficialis; for duration of stay
Fe	iron; female
FEC	forced expiratory capacity
FEF	forced expiratory flow
FEL	familial erythrophagocytic lymphohistiocytosis
FEM	femoral
Fem-pop	femoral popliteal (bypass)
FEN	fluid, electrolytes, nutrition
FENa	fractional extraction of sodium
FEP	free erythrocyte protoporphyrin
FEV	forced expiratory volume

FF	filtration fraction; fundus firm; flat feet; fat free; force fluids
FFA	free fatty acid
F factor	fertility/sex factor
FFP	fresh frozen plasma
FFT	fast-Fourier transforms
FGF	fibroblast growth factor
FH	family history; fetal heart; fundal height
FHF	fulminant hepatic failure
FHH	familial hypocalciuric hypercalcemia
FHI	Fuchs heterochromic iridocyclitis
FHR	fetal heart rate
FHS	fetal heart sounds; fetal hydantoin syndrome
FHT	fetal heart tone
FiCO$_2$	fraction of inspired carbon dioxide
FIM	functional independent measure
FiO$_2$	fraction of inspired oxygen
FL	fluid
FLK	funny looking kid
FLS	flashing lights and/or scotoma
FM	fetal movements; face mask
F & M	firm and midline (uterus)
FMC	fetal movement count
FMD	foot and mouth disease
FME	full mouth extraction
FMF	forced midexpiratory flow; familial Mediterranean fever
FMG	foreign medical graduate; fine mesh gauze
FMH	family medical history; fibromuscular hyperplasia
FMP	fasting metabolic panel
FMX	full mouth X ray
FN	false negative; finger-to-nose
FNAB	fine-needle aspiration biopsy
FNAC	fine-needle aspiration cytology
FNCJ	fine needle catheter jejunostomy
FNH	focal nodular hyperplasia; febrile nonhemolytic reaction
FNR	false negative rate
FNS	functional neuromuscular stimulation
FOB	foot of bed; fiberoptic bronchoscope; father of baby
FOBT	fecal occult blood test
FOC	father of child
FOD	free of disease
FOI	flight of ideas
FOOB	fell out of bed
FP	family planning; family practice; frozen plasma; flat plate; false positive
FPAL	full-term, premature, abortion, living
FPB	flexor pollicis brevis
FPD	feto-pelvic disproportion; fixed partial denture
FPG	fasting plasma glucose
FPIA	fluorescence-polarization immunoassay
FPL	flexor pollicis longus
FPNA	first-pass nuclear angiocardiography
FR	flow rate
F & R	flow and rhythm (pulse)

FRC	functional residual capacity
FRJM	full range of joint motion
FROM	full range of movement
FS	frozen section; flexible sigmoidoscopy
FSB	fetal scalp blood
FSBM	full-strength breast milk
FSE	fetal scalp electrode
FSG	focal and segmental
FSGS	focal and segmental glomerulosclerosis
FSH	follicle stimulating hormone; facioscapulohumeral
FSHMD	facioscapulohumeral muscular dystrophy
FSHRF	follicle stimulating hormone releasing factor
FSP	fibrin split products
FT	full term
FTA	fluorescent treponemal/titer antibody
FTD	failure to descend
FTI	free thyroxine index
FTLFC	full-term living female child
FTLMC	full-term living male child
FTN	finger-to-nose; full-term nursery
FTND	full-term normal delivery
FTP	failure to progress
FTR	for the record
FTSG	full-thickness skin graft
FTT	failure to thrive
F & U	flanks and upper quadrants
F/U	followup; fundus at umbilicus
FUB	functional uterine bleeding
FUN	followup note
FUO	fever of undetermined origin
FVC	forced vital capacity
FVH	focal vascular headache
FVL	flow volume loop
FWB	full weight bearing
FWS	fetal warfarin syndrome
FWW	front wheel walker
Fx	fracture; fractional urine
Fx-dis	fracture-dislocation
FXN	function
FXR	fracture
G	gauge; gravida; gram; gallop
G1-4	grade 1–4
GA	gastric analysis; general appearance; general anesthesia; gestational age
GABA	gamma-aminobutyric acid
GABHS	group A beta hemolytic streptococci
GAD	generalized anxiety disorder
GAF	Global Assessment of Functioning (Scale)
GAS	general adaptation syndrome
GAT	group adjustment therapy
GB	gallbladder
GBM	glomerular basement membrane

GBP	gastric bypass
GBS	gallbladder series; Guillain-Barré syndrome; group B streptococci
GC	gonococci (gonorrhea); geriatric chair
G− C	gram-negative cocci
G+C	gram-positive cocci
GCA	giant cell arteritis
GCDFP	gross cystic disease fluid protein
GCIIS	glucose control insulin infusion system
GCS	Glasgow coma scale
GCT	giant cell tumor
GD	Graves disease
G & D	growth and development
GDF	gel diffusion precipitin
GDM	gestational diabetes mellitus
GE	gastroenteritis
GEP	gastroenteropancreatic
GER	gastroesophageal reflux
GERD	gastroesophageal reflux disease
GETA	general endotracheal anesthesia
GF	grandfather; gluten-free; gastric fistula
GFR	glomerular filtration rate
GG	gamma globulin
GGE	generalized glandular enlargement
GGT	gamma glutamyl transpeptidase
GGTP	gamma glutamyl transpeptidase
GH	growth hormone; glycosylated hemoglobin
GHb	glycosylated hemoglobin
GHD	growth hormone deficiency
GHQ	general health questionnaire
GI	gastrointestinal; granuloma inguinale
GIB	gastric ileal bypass
GIC	general immunocompetence
GIFT	gamete intrafallopian treatment
GIP	giant cell interstitial pneumonia; gastric inhibitory peptide
GIS	gastrointestinal series
GIT	gastrointestinal tract
GJ	gastrojejunostomy
GL	greatest length
GLA	gingivolinguoaxial
GLNH	giant lymph node hyperplasia
GM	gram; grandmother
GMC	general medicine clinic
GMTs	geometric mean antibody titers
GN	glomerulonephritis; gram-negative; graduate nurse
GnRH	gonadotropin-releasing hormone
GOT	glucose oxidase test
GP	general practitioner; gutta percha
G/P	gravida/para
GPC	gram-positive cocci; giant papillary conjunctivitis
G6PD	glucose-6-phosphate dehydrogenase
GPMAL	gravida, para, multiple births, abortions, and live births
GPN	graduate practical nurse

gr	grain
G−R	gram-negative rods
G+R	gram-positive rods
grav	gravid (pregnant)
GRD	gastroesophageal reflux disease
GRN	granules
GSC	Glasgow coma scale
GSD	glycogen storage disease
GSD-1	glycogen storage disease, type 1
GSE	grip strong and equal; gluten sensitive enteropathy
GSI	genuine stress incontinence
GSP	general survey panel
GSPN	greater superficial petrosal neurectomy
GSR	galvanic skin resistance
GSW	gunshot wound
GT	gastrotomy tube; gait training
GTN	gestational trophoblastic neoplasms
GTT	glucose tolerance test; drop
GU	genitourinary
GUS	genitourinary sphincter; genitourinary system
GVF	good visual fields
GVHD	graft-versus-host disease
G & W	glycerin and water
GW	glucose in water
GWA	gunshot wound of the abdomen
GWT	gunshot wound of the throat
GXT	graded exercise testing
GYN	gynecology
H	hypodermic; hydrogen; hour; husband
H2	histamine
HA	headache; hyperalimentation; hypothalamic amenorrhea; hearing aid; hemolytic anemia; hospital admission; hepatitis, type A; hemagglutination assay
HAA	hepatitis-associated antigen
HAE	hereditary angioedema; hepatic artery embolization; hearing aid evaluation
HAI	hepatic arterial infusion
HAL	hyperalimentation
HAN	heroin associated nephropathy
HANE	heredity angioneurotic edema
HAPS	hepatic arterial perfusion scintigraphy
HAQ	Headache/Health Assessment Questionnaire
HAS	hyperalimentation solution
HASHD	hypertensive arteriosclerotic heart disease
HAT	head, arms, and trunk
HAV	hepatitis A virus; hallux abducto valgus
HB	hemoglobin; heart block; hepatitis, type B; hold breakfast
HBBW	hold breakfast blood work
HBD	has been drinking
HBGM	home blood glucose monitoring
HBI	hemibody irradiation
HBIG	hepatitis B immune globulin
HbAIc	glycosylated hemoglobin

HBF	hepatic blood flow
HBO	hyperbaric oxygen
HBP	high blood pressure
HBS	Health Behavior Scale
HBsAg	hepatitis B surface antigen
HBV	hepatitis B virus; hepatitis B vaccine; honeybee venom
HC	home care; head circumference; heel cord; house call; Hickman catheter
HCA	health care aide
HCC	hepatocellular carcinoma
HCFA	Health Care Financing Administration
HCG	human chorionic gonadotropin
HCL	hair cell leukemia
HCLs	hard contact lenses
HCM	health care maintenance; hypertropic cardiomyopathy
HCP	hereditary coprophemia
HCT	hematocrit; histamine challenge test
HCV	hepatitis C virus
HCVD	hypertensive cardiovascular disease
HD	Hodgkin's disease; Huntington's disease; hearing distance; hemodialysis; heloma mole; hip disarticulation; high dose
HDC	high-dose chemotherapy
HDCV	human diploid cell vaccine
HDL	high-density lipoprotein
HDLW	hearing distance for watch in left ear
HDRW	hearing distance for watch in right ear
HDN	hemolytic disease of the newborn
HDPAA	heparin-dependent, platelet-associated antibody
HDRS	Hamilton Depression Rate Scale
HDV	hepatitis D virus
H & E	hemorrhage and exudate; hematoxylin and eosin
HEENT	head, eyes, ears, nose, and throat
HEK	human embryonic kidney
HEL	human embryonic lung
hemi	hemiplegia
HEMPAS	hereditary erythrocytic multinuclearity with positive acidified serum test
HEP	histamine equivalent prick; hepatic
HES	hypereosinophilic syndrome
HEV	hepatitis E virus
HF	heart failure
HFD	high forceps delivery
HFHL	high frequency hearing loss
Hbg	hemoglobin
HGH	human growth hormone
HH	hiatal hernia; hypogonadotropic hypogonadism; home health; hard of hearing
H & H	hematocrit and hemoglobin
HHC	home health care
HHD	hypertensive heart disease
HHFM	high-humidity face mask
HHN	hand-held nebulizer
HHNK	hyperglycemic hyperosmolar nonketotic (coma)
HHT	hereditary hemorrhagic telangiectasis
HHV-6	human herpes virus 6

HI	hemagglutination inhibition; head injury
HIA	hemagglutination inhibition antibody
HIB	Haemophilus influenzae type B (vaccine)
HID	headache, insomnia, depression
HIE	hypoxic-ischemic encephalopathy
HIF	higher integrative functions
HIL	hypoxic-ischemic lesion
HIR	head injury routine
HIS	Health Intention Scale
Histo	histoplasmin skin test
HIT	heparin-induced thrombocytopenia; histamine inhalation test
HIV	human immunodeficiency virus
HIVD	herniated intervertebral disc
HJR	hepato-jugular reflex
H-K	hand to knee
HKAFO	hip-knee-ankle-foot orthosis
HKO	hip-knee orthosis
HL	heparin lock; harelip; hairline; hearing level; Hickman line
HLA	human lymphocyte/leukocyte antigen
HLD	herniated lumbar disc
HLHS	hypoplastic left heart syndrome
HLV	hypoplastic left ventricle
HM	hand motion
HMD	hyaline membrane disease
HMG	human menopausal gonadotropin
HMI	healed myocardial infarction
HMO	health maintenance organization
HMP	hot moist packs
HMR	histiocytic medullary reticulosis
HMX	heat massage exercise
HN	high nitrogen
H & N	head and neck
HNP	herniated nucleus pulposus
hnRNA	heterogeneous nuclear ribonucleic acid
HNV	has not voided
HO	house officer
H/O	history of
H2O	water
HOB	head of bed
HOB UPSOB	head of bed up for shortness of breath
HOC	Health Officer Certificate
HOCM	hypertrophic obstructive cardiomyopathy
HOG	halothane, oxygen, and gas (nitrous oxide)
HOH	hard of hearing
HOPI	history of present illness
HP	hemiplegia; hemipelvectomy; hot packs
H & P	history and physical
HPA	human papilloma virus; hypothalamic-pituitary-adrenal (axis)
HPF	high-power field
HPFH	hereditary persistence of fetal hemoglobin
HPI	history of present illness
HPL	human placenta lactogen

HPLC	high-pressure (performance) liquid chromatography
HPG	human pituitary gonadotropin
HPL	hyperpexia; human placental lactogen
HPM	hemiplegic migraine
HPN	home parenteral nutrition
HPO	hypertrophic pulmonary osteoarthropathy; hydrophilic ointment
HPT	hyperparathyroidism
HPZ	high-pressure zone
HR	heart rate; hour; hallux rigidus; hospital record; Harrington rod
HRA	histamine releasing activity
HRLA	human retrovirus-like agent
HRS	hepatorenal syndrome
HRT	hormone replacement therapy
HS	bedtime; hereditary spherocytosis; heel spur; heel stick; herpes simplex; Hartmann's (lactated Ringer's) solution
H>S	heel to shin
HSA	human serum albumin; hypersomnia-sleep apnea; health systems agency
HSBG	heel stick blood gas
HSE	herpes simplex encephalitis
HSG	hysterosalpingogram
HSM	hepato-splenomegaly; holosystolic murmur
HSP	Henoch-Schönlein purpura
HSR	heated serum reagin
HSSE	high soap suds enema
HSV	herpes simplex virus
HT	hypertension; hypermetropia; height; heart; hammertoe; hyperopia; Hubbard tank
ht aer	heated aerosol
HTAT	human tetanus antitoxin
HTC	hypertensive crisis
HTF	house tube feeding
HTL	human thymic leukemia
HTLC	human T-cell leukemia virus
HTLV III	human T-cell lymphotrophic virus type III
HTN	hypertension
HTP	House-Tree-Person test
HTR	acute hemolytic transfusion reaction
HTVD	hypertensive vascular disease
HUIFM	human leukocyte interferon meloy
HUR	hemolytic uremic syndrome
HUS	hemolytic uremic syndrome
HV	hallux valgus; has voided
H & V	hemigastrectomy and vagotomy
HW	heparin well; housewife
hwb	hot water bottle
Hx	history; hospitalization
Hz	Hertz
HZ	herpes zoster
HZO	herpes zoster ophthalmicus
I	independent; impression; incisal; one
IA	intra-amniotic
IAA	interrupted aortic arch

IABC	intra-aortic balloon counterpulsation
IABP	intra-aortic balloon pump
IAC	internal auditory canal
IAC-CPR	interposed abdominal compressions-cardiopulmonary resuscitation
IACP	intra-aortic counterpulsation
IADH	inappropriate antidiuretic hormone
IA DSA	intra-arterial subtraction arteriography
IAHA	immune adherence hemagglutination
IAI	intra-abdominal infection
IAM	internal auditory meatus
IAN	intern admission note
IAP	intermittent acute porphyria
IASD	interatrial septal defect
IAT	indirect antiglobulin test
IB	isolation bed
IBC	iron binding capacity
IBD	inflammatory bowel disease
IBI	intermittent bladder irrigation
ibid	at the same place
IBNR	incurred but not reported
IBS	irritable bowel syndrome
IBW	ideal body weight
IC	irritable colon; intercostal; intracranial; individual counseling; inspiratory capacity
ICA	internal carotid artery; islet cell antibodies
ICBT	intercostobronchial trunk
ICCE	intracapsular cataract extraction
ICCU	intermediate coronary care unit
ICD	instantaneous cardiac death
ICD 9 CM	International Classification of Diseases, 9th Revision, Clinical Modification
ICF	intracellular fluid; intermediate care facility
ICG	indocyanine green
ICH	intracranial hemorrhage
ICM	intracostal margin
ICN	intensive care nursery
ICP	intracranial pressure
ICPP	intubated continuous positive pressure
ICS	intracostal space
ICSH	interstitial cell-stimulating hormone
ICT	intensive conventional therapy; inflammation of connective tissue
ICU	intensive care unit
ICVH	ischemic cerebrovascular headache
ICW	intercellular water
ID	intradermal; initial dose; infectious disease; identification; immunodiffusion; identify
I & D	incision and drainage
IDE	Investigational Device Exemption
IDDM	insulin-dependent diabetes mellitus
IDDS	implantable drug delivery system
IDFC	immature dead female child
IDM	infant of a diabetic mother
IDMC	immature dead male child
IDS	Infectious Disease Service

IDV	intermittent demand ventilation
IEC	inpatient exercise center
IEF	iso-electric focusing
IEM	immune electron microscopy
IEP	individualized education program; immunoelectrophoresis
IF	intrinsic factor; immunofluorescence; involved field
IFA	indirect fluorescent antibody test
IFE	immunofixation electrophoresis
IgA	immunoglobulin A
IgD	immunoglobulin D
IgE	immunoglobulin E
IGF	insulin-like growth factor
IgG	immunoglobulin G; immune gammaglobulin
IGIV	immune globulin intravenous
IgM	immunoglobulin M
IGR	intrauterine growth retardation
IGT	impaired glucose tolerance
IH	infectious hepatitis; inguinal hernia; indirect hemagglutination
IHA	immune hemagglutination assay
IHC	immobilization hypercalcemia
IHD	ischemic heart disease; intrahepatic duct
IHH	idiopathic hypogonadotropic hypogonadism
IHS	Idiopathic Headache Score
IHs	iris hamartomas
IHSS	idiopathic hypertrophic subaortic stenosis
IHT	insulin hypoglycemia test
IICP	increased intracranial pressure
IICU	infant intensive care unit
IIT	intensive insulin therapy
IJ	internal jugular; ileojejunal
IL	independent living
ILD	ischemic leg disease
ILFC	immature living female child
ILM	internal limiting membrane
ILMC	immature living male child
ILMI	inferolateral myocardial infarct
IM	intramuscular; infectious mononucleosis; intermetatarsal; internal medicine
IMA	inferior mesenteric artery; internal mammary artery
IMAG	internal mammary artery graft
IMB	intermenstrual bleeding
IMF	intermaxillary fixation
IMG	internal medicine group (practice)
IMH	indirect microhemagglutination (test)
IMI	inferior myocardial infarction; imipramine
IMIG	intramuscular immunoglobulin
IMN	internal mammary (lymph) node
IMP	impression; impacted
IMV	intermittent mandatory ventilation
IN	interstitial nephritis
INB	intermittent nebulized beta-agonists
INC	incomplete; incontinent; inside-the-needle catheter
IND	investigational new drug

INDM	infant of nondiabetic mother
INF	inferior; infusion; infant; infected
ING	inguinal
inj	injection; injury
INS	insurance
INST	instrumental delivery
int	internal
int-rot	internal rotation
inver	inversion
I & O	intake and output
IO	intraocular pressure; inferior oblique; initial opening
IOC	intern on call; intraoperative cholangiogram
IOD	interorbital distance
IOF	intraocular fluid
IOFB	intraocular foreign body
IOH	idiopthic orthostatic hypotension
IOL	intraocular lens
ION	ischemic optic neuropathy
IOP	intraocular pressure
IORT	intraoperative radiation therapy
IOS	intraoperative sonography
IOV	initial office visit
IP	intraperitoneal
IPA	invasive pulmonary aspergillosis; individual practice association
IPCD	infantile polycystic disease
IPD	immediate pigment darkening; intermittent peritoneal dialysis
IPFD	intrapartum fetal distress
IPG	impedance plethysmography; individually polymerized grass
IPJ	interphalangeal joint
IPK	intractable plantar keratosis
IPMI	inferoposterior myocardial infarct
IPN	infantile periarteritis nodosa; intern's progress note
IPP	inflatable penile prosthesis
IPPA	inspection, palpation, percussion, and auscultation
IPPB	intermittent positive pressure breathing
IPPV	intermittent positive pressure ventilation
IPV	inactivated polio vaccine
IQ	intelligence quotient
IR	internal rotation; infrared
IRBBB	incomplete right bundle branch block
IRMA	intraretinal microvascular abnormalities
IRR	intrarenal reflux
IRV	inspiratory reserve volume
IS	intercostal space; incentive spirometer; induced sputum
ISB	incentive spirometry breathing
ISCs	irreversible sickle cells
ISG	immune serum globulin
ISH	isolated systolic hypertension
ISMA	infantile spinal muscular atrophy
ISS	Injury Severity Score
IST	insulin sensitivity test; insulin shock therapy
ISW	interstitial water

IT	intrathecal; inhalation therapy; intertuberous
ITCP	idiopathic thrombocytopenia purpura
ITE	insufficient therapeutic effect
ITP	idiopathic thrombocytopenic purpura; interim treatment plan
ITVAD	indwelling transcutaneous vascular access device
IU	international unit
IUCD	intrauterine contraceptive device
IUD	intrauterine device; intrauterine death
IUFD	intrauterine fetal death
IUGR	intrauterine growth retardation
IUP	intrauterine pregnancy
IUPD	intrauterine pregnancy delivered
IV	intravenous
IVC	intravenous cholangiogram; inferior vena cava; intraventricular catheter
IVD	intervertebral disk; intravenous drip
IVDA	intravenous drug abuse
IVF	*in vitro* fertilization; intravenous fluid
IVFE	intravenous fat emulsion
IVF-ET	*in vitro* fertilization, embryo transfer
IVGTT	intravenous glucose tolerance test
IVH	intravenous hyperalimentation; intraventricular hemorrhage
IVIG	intravenous immunoglobulin
IVLBW	infant of very low birth weight
IVP	intravenous pyelogram; intravenous push
IVPB	intravenous piggyback
IVR	idioventricular rhythm
IVS	intraventricular septum
IVSD	intraventricular septal defect
IVSP	intravenous syringe pump
IVT	intravenous transfusion
IVU	intravenous urography
IWL	insensible water loss
IWMI	inferior wall myocardial infarct
J	joint
JAMG	juvenile autoimmune myasthenia gravis
JC	junior clinicians
JDMS	juvenile dermatomyositis
JE	Japanese encephalitis
JF	joint fluid
JI	jejunoileal
JIB	jejunoileal bypass
JJ	jaw jerk
JMS	junior medical student
JODM	juvenile onset diabetes mellitus
JP	Jobst pump; Jackson-Pratt (drain)
JRA	juvenile rheumatoid arthritis
JSPN	junior student progress note
jt	joint
juv	juvenile
JVD	jugular venous distention

JVP	jugular venous pulse; jugular venous pressure
JVPT	jugular venous pulse tracing
KA	ketoacidosis
KAFO	knee-ankle-foot orthosis
KAO	knee-ankle orthosis
KAS	Katz Adjustment Scale
KBM	a below-knee prosthesis
K Cal	kilocalorie
KCS	keratoconjunctivitis sicca
KD	Kawasaki's disease; knee disarticulation; Keto Diastex®
KDA	known drug allergies
KDDM	kidney disease of diabetes mellitus
KF	kidney function
KFD	Kyasanur Forrest disease
kg	kilogram
K24H	potassium, urine 24 hour
KI	karyopyknotic index
KID	keratitis, ichthyosis, deafness
KILO	kilogram
KISS	saturated solution of potassium iodide
KJ	knee jerk
KK	knee kick
KLH	keyhole limpet hemocyanin (antibody)
KNO	keep needle open
KO	keep open
KP	keratoprecipitate; hot pack
KS	ketosteroids; Kaposi's sarcoma
17-KS	17-ketosteroids
KTU	kidney transplant unit
KUB	kidney, ureter, bladder
KVO	keep vein open
KW	Kimmelstiel-Wilson (disease); Keith-Wagener (ophthalmoscopic finding)
K-wire	Kirschner wire
L	left; liter; lumbar; lingual; lymphocyte; fifty
L2	second lumbar vertebra
LA	left atrium; local anesthesia; long acting; left arm; Latin American
L+A	light and accommodation
lab	laboratory
LAC	laceration; long arm cast
LAD	left anterior descending; left axis deviation
LAD-MIN	left axis deviation minimal
LAE	left atrial enlargement
LAF	lymphocyte-activating factor; laminar air flow; Latin American female
LAG	lymphangiogram
LAH	left atrial hypertrophy
LAL	left axillary line; limulus amebocyte lysate
LAM	Latin American male
LAN	lymphadenopathy
LAO	left anterior oblique

LAP	laparotomy; laparoscopy; left arterial pressure; leukocyte; leucine amino peptidase
LAPMS	long arm posterior molded splint
LAR	late asthmatic response
LAT	left anterior thigh; lateral
LATS	long-acting thyroid stimulator
LAV	lymphadenopathy associated virus
LAVH	laparoscopic-assisted vaginal hysteroscopy
LB	low back; left buttock; large bowel; left breast; pound
LBB	left breast biopsy
LBBB	left bundle branch block
LBCD	left border of cardiac dullness
LBD	left border dullness
LBF	*Lactobacillus bulgaricus* factor
LBM	lean body mass; loose bowel movement
LBO	large bowel obstruction
LBP	low back pain; low blood pressure
LBT	lupus band test
LBV	left brachial vein
LBW	low birth weight; lean body weight
LC	living children; low calorie
LCA	left coronary artery; Leber's congenital amaurosis
LCCA	leukocytoclastic angitis; left common carotid artery
LCCS	low cervical Cesarean section
LCD	liquor carbonis detergens (coal tar solution); localized collagen dystrophy
LCGU	local cerebral glucose utilization
LCH	local city hospital
LCLC	large cell lung carcinoma
LCM	left costal margin; lymphocytic choriomeningitis
LCR	late cutaneous reaction
LCS	low constant suction; low continuous suction
LCT	long chain triglyceride; low cervical transverse; lymphocytotoxicity
LCV	low cervical vertical
LCX	left circumflex coronary artery
LD	lethal dose; loading dose; liver disease; labor and delivery
LDA	left dorsoanterior position
LDB	Legionnaires disease bacterium
LDDS	local dentist
LDH	lactic dehydrogenase
LDL	low-density lipoprotein
LDP	left dorsoposterior position
LDV	laser Doppler velocimetry
LE	lupus erythematosus; lower extremities; left eye
LED	lupus erythematosus disseminatus
LEEP	loop electrocautery excision procedure
LEHPZ	lower esophageal high-pressure zone
L-ERX	leukoerythroblastic reaction
LES	lower esophageal sphincter; local excitatory state
LESP	lower esophageal sphincter pressure
LET	linear energy transfer
LF	low forceps; left foot
LFA	left fronto-anterior; low friction arthroplasty
LFC	living female child

LFD	low fat diet; low forceps delivery; lactose free diet
LFP	left frontoposterior
LFS	liver function studies
LFT	liver function test; left frontotransverse; latex flocculation test
lg	large; left gluteus
LG	lymph glands
LGA	large for gestational age
LGL	Lown-Ganong-Levine (syndrome)
LGV	lymphogranuloma venereum
LH	luteinizing hormone; left hyperphoria; left hand
LHF	left heart failure
LHL	left hemisphere lesions
LHP	left hemiparesis
LHR	leukocyte histamine release
LHRH	luteinizing hormone-releasing hormone
LHT	left hypertropia
LIB	left in bottle
LIC	left iliac crest; left internal carotid
LICA	left internal carotid artery
LIF	left iliac fossa; liver inhibitory factor
lig	ligament
LIH	left inguinal hernia
LIMA	left internal mammary artery (graft)
LIP	lymphocytic interstitial pneumonia
LIQ	lower inner quadrant; liquid
LIS	low intermittent suction
LISREL	(computer program that performs structural equation modeling)
LISS	low ionic strength saline
LK	left kidney
LKKS	liver, kidneys, spleen
LKS	liver, kidneys, spleen
LL	large lymphocyte; lumbar length; lymphoblastic lymphoma; left leg; lower lip
LLB	long leg brace
LLC	long leg case
LLE	left lower extremity
LLETZ	large loop excision of transformation zone (of cervix)
LL-GXT	low-level graded exercise test
LLL	left lower lobe; left lower lid
LLO	Legionella-like organism
LLQ	left lower quadrant
LLS	lazy leukocyte syndrome
LLSB	left lower sternal border
LLT	left lateral thigh
LMA	left mento-anterior; liver membrane autoantibody
LMB	Laurence-Moon-Biedl syndrome
LMC	living male child
LMCA	left main coronary artery
LMD	low molecular weight dextran
LMEE	left middle ear exploration
L/min	liters per minute
LML	left medial lateral/lobe
LMM	lentigo maligna melanoma

LMP	last menstrual period; left mentoposterior
LMT	left mentotransverse
LMWD	low molecular weight dextran
LN	lymph nodes
LND	lymph node dissection
LNMP	last normal menstrual period
LO	lateral oblique
LOA	left occiput anterior; leave of absence
LOC	loss of consciousness; level of consciousness; level of care; laxative of choice; local
LOD	line of duty
LOM	limitation of motion; left otitis media
LoNa	low sodium
LOP	left occiput posterior; leave on pass
LOQ	lower outer quadrant
LORS	Level of Rehabilitation Scale
LOS	length of stay
LOT	left occiput transverse
LOV	loss of vision
loz	lozenge
LP	lumbar puncture; light perception
LPC	laser photocoagulation
LPD	luteal phase defect
LPF	low power field
LPH	left posterior hemiblock
LPN	licensed practical nurse
LPO	left posterior oblique; light perception only
LPP	lipoprotein lipase
LR	light reflex; labor room; left-right
L>R	left to right
LRD	living renal donor
LRND	left radical neck dissection
LRQ	lower right quadrant
L-S	lumbo-sacral
L/S	lecithin-sphingomyelin ratio
LSA	left sacrum anterior; lipid-bound sialic acid; lymphosarcoma
LSB	left sternal border
LS BPS	laparoscopic bilateral partial salpingectomy
LSD	low-salt diet
LSE	local side effects
LSF	low saturated fat
LSKM	liver-spleen-kidney-megalgia
LSM	late systolic murmur
LSO	left salpingo-oophorectomy
LSP	left sacrum posterior; liver-specific (membrane) lipoprotein
L/S ratio	lecithin/sphingomyelin ratio
LSS	liver-spleen scan
LST	left sacrum transverse
LSTL	laparoscopic tubal ligation
LT	light; left; left thigh; lumbar traction; Levin tube; leukotrienes
LTB	laparoscopic tubal banding; laryngotracheobronchitis
LTC	long-term care; left to count; lean tissue compartment

LTCF	long-term care facility
LTCS	low transverse cesarean section
LTGA	left transposition of great artery
LTL	laparoscopic tubal ligation
LTT	lymphocyte transformation test
L & U	lower and upper
LUE	left upper extremity
LUL	left upper lobe
LUQ	left upper quadrant
LUSB	left upper sternal border
LV	left ventricle
LVA	left ventricular aneurysm
LVAD	left ventricular assist device
LVE	left ventricular enlargement
LVEDP	left ventricular end diastolic pressure
LVEDV	left ventricular end diastolic volume
LVEF	left ventricular ejection fraction
LVF	left ventricular failure
LVFP	left ventricular filling pressure
LVH	left ventricular hypertrophy
LVL	left vastus lateralis
LVMM	left ventricular muscle mass
LVN	licensed vocational nurse
LVP	left ventricular pressure; large volume parenteral
LVPW	left ventricular posterior wall
LVSWI	left ventricular stroke work index
LVV	left ventricular volume
L & W	living and well
LWCT	Lee-White clotting time
LYG	lymphomatoid granulomatosis
lymphs	lymphocytes
lytes	electrolytes
M	murmur; meter; minimum; medial; myopia; monocytes; male; molar; married; thousand
M1	first mitral sound
M2	square meters (body surface)
MA	mental age; medical assistance; milliamps; menstrual age; Miller-Abbott (tube)
M/A	mood and/or affect
MAA	macroaggregates of albumin
MAB	monoclonal antibody
MABP	mean arterial blood pressure
MAC	maximum allowable concentration; midarm circumference; minimum alveolar concentration; mycobacterium avium complex
MAE	moves all extremities
MAEEW	moves all extremities equally well
MAFAs	movement-associated fetal (heart rate) accelerations
MAHA	microangiopathic hemolytic anemia
MAI	mycobacterium avium-intracellulare
MAL	midaxillary line
MALT	mucosa-associated lymphoid tissue
MAMC	mid-arm muscle circumference

mammo	mammography
MAOI	monoamine oxidase inhibitor
mand	mandibular
MAP	mean arterial pressure
MAS	meconium aspiration syndrome; mobile arm support
MAST	military antishock trousers
MAT	multifocal atrial tachycardia
max	maximal; maxillary
M-BACOD	a drug combination protocol
MBC	maximum breathing capacity; minimal bacteriocidal concentration
MB-CK	a creatinine kinase isoenzyme
MBD	minimal brain damage; minimal brain dysfunction
MBI	methylene blue installation
MBM	mother's breast milk
MC	mixed cellularity; metatarso-cuneiform
MCA	middle cerebral aneurysm; middle cerebral artery; motorcycle accident; monoclonal antibodies
MCC	midstream clean-catch
MCCU	midstream clean-catch urine
MCD	minimal change disease
mcg	microgram
MCGN	minimal change glomerular nephritis
MCH	mean corpuscular hemoglobin; muscle contraction headache
MCHC	mean corpuscular hemoglobin concentration
MCL	midclavicular line; midcostal line
MCLNS	mucocutaneous lymph node syndrome
MCP	metacarpophalangeal joint
MCS	microculture and sensitivity
MCSA	minimal cross-sectional area
MCT	medium chain triglyceride; mean circulation time
MCTD	mixed connective tissue disease
MCV	mean corpuscular/cell volume
MD	medical doctor; mental deficiency; muscular dystrophy; manic depression
MDA	manual dilation of the anus; micrometastases detection assay
MDC	medial dorsal cutaneous (nerve); major diagnostic category
MDD	manic-depressive disorder; major depressive disorder
MDF	myocardial depressant factor
MDI	multiple daily injection; metered dose inhaler
MDII	multiple daily insulin injection
MDM	mid-diastolic murmur; minor determinant mix
MDR	minimum daily requirement
MDS	maternal deprivation syndrome; minimum data set
MDTP	multidisciplinary treatment plan
ME	macula edema; medical examiner; middle ear
MEA-I	multiple endocrine adenomatosis type I
mec	meconium
MED	median erythrocyte diameter; medial; medical; medication; medicine; minimum erythema dose; medium
MEDAC	multiple endocrine deficiency-autoimmune-candidiasis
MEE	middle ear effusion
MEF	maximum expired flow rate
MEFV	maximum expiratory flow volume

MEN (II)	multiple endocrine neoplasia (type II)
MEOS	microsomal ethanol oxidizing system
mEq	milliequivalent
M/E ratio	myeloid/erythroid ratio
META	metamyelocytes
METS	metabolic equivalents (multiples of resting oxygen uptake); metastases
MF	myocardial fibrosis; mycosis fungoides; midcavity forceps
M & F	mother and father; male and female
MFA	mid-forceps delivery
MFAT	multifocal atrial tachycardia
MFEM	maximal forced expiratory maneuver
MFH	malignant fibrous histiocytoma
MFR	mid-forceps rotation
MG	myasthenia gravis; milligram; Marcus Gunn
MGF	maternal grandfather
MGM	maternal grandmother
MGN	membranous glomerulonephritis
MGUS	monoclonal gammopathies of undetermined significance
M-GXT	multistage graded exercise test
MH	marital history; menstrual history; mental health; malignant hyperthermia
MHA	microangiopathic hemolytic anemia
MHB	maximum hospital benefit
MHC	major histocompatibility complex; mental health center
MH/MR	mental health and mental retardation
MI	myocardial infarction; mitral insufficiency; mental institution
MIA	medically indigent adult; missing in action
MIC	minimum inhibitory concentration; maternal and infant care
MICN	mobile intensive care nurse
MICU	medical intensive care unit; mobile intensive care unit
MID	multi-infarct dementia
MIDD	monoclonal immunoglobulin deposition
MIF	migration inhibitory factor
MIH	migraine with interparoxysmal headache
min	minimum; minute; minor
MIO	minimum identifiable odor
MIRP	myocardial infarction rehabilitation program
mix mon	mixed monitor
MJT	Mead Johnson tube
MKAB	may keep at bedside
ML	midline; milliliter; middle lobe
mL	milliliter
MLC	mixed lymphocyte culture; minimal lethal concentration
MLD	metachromatic leukodystrophy; minimal lethal dose
MLF	median longitudinal fasciculus
MLNS	mucocutaneous lymph node syndrome
MLR	mixed lymphocyte reaction
MM	millimeter; mucous membrane; multiple myeloma
mM	millimole
M & M	milk and molasses; morbidity and mortality
MMA	monocyte monolayer assay
MMECT	multiple monitor electroconvulsive therapy
MMEFR	maximal midexpiratory flow rate

MMF	mean maximum flow
MMFR	maximal midexpiratory flow rate
mmHg	millimeters of mercury
MMK	Marshall-Marchetti-Krantz (cystourethropexy)
MMOA	maxillary mandibular odontectomy alveolectomy
mmol	millimole
MMPI	Minnesota Multiphasic Personality Inventory
MMR	measles, mumps, rubella; midline malignant reticulosis
MMS	Mini-Mental State (examination)
MMT	manual muscle test
MMWR	Morbidity & Mortality Weekly Report
MN	midnight
M & N	morning and night
MNC	mononuclear leukocytes
MNG	multinodular goiter
MNR	marrow neutrophil reserve
Mn SSEPS	median nerve somatosensory evoked potentials
MNTB	medial nucleus of the trapezoid body
MO	month; medial oblique
MOA	mechanism of action
MOB	medical office building
MOD	medical officer of the day; moderate
MODY	maturity onset diabetes of youth
MOF	multiple organ failure
mono	monocyte; infectious mononucleosis
mOsm	milliosmole
mOsmol	milliosmole
MP	metacarpal phalangeal joint
MPGN	membranoproliferative glomerulonephritis
MPH	Master of Public Health
MPJ	metacarpophalangeal joint
MPL	maximum permissible level
MPR	multifetal pregnancy reduction
MPS	mucopolysaccharidosis
MPTR	motor, pain, touch reflex deficit
MQ	memory quotient
MR	mental retardation; may repeat; magnetic resonance; mitral regurgitation
MR × 1	may repeat times one
MRA	medical record administrator; magnetic resonance angiography
MRAN	medical resident admitting note
MRD	Medical Records Department
MRG	murmurs, rubs and gallops
MRI	magnetic resonance imaging
mRNA	messenger ribonucleic acid
MRS	magnetic resonance spectroscopy
MRSA	methicillin resistant *Staphylococcus aureus*
MS	multiple sclerosis; mitral stenosis; musculoskeletal; medical student; minimal support; muscle strength; mental status
M & S	microculture and sensitivity
MSAF	meconium stained amniotic fluid
MSAFP	maternal serum alpha fetoprotein
MSC	medical social consultant

MSE	Mental Status Examination
MSH	melanocyte-stimulating hormone
MSK	medullary sponge kidney
MSL	midsternal line
MSR	muscle stretch reflexes
MSS	minor surgery suite; muscular subaortic stenosis; Marital Satisfaction Scale
MST	mean survival time
MSTA®	mumps skin test antigen
MSU	midstream urine
MSUD	maple syrup urine disease
MSW	multiple stab wounds; Master of Social Work
MT	music therapy; medical technologist
MTAL	medullary thick ascending limb
MTD	Monro Tidal drainage
MTI	malignant teratoma interminate
MTM	modified Thayer-Martin medium
MTP	metatarsal phalangeal
MTU	malignant teratoma undifferentiated
MU	million units
MUDPIES	methanol, uremia, diabetic ketoacidosis, paraldehyde, idiopathic, ethylene glycol, salicylate (cause of metabolic acidosis)
MULEPAK	methanol, uremia, lactic acidosis, ethylene glycol, paraldehyde, aspirin, diabetic ketoacidosis (cause of metabolic acidosis)
MUGA	multiple gated acquisition
MUGX	multiple gated acquisition exercise
MVA	motor vehicle accident; malignant ventricular arrhythmias
MVB	mixed venous blood
MVC	maximal voluntary contraction
MVI®	parenteral multivitamins
MVO$_2$	myocardial oxygen consumption
MVP	mitral valve prolapse
MVR	mitral valve replacement; mitral valve regurgitation
MVS	mitral valve stenosis
MVV	maximum voluntary ventilation; mixed vespid venom
MWS	Mickey-Wilson syndrome
My	myopia
myelo	myelocyte
N	normal; negative; Negro
5'-N	5'-Nucleotidase
NA	nursing assistant; nurse anesthetist; not applicable
NAA	neutron activation analysis
NABS	normoactive bowel sounds
NAD	no acute distress; no apparent distress; no appreciable disease; normal axis deviation; nothing abnormal detected
NAEP	National Asthma Education Program
NAG	narrow angle glaucoma
NANB	non-A, non-B hepatitis
NANC	nonadrenergic, noncholinergic
NAS	no added salt; neonatal abstinence syndrome
NAT	no action taken
NB	newborn; note well; needle biopsy

NBM	no bowel movement; normal bowel movement; nothing by mouth
NBN	newborn nursery
NBS	normal bowel sound; no bacteria seen
NBT	nitroblue tetrazolium reduction test
NBTE	nonbacterial thrombotic endocarditis
NC	neurologic check; no complaints; not completed; nasal cannula
NCA	neurocirculatory asthenia
NC/AT	normal cephalic atraumatic
NCB	no code blue
NCD	normal childhood diseases; not considered disabling
NCF	neutrophilic chemotactic factor
NCI	National Cancer Institute
NCJ	needle catheter jejunostomy
NCL	neuronal ceroid lipofuscinosis
NCM	nailfold capillary microscopy
NCNC	normochromic, normocytic
NCPR	no cardiopulmonary resuscitation
NCS	no concentrated sweets; nerve conduction studies
NCV	nerve conduction velocity
ND	normal delivery; normal development; not done; not diagnosed; nasal deformity
NDA	new drug application
NDD	no dialysis days
NDT	neurodevelopmental treatment
NDV	Newcastle disease virus
NE	norepinephrine; not elevated; not examined
NEC	necrotizing enterocolitist elsewhere classified
NED	no evidence of disease
NEG	negative
NEMD	nonspecific esophageal motility disorder
NET	naso-endotracheal tube
neut	neutrophil
NF	Negro female; not found; neurofibromatosis
NFL	nerve fiber layer
NFTD	normal full-term delivery
NFTT	nonorganic failure to thrive
NFW	nursed fairly well
NG	nasogastric; nanogram
NGF	nerve growth factor
NGR	nasogastric replacement
NGT	nasogastric tube
NGU	nongonococcal urethritis
NH	nursing home
NHD	normal hair distribution
NHL	non-Hodgkin's lymphoma; nodular histiocytic lymphoma
NHP	nursing home placement
NCC	neonatal intensive care center
NICU	neurosurgical intensive care unit; neonatal intensive care unit
NIDD	non-insulin-dependent diabetes
NIDDM	non-insulin-dependent diabetes mellitus
NIF	negative inspiratory force
NIH	National Institutes of Health
NINVS	noninvasive neurovascular studies

NJ	nasojejunal
NK	natural killer (cells)
NKA	no known allergies
NKDA	no known drug allergies
NKHS	nonketotic hyperosmolar syndrome
NKMA	no known medication allergies
NL	normal; normal limits
NLD	necrobiosis lipoidica diabeticorum; nasolacrimal duct
NLF	nasolabial fold
NLP	nodular liquefying panniculitis; no light perception
NLT	not later than; not less than
NM	Negro male; neuromusculardular melanoma
NMD	normal muscle development
NMR	nuclear magnetic resonance
NMI	no middle initial
NMS	neuroleptic malignant syndrome
NMT	no more than
NN	neonatal; nursing notes
NND	neonatal death
NNE	neonatal necrotizing enterocolitis
NNM	Nicole-Novy-MacNeal (media)
NNO	no new orders
NNP	neonatal nurse practitioner
NNU	net nitrogen utilization
no	number
noc	night
noct	nocturnal
NOD	notify of death
NOMI	nonocclusive mesenteric infarction
NOOB	not out of bed
NOS	not otherwise specified
NOSIE	Nurse Observation Scale for Inpatient Evaluation
NP	neuropsychiatric; nasopharyngeal; newly presented; no pain; not pregnant; not present; nursed poorly; nasal prongs; nurse practitioner
NPA	near point of accommodation
NPC	near point convergences; nodal premature contractions; nonpatient contact
NPDL	nodular poorly differentiated lymphocytic
NPDR	nonproliferative diabetic retinopathy
NPH	normal pressure hydrocephalus; no previous history; neutral protamine Hagedorn (insulin)
NPO	nothing by mouth
NPR	noncardiogenic pulmonary reaction
NPT	normal pressure and temperature; nocturnal penile tumescence
NR	nonreactive
NRBS	non-rebreathing system
NRC	normal retinal correspondence
NREM	nonrapid eye movement
NREMS	nonrapid eye movement sleep
NRT	neuromuscular reeducation techniques
NS	nephrotic syndrome; nuclear sclerosis; not seen; not significant; nylon suture
NSA	normal serum albumin; no significant abnormality
NSABP	National Surgical Adjuvant Breast Project

NSC	no significant change; not service connected
NSCLC	non-small-cell lung cancer
NSD	normal spontaneous delivery; nominal standard dose
NSDA	non-steroid-dependent asthmatic
NSE	neuron-specific enolase
NSFTD	normal spontaneous full-term delivery
NSG	nursing
NSILA	nonsuppressible insulin-like activity
NSN	nephrotoxic serum nephritis
NSPVT	nonsustained polymorphic ventricular tachycardia
NSR	normal sinus rhythm; not seen regularly; nonspecific reaction; nasoseptal repair
NSSTT	nonspecific ST and T wave
NST	nutritional support team; nonstress test; not sooner than
NSU	nonspecific urethritis
NSV	nonspecific vaginitis
NSVD	normal spontaneous vaginal delivery
NT	not tested; nasotracheal; not tender
N & T	nose and throat
NTC	neurotrauma center
NTD	neural tube defects
NTE	not to exceed
NTF	normal throat flora
NTG	nontreatment group
NTMB	nontuberculous mycobacteria
NTMI	nontransmural myocardial infarction
NTP	normal temperature and pressure
NTS	nasotracheal suction; nucleus tractus solitarii
NTT	nasotracheal tube
NUD	nonulcer dyspepsia
nullip	nullipara
NV	neurovascular
N & V	nausea and vomiting
NVD	nausea, vomiting, and diarrhea; neck vein distention; no venereal disease; neuro-vesicle dysfunction; nonvalvular disease; neovascularization of the disc
NVE	neovascularization elsewhere
NVG	neovascular glaucoma
NVS	neurological vital signs
NWB	non-weight bearing
NWTS	National Wilms' Tumor Study
NYD	not yet diagnosed
NZ	enzyme
O	oxygen; objective finding; eye; oral; open; obvious; often; other; occlusal
1O2	singlet oxygen
O2	oxygen; both eyes
O2v	superoxide
OA	oral alimentation; occiput anterior; osteoarthritis; Overeaters Anonymous
O & A	observation and assessment
OAF	osteoclast activating factor
Ob	obstetrics
OB	occult blood
OBE-CALP	placebo capsule or tablet

Ob-Gyn	obstetrics and gynecology
OBS	organic brain syndrome
OC	oral contraceptive; obstetrical conjugate; oral care; on call; office call
OCA	oculocutaneous albinism
OCCC	open chest cardiac compression
OCCM	open chest cardiac massage
OCD	obsessive-compulsive disorder
OCG	oral cholecystogram
OCP	ova, cysts, parasites
OCT	oxytocin challenge test; optical coherence tomography
OCU	observation care unit
OD	right eye; overdose; on duty; Doctor of Optometry
OER	oxygen enhancement ratios
OFC	occipital-frontal circumference
OG	orogastric (feeding)
OGTT	oral glucose tolerance test
OH	occupational history; open heart
OHA	oral hypoglycemic agents
OHD	organic heart disease
OHF	omsk hemorrhage fever
OHG	oral hypoglycemic
OHP	oxygen under hyperbaric pressure
OHRR	open heart recovery room
OHS	open heart surgery
OI	osteogenesis imperfecta
OIF	oil-immersion field
OJ	orthoplast jacket; orange juice
OKAN	optokinetic after nystagmus
OKN	optokinetic nystagmus
OLA	occiput left anterior
OM	otitis media; every morning
OME	Office of the Medical Examiner; otitis media with effusion
OMI	old myocardial infarct
OMR	operative mortality rate
OMSC	otitis media secretory/suppurative chronic
ON	overnight; every night
ONC	over-the-needle catheter
OOB	out of bed
OOBBRP	out of bed with bathroom privileges
OOC	out of control
OOP	out on pass; out of pelvis
OOR	out of room
OOT	out of town
OP	outpatient; operation; occiput posterior; open
O & P	ova and parasites
OPB	outpatient basis
OPC	outpatient clinic
OPCA	olivopontocerebellar atrophy
OPD	outpatient department
OPG	ocular plethysmography
OPM	occult primary malignancy
OPPG	oculopneumoplethysmography

OPS	operations
OPV	oral polio vaccine
OR	operating room; oil retention
ORIF	open reduction internal fixation
ORL	otorhinolaryngology
OS	left eye; mouth; opening snap
OSA	obstructive sleep apnea
OSD	overside drainage
OSM S	osmolarity serum
OSM U	osmolarity urine
OSN	off service note
OSS	osseous
OT	old tuberculin; occupational therapy/therapist
OTC	over-the-counter
OTD	out the door
OTO	otology
OTR	Occupational Therapist, Registered
OTS	orotracheal suction
OTT	orotracheal tube
OU	both eyes
OV	office visit; ovum; ovary
OW	out of wedlock
oz	ounce
P	plan; protein; pint; pulse; peripheral; phosphorous; para
p	after
P2	pulmonic second heart sound
PA	posterior-anterior; pulmonary artery; pernicious anemia; physician assistant; presents again; psychiatric aide; professional association
P & A	percussion and auscultation
PAB	premature atrial beat
PAC	premature atrial contraction
PACH	pipers to after coming head
PACO	pivot ambulating crutchless orthosis
PaCO2	arterial carbon dioxide tension
PADP	pulmonary artery diastolic pressure
PAF	paroxysmal atrial fibrillation; platelet activating factors
PAGE	polyacrylamide gel electrophoresis
PAIVS	pulmonary atresia with intact ventricle septum
Pa Line	pulmonary artery line
PALN	para-aortic lymph node
PAN	periodic alternating nystagmus; polyarteritis nodosa
PAO$_2$	arterial oxygen tension
PAOG	primary open angle glaucoma
PAOP	pulmonary artery occlusion pressure
PAP	pulmonary artery pressure; prostatic acid phosphatase
Pap smear	Papanicolaou smear
PA/PS	pulmonary atresia/pulmonary stenosis
PAR	postanesthetic recovery; platelet aggregate ratio
PARA	number of pregnancies
para	paraplegic
PARU	postanesthetic recovery unit

PAS	periodic acid-Schiff (reagent); peripheral anterior synechia; pulmonary artery stenosis
PasEx	passive exercise
PAT	paroxysmal atrial tachycardia; preadmission testing; percent acceleration time
Path	pathology
PAWP	pulmonary artery wedge pressure
Pb	lead
PB	powder board; paraffin bath
PBA	percutaneous bladder aspiration
PBC	point of basal convergence; primary biliary cirrhosis
PBD	percutaneous biliary drainage
PBL	peripheral blood lymphocyte
PBMC	peripheral blood mononuclear cell
PBMNC	peripheral blood mononuclear cell
PBO	placebo
PC	after meal; packed cells; professional corporation; platelet concentrate
PCA	patient care assistant/aide; patient-controlled analgesia; posterior cerebral artery; procoagulation activity; passive cutaneous anaphylaxis
PCCU	postcoronary care unit
PCG	phonocardiogram
PCH	paroxysmal cold hemoglobinuria
PCI	prophylactic cranial irradiation
PCIOL	posterior chamber intraocular lens
PCL	posterior chamber lens; posterior cruciate ligament
PCM	protein-calorie malnutrition
PCO	polycystic ovary
PCO$_2$	carbon dioxide pressure/tension
PCOD	polycystic ovarian disease
PCP	pneumonocystis carinii pneumonia; pulmonary capillary pressure
PCR	protein catabolic/caloric rate; polymerase chain reaction
PCT	porphyria cutanea
PCTA	percutaneous transluminal angioplasty
PCU	progressive care unit
PCV	packed cell volume
PCWP	pulmonary capillary wedge pressure
PD	peritoneal dialysis; postural drainage; Parkinson's disease; interpupillary distance; percutaneous drain
P/D	packs per day (cigarettes)
PDA	patent ductus arteriosus
PDE	paroxysmal dyspnea on exertion; pulsed Doppler echocardiography
PDFC	premature dead female child
PDGF	platelet-derived growth factor
PDL	poorly differentiated lymphocytic
PDL-D	poorly differentiated lymphocytic-diffuse
PDL-N	poorly differentiated lymphocytic-nodular
PDMC	premature dead male child
PDN	private duty nurse
PDR	proliferative diabetic retinopathy; *Physician's Desk Reference*
PDS	pain dysfunction syndrome
PDGXT	predischarge graded exercise test
PDT	photodynamic therapy
PDU	pulsed Doppler ultrasonography

PE	physical examination; pulmonary embolism; pressure equalization; pleural effusion
PECHO	prostatic echogram
PECO$_2$	mixed expired carbon dioxide tension
Peds	pediatrics
PEEP	positive end-expiratory pressure
PEER	peak expiratory flow rate
PEG	pneumoencephalogram; percutaneous endoscopic gastrostomy
PEN	parenteral and enteral nutrition
PENS	percutaneous epidural nerve stimulator
PEP	protein electrophoresis; pre-ejection period; Parkinson's educational program
PER	pediatric emergency room
perf	perforation
PERL	pupils equal, reactive to light
per os	by mouth
PERR	pattern evoked retinal response
PERRLA	pupils equal, round, reactive to light and accommodation
PES	pre-excitation syndrome
PET	positron-emission tomography; pre-eclamptic toxemia; pressure equalizing tubes
PF	power factor
PFC	persistent fetal circulation
PFM	porcelain fused to metal
PFR	peak flow rate; parotid flow rate
PFT	pulmonary function test
PFU	plaque-forming unit
PG	pregnant
PGF	parenteral grandfather
PGH	pituitary growth hormones
PGL	persistent generalized lymphadenopathy
PGM	paternal grandmother
PgR	progesterone receptor
PGU	postgonococcal urethritis
pH	hydrogen ion concentration
PH	past history; poor health; public health
PHA	passive hemagglutinating; phytohemagglutinin; arterial pH; phytohemagglutinin antigen; peripheral hyperalimentation
Pharm	pharmacy
PHC	primary hepatocellular carcinoma
PHH	posthemorrhagic hydrocephalus
PHN	public health nurse; postherpetic neuralgia
PHPT	primary hyperparathyroidism
PHPV	persistent hyperplastic primary vitreous
Phx	pharynx
PI	present illness; pulmonary infarction; peripheral iridectomy
PIAT	Peabody Individual Achievement Test
PICA	posterior inferior communicating artery; posterior inferior cerebellar artery
PICU	pediatric intensive care unit
PID	pelvic inflammatory disease; prolapsed intervertebral disc
PIE	pulmonary infiltration with eosinophilia; pulmonary interstitial emphysema
PIFR	peak inspiratory flow rate
PIH	pregnancy-induced hypertension
PIOK	poikilocytosis

PIP	proximal interphalangeal joint; postinspiratory pressure
PISA	phase invariant signature algorithm
PITR	plasma iron turnover rate
PIV	peripheral intravenous
PIVD	protruded intervertebral disc
PJB	premature junctional beat
PJC	premature junctional contractions
PJS	Peutz-Jeghers syndrome
PK	penetrating keratoplasty
PKD	polycystic kidney disease
PK test	Prausnitz-Kustner transfer test
PKU	phenylketonuria
PL	plantar; place; light perception
PLAP	placental alkaline phosphatase
PLFC	premature living female child
PLH	paroxysmal localized hyperhidrosis
PLL	prolymphocytic leukemia
PLMC	premature living male child
PLN	pelvic lymph node; popliteal lymph node
PLS	primary lateral sclerosis
plts	platelets
PM	postmortem; evening; pretibial myxedema; primary motivation; presents mainly
PMA	Prinzmetal's angina; premenstrual asthma
PMB	postmenopausal bleeding; polymorphonuclear basophils
PMC	pseudomembranous colitis
PMD	private medical doctor
PME	postmenopausal estrogen
PMF	progressive massive fibrosis
PMH	past medical history
PMI	point of maximal impulse; patient medication instructions
PML	progressive multifocal leukoencephalopathy
PMN	polymorphonuclear neutrophil
PMP	pain management program; previous menstrual period
PMR	polymyalgia rheumatica; polymorphic reticulosis
PM & R	physical medicine and rehabilitation
PMS	premenstrual syndrome
PMT	premenstrual tension
PMTS	premenstrual tension syndrome
PMV	prolapse of mitral valve
PMW	pacemaker wires
PN	parenteral nutrition; progress note; percussion note
PNAS	prudent no added salt
PNB	premature nodal beat
PNC	premature nodal contraction; peripheral nerve conduction
PND	paroxysmal nocturnal dyspnea; postnasal drip
PNET-MB	primitive neuroectodermal tumors—medulloblastoma
PNF	proprioceptive neuromuscular fasciculation reaction
PNH	paroxysmal nocturnal hemoglobinuria
PNI	prognostic nutrition index; peripheral nerve injury
PNMG	persistent neonatal myasthenia gravis
PNP	Pediatric Nurse Practitioner; progressive nuclear palsy
PNS	peripheral nervous system; partial nonprogressing stroke; practical nursing student

PNT	percutaneous nephrostomy tube
PNU	protein nitrogen units
PNV	prenatal vitamins
Pnx	pneumothorax
PO	postoperative; phone order; by mouth (per os)
PO$_2$	partial pressure of oxygen
POA	pancreatic oncofetal antigen
POAG	primary open-angle glaucoma
POC	product of conception; postoperative care
POD 1	postoperative day one
POEMS	plasma cell dyscrasia with polyneuropathy, organomegaly, endocrinopathy, monoclonal (M)-protein, skin changes
POG	Pediatric Oncology Group
POIK	poikilocytosis
POL	premature onset of labor
POLY	polymorphonuclear leukocyte
POMR	problem-oriented medical record
poplit	popliteal
PORT	postoperative respiratory therapy
POS	parosteal osteosarcoma; point of service
POSM	patient-operated selector mechanism
post	postmortem examination (autopsy)
post op	postoperative
PP	postpartum; postprandial; paradoxical pulse; pin prick; patient profile; protoporphyria; proximal phalanx; private patient; near point of accommodation
P & P	pins and plater
PPB	parts per billion
PPBG	postprandial blood glucose
PPBS	postprandial blood sugar
PPC	progressive patient care
PPD	packs per day; postpartum day; posterior polymorphous dystrophy; purified protein derivative
P & PD	percussion and postural drainage
PPD-B	purified protein derivative, Battey
PPD-S	purified protein derivative, standard
PPF	plasma protein fraction
PPG	photoplethysmography
PPH	postpartum hemorrhage
PPHN	persistent pulmonary hypertension of the newborn
PPI	patient package insert
PPL	pars planus lensectomy
PPLO	pleuro-pneumonia-like organisms
PPM	parts per million
PPN	peripheral parenteral nutrition
PPNG	penicillinase producing Neisseria gonorrhoeae
PPO	preferred provider organization
PPP	postpartum psychosis
PPPG	postprandial plasma glucose
PPPBL	peripheral pulses palpable both legs
PPROM	prolonged premature rupture of membranes
PPS	postpartum sterilization; pneumococcal polysaccharide (vaccine)
PPTL	postpartum tubal ligation

PPVT	Peabody Picture Vocabulary Test
PR	per rectum; pulse rate; profile; Puerto Rican; far point of accommodation
P & R	pulse and respiration; pelvic and rectal
PRA	plasma renin angiotensin
PRAT	platelet radioactive antiglobulin test
PRBC	packed red blood cells
PRCA	pure red cell aplasia
PRE	progressive/passive resistive exercise
pre-op	before surgery
prep	prepare for surgery
PRG	phleborrheogram
PRIMP	primipara (first pregnancy)
PRN	as needed
PRO	protein; peer review organization
prob	probable
PROC-TO	proctology; proctoscopic
prog	prognosis; prognathism
PROM	passive range of motion; premature rupture of membranes
ProMACE	a drug protocol combination
prov	provisional
PRP	panretinal photocoagulation
PRRE	pupils round, regular, equal
PRSs	positive rolandic spikes
PRTH-C	prothrombin time control
PRV	polycythemia rubra vera
PRVEP	pattern reversal visual evoked potentials
PRW	polymerized ragweed
PS	pulmonary stenosis; paradoxic sleep; pathologic stage; plastic surgery; serum from pregnant women; performance status
P & S	paracentesis and suction; pain and suffering
PSA	prostate-specific antigen
PS I	healthy patient with localized pathological process
PS II	patient with mild to moderate systemic disease
PS III	patient with severe systemic disease limiting activity, but not incapacitating
PS IV	patient with incapacitating systemic disease
PS V	moribund patient not expected to live
PsA	psoriatic arthritis
PSC	posterior subcapsular cataract; primary sclerosing cholangitis
PSE	portal systemic encephalopathy
PSF	posterior spinal fusion
PSG	polysomnography
PSGN	poststreptococcal glomerulonephritis
PSH	postspinal headache
PSI	pounds per square inch
PSM	presystolic murmur
PSP	pancreatic spasmolytic peptide; progressive supranuclear palsy
PSRBOW	premature spontaneous rupture of bag of waters
PSS	progressive systemic sclerosis; physiologic saline solution
PSW	psychiatric social worker
PSVT	paroxysmal supraventricular tachycardia
PT	physical therapy/therapist; patient; prothrombin time; pine tar; posterior tibial; pint

PTA	prior to admission; plasma thromboplastin antecedent; pretreatment anxiety; puretone average; physical therapy assistant; percutaneous transluminal angioplasty
PTB	patellar tendon bearing
PTBD-EF	percutaneous transhepatic biliary drainage—enteric feeding
PTC	plasma thromboplastin components; percutaneous transhepatic cholangiography
PTCA	percutaneous transluminal coronary angioplasty
PTD	period to discharge; permanent and total disability
PTE	proximal tibial epiphysis; pulmonary thromboembolism; pretibial edema
PTF	plasma thromboplastin factor
PTH	post transfusion hepatitis; parathyroid hormone
PTL	pre-term labor
PTMDF	pupils, tension, media, disc, fundus
pTNM	postsurgical resection—pathologic staging of cancer
PTPM	posttraumatic progressive myelopathy
PTPN	peripheral (vein) total parenteral nutrition
PTS	prior to surgery
PTSD	posttraumatic stress disorder
PTT	partial thromboplastin time
PTX	pneumothorax
PU	peptic ulcer; pregnancy urine
PUBS	percutaneous umbilical blood sampling
PUD	peptic ulcer disease
PUFA	polyunsaturated fatty acids
pul	pulmonary
PUN	plasma urea nitrogen
PUO	pyrexia of undetermined origin
PUPPP	pruritic urticarial papules and plaques of pregnancy
PUVA	psoralen-ultraviolet light
PV	polycythemia vera; polio vaccine; portal vein; pulmonary vein; per vagina
P & V	pyloroplasty and vagotomy
PVB	premature ventricular beat
PVC	premature ventricular contraction; pulmonary venous congestion
PVD	patient very disturbed; peripheral vascular disease; posterior vitreous detachment
PVE	premature ventricular extrasystole; perivenous encephalomyelitis
PVO	peripheral vascular occlusion; pulmonary venous occlusion
PVOD	pulmonary vascular obstructive disease
PVP	peripheral venous pressure
PVR	peripheral vascular resistance; postvoiding residual; proliferative vitreoretinopathy; pulse-volume recording
PVS	peritoneovenous shunt; pulmonic valve stenosis; percussion, vibration, and suction
PVT	paroxysmal ventricular tachycardia; private
PWB	partial weight bearing
PWLV	posterior wall of left ventricle
PWM	pokeweed mitogens
PWP	pulmonary wedge pressure
PWV	polistes wasp venom
Px	physical exam; prognosis; pneumothorax; practice
PXE	pseudoxanthoma elasticum
PTx	parathyroidectomy
PY	pack years

q	every
QA	quality assurance
QAM	every morning
QCA	quantitative coronary angiography
qd	every day
QEEG	quantitative electroencephalogram
q4h	every four hours
qh	every hour
qhs	every night
qid	four times daily
qn	every night
qns	quantity not sufficient
qod	every other day
qoh	every other hour
qon	every other night
qpm	every evening
QRS	principal deflection in an electrocardiogram
QS	sufficient quantity; every shift
QUART	quadrantectomy, axillary dissection, and radiotherapy
qwk	once a week
R	respiration; right; rectum; regular; rate; regular insulin
RA	rheumatoid arthritis; right atrium; right auricle, right arm; room air
RABG	room air blood gas
RAC	right atrial catheter
RAD	right axis deviation; radical
RAE	right atrial enlargement
RAEB	refractory anemia, erythroblastic
RAG	room air gas
RAI	resident assessment instrument
RAIU	radioactive iodine uptake
RALT	routine admission laboratory tests
RAM	rapid alternating movements
RAN	resident admission notes
RAO	right anterior oblique
RAP	right atrial pressure; resident assessment protocol
RAPD	relative afferent pupillary defect
RAS	renal artery stenosis
RAST	radioallergosorbent test
RAT	right anterior thigh
RA test	test for rheumatoid factor
R(AW)	airway resistance
RB	retrobulbar; right buttock
R & B	right and below
RBA	right brachial artery
RBB	right breast biopsy
RBBB	right bundle branch block
RBCD	right border cardiac dullness
RBC	red blood cell/count
RBD	right border of dullness
RBE	relative biologic effectiveness
RBF	renal blood flow

RBOW	rupture bag of water
RBP	retinol-binding protein
RBV	right brachial vein
R/C	reclining chair
RCA	right coronary artery; radionuclide cerebral angiogram; regional citrate anticoagulation
RCC	renal cell carcinoma
RCD	relative cardiac dullness
RCM	right costal margin; radiographic contrast media
RCR	replication-competent retrovirus
RCS	reticulum cell sarcoma
RCT	root canal therapy
RCV	red cell volume
RD	registered dietitian; renal disease; retinal detachment; respiratory disease
RDA	recommended daily allowance
RDPE	reticular degeneration of pigment epithelium
RDH	Registered Dental Hygienist
RDI	respiratory disturbance/distress index
RDS	respiratory distress syndrome
RDT	regular dialysis/hemodialysis treatment
RDVT	recurrent deep vein thrombosis
RDW	red cell size distribution width
RE	reticuloendothelial; rectal examination; regional enteritis; right eye; concerning
REE	resting energy expenditure
REF	renal erythropoietic factor; referred
rehab	rehabilitation
Rel	religion
REM	rapid eye movement
REMS	rapid eye movement sleep
REP	repeat; report; repair
repol	repolarization
RER	renal excretion rate
RES	reticuloendothelial system; resident; rehabilitation evaluation system
RESC	resuscitation
resp	respiratory; respiration
retic	reticulocyte
REV	revolutions; review; reverse
RF	rheumatoid factor; rheumatic fever; renal failure
RFA	right fronto-anterior; right femoral artery
RFL	right frontolateral
RFP	right frontoposterior
RFT	right frontotransverse
RG	right gluteal
RGM	right gluteus medius
Rh	Rhesus factor in blood
RH	right hyperphoria; right hand; reduced haloperidol; room humidifier
RHB	raise head of bed
RHC	respiration has ceased
RHD	rheumatic heart disease; relative hepatic dullness
RHE	recombinant human erythropoietin
RHF	right heart failure

RHL	right hemisphere lesions
R-HuEPO	recombinant human erythropoietin
RHT	right hypertropia
RIA	radioimmunoassay
RIC	right iliac crest; right internal carotid (artery)
RICE	rest and immobilization, ice, compression, elevation
RICS	right intercostal space
RICU	respiratory intensive care unit
RID	radial immunodiffusion
RIF	rigid internal fixation; right iliac fossa
RIH	right inguinal hernia
RIMA	right internal mammary anastomosis
RIND	reversible ischemic neurologic defect
RIP	radioimmunoprecipitin test; rapid infusion pump
RISA	radioactive iodinated serum albumin
RIST	radioimmunosorbent test
RK	radial keratotomy
RL	right leg; right lung; right lateral
R-L	right to left
RLE	right lower extremity
RLF	retrolental fibroplasia
RLL	right lower lobe
RLQ	right lower quadrant
RLR	right lateral rectus
RLT	right lateral thigh
RM	repetitions maximum; room; radical mastectomy; respiratory movement
R & M	routine and microscopic
RMA	right meno-anterior
RMCA	right main coronary artery
RMCL	right midclavicular line
RMD	rapid movement disorder
RME	right mediolateral episiotomy
RMEE	right middle ear exploration
RMI	repetitive motion injuries
RML	right middle lobe
RMP	right mentoposterior
RMR	right medial rectus; resting metabolic rate
RMSF	Rocky Mountain spotted fever
RMT	right mentotransverse; registered music therapist
RN	registered nurse
RNA	radionuclide angiography
RND	radial neck dissection
RNEF	resting/radionuclide ejection fraction
RO	rule out; routine order
ROA	right occiput anterior
ROM	range of motion
ROP	right occiput posterior; retinopathy of prematurity
ROS	review of systems
ROSC	restoration of spontaneous circulation
RoRx	radiation therapy
ROT	right occipital transverse; remedial occupational therapy

RP	retinitis pigmentosa; retrograde pyelogram; Raynaud's phenomenon
RPA	right pulmonary artery; radial photon absorptiometry; registered physician assistant/associate
RPCF	Reiter protein complement fixation
RPD	removable partial denture
RPE	retinal pigment epithelium; rating of perceived exertion
RPF	renal plasma flow; relaxed pelvic floor
RPGN	rapidly progressive glomerulonephritis
RPH	retroperitoneal hemorrhage; registered pharmacist
RPICCE	round pupil intracapsular cataract extraction
RPLND	retroperitoneal lymphadenectomy
RPM	renal parenchymal malacoplakia
RPN	renal papillary necrosis
RPO	right posterior oblique
RPP	rate-pressure product
RPR	rapid plasma reagin; Reiter protein reagin
RPT	registered physical therapist
RQ	respiratory quotient
RR	recovery room; respiratory rate; regular respirations
R & R	rate and rhythm
RRE	round, regular, and equal
RREF	resting radionuclide ejection fraction
rRNA	ribosomal ribonucleic acid
RRND	right radical neck dissection
RRR	regular rhythm and rate
RRRN	round, regular, react normally
RS	Reiter's syndrome; Reye's syndrome; rhythm strip; right side
RSA	right sacrum anterior; right subclavian artery
RSDS	reflex-sympathetic dystrophy syndrome
RSI	repetitive stress injury
R-SICU	respiratory-surgical intensive care unit
RSO	right salpingo-oophorectomy; radiation safety officer
RSP	right sacroposterior
RSR	regular sinus rhythm; relative survival rate
RSTs	Rodney Smith tubes
RSV	respiratory syncytial virus
RSW	right-sided weakness
RT	right; radiation therapy; recreational therapy; renal transplant; running total; respiratory therapist; radiologic technician
R/t	related to
RTA	renal tubular acidosis
RTC	return to clinic; round the clock
RTL	reactive to light
rTNM	retreatment staging of cancer
RTO	return to office
RTOG	Radiation Therapy Oncology Group
rtPA	recombinant tissue-type plasminogen
RTRR	return to recovery room
RTS	real time scan
RT3U	resin triiodothyronine uptake
RTx	radiation therapy
RUA	routine urine analysis

RUE	right upper extremity
RUG	retrograde urethrogram
RUL	right upper lobe
rupt	ruptured
RUQ	right upper quadrant
RURTI	recurrent upper respiratory tract infection
RUSB	right upper sternal border
RV	right ventricle; residual volume; rectovaginal; rubella vaccine
RVD	relative vertebral density
RVE	right ventricular enlargement
RVET	right ventricular ejection time
RVG	radionuclide ventriculography
RVH	right ventricular hypertrophy; renovascular hypertension
RVL	right vastus lateralis
RVO	retinal vein occlusion; relaxed vaginal outlet
RVOT	right ventricular outflow tract
RVR	rapid ventricular response
RVSWI	right ventricular stroke work index
RV/TLC	residual volume to total lung capacity ratio
RVV	rubella vaccine virus
Rx	therapy; drug; medication; treatment; take
RXN	reaction
S	subjective findings; serum; suction; sacral; single; sister
S1	first heart sound; sacral vertebrae 1
S2	second heart sound
SA	sinoatrial; salicylic acid; sustained action; surface area; Spanish American
S/A	sugar and acetone
SAARD	slow-acting antirheumatic drugs
SAB	subarachnoid block/bleed
SAC	short arm cast
SACH	solid ankle cushion heel
SAD	sugar and acetone determination; seasonal affective disorder
SAE	signal-averaged electrocardiogram
SAF	self-articulating femoral
SAFE	stationary attachment and flexible endoskeletal (prosthesis)
Sag D	sagittal diameter
SAH	subarachnoid hemorrhage; systemic arterial hypertension
SAL 12	sequential analysis of 12 chemistry constituents
SAM	systolic anterior motion; self-administered medication
SAN	sinoatrial node
sang	sanguinous
SAPD	self-administration of psychotropic drugs
SAPHO	synovitis, acne, pustulosis, hyperostosis, osteitis
SAS	sleep apnea syndrome
SAT	subacute thyroiditis; saturation
SAVD	spontaneous assisted vaginal delivery
SB	stillbirth; stillborn; spina bifida; sternal border; Sengstaken-Blakemore (tube); sinus bradycardia; small bowel
SBE	subacute bacterial endocarditis
SBFT	small bowel follow through
SBGM	self blood glucose monitoring

SBI	systemic bacterial infection
SB-LM	Stanford Binet Intelligence Test—Form LM
SBO	small bowel obstruction
SBP	systolic blood pressure; spontaneous bacterial peritonitis
SBR	strict bed rest
SBT	serum bacterial titers
SC	subcutaneous; subclavian; sternoclavicular; sickle-cell; sulfur colloid; service connected
SCA	subcutaneous abdominal (block)
SCB	strictly confined to bed
SCBC	small cell bronchogenic carcinoma
SCC	squamous cell carcinoma; sickle cell crisis
SCCa	squamous cell carcinoma
SCCA	semi-closed circle absorber
SCD	sudden cardiac death; sickle cell disease; subacute combined degeneration; service connected disability; spinal cord disease
SCE	sister chromatic exchange
SCI	spinal cord injury
SCID	severe combined immunodeficiency disorder
SCIV	subclavian intravenous
SCLC	small-cell lung cancer
SCLE	subcutaneous lupus erythematosis
SCLs	soft contact lenses
SCM	sternocleidomastoid; spondylitic caudal myelopathy
SCR	spondylitic caudal radiculopathy
SC/SP	supracondylar/suprapatellar prosthesis
SCT	sickle cell trait; sugar coated tablet; sentence completion test
SCUT	schizophrenia chronic undifferentiated type
SCV	subcutaneous vaginal (block)
SD	senile dementia; scleroderma; spontaneous delivery; sterile dressing; surgical drain
S & D	stomach and duodenum
SDA	steroid-dependent asthmatic; Seventh-Day Adventist
SDAT	senile dementia of Alzheimer's type
SDH	subdual hematoma
SDL	serum digoxin level
SDS	same day surgery
SDT	speech detection threshold
SE	side effect
sec	secondary
sed	sedimentation
sed rt	sedimentation rate
SEER	Surveillance, Epidemiology, and End Results (program)
seg	segment; segmented neutrophil
SEM	systolic ejection murmur; scanning electron microscopy; standard error of mean
SEMI	subendocardial myocardial infarction
SENS	sensorium
SEP	systolic ejection period; somatosensory evoked potential; separate
SER-IV	supination external rotation, type 4 fracture
SERs	somatosensory-evoked responses
SES	socioeconomic status
SF	scarlet fever; sugar free; salt free; symptom free; spinal fluid

SFA	superficial femoral artery; saturated fatty acids
SFC	spinal fluid count
SFEMG	single-fiber electromyography
SFP	spinal fluid pressure
SFPT	standard fixation preference test
SG	specific gravity; serum glucose; Swan-Ganz
SGA	small for gestational age
SGD	straight gravity drainage
SGE	significant glandular enlargement
s gl	without correction/glasses
SGOT	serum glutamic oxaloacetic transaminase
SGPT	serum glutamic pyruvic transaminase
SH	serum hepatitis; social history; shower; short; shoulder
S & H	speech and hearing
S/H	suicidal/homicidal ideation
SHA	super heater aerosol
S Hb	sickle hemoglobin screen
SHEENT	skin, head, eyes, ears, nose throat
SHS	Student Health Service
SI	sacroiliac
SIADH	syndrome of inappropriate antidiuretic hormone secretion
S & I	suction and irrigation
SIB	self-injurious behavior
sibs	siblings
SICT	selective intracoronary thrombolysis
SICU	surgical intensive care unit
SIDS	sudden infant death syndrome
sig	let it be marked
SIJ	sacroiliac joint
SIMV	synchronized intermittent mandatory ventilation
SISI	short increment sensitivity index
SIT	sperm immobilization test; Slossen Intelligence Test
SIW	self-inflicted wound
SJS	Stevens-Johnson syndrome
SK	SmithKline®
SL	sublingual; slight
SLB	short leg brace
SLC	short leg cast
SLE	systemic lupus erythematosus; slit lamp examination
SLGXT	symptom limited graded exercise test
SLK	superior limbic keratoconjunctivitis
SLR	straight leg raising
SLRT	straight leg raising cast
SLWC	short leg walking cast
SM	systolic murmur; small
SMA	sequential multiple analyzer; simultaneous multichannel autoanalyzer; superior mesenteric artery; spinal muscular atrophy
SMC	special mouth care; somatomedin-C
SMD	senile macular degeneration
SMI	small volume infusion; sustained maximal inspiration
SMON	subacute myelopticoneuropathy
SMP	self-management program

SMR	submucosal resection; standardized mortality ratio; skeletal muscle relaxant; senior medical resident
SMS	senior medical student
SMVT	sustained monomorphic ventricular tachycardia
SN	student nurse
SNAP	sensory nerve action potential
SNCV	sensory nerve conduction velocity
SND	sinus node dysfunction
SNE	subacute necrotizing encephalomyelopathy
SNGFR	single nephron glomerular filtration rate
SNT	Suppan nail technique
S-O	salpingo-oophorectomy
SOA	swelling of ankles; supraorbital artery
SOAA	signed out against advice
SOAP	subjective, objective, assessment, and plan
SOB	shortness of breath
S & OC	signed and on chart (permission)
SOD	surgical officer of the day; superoxide dismutase
SOFAS	Social and Occupational Functioning Assessment Scale
sol	solution
SOM	serous otitis media
SOMI	sterno-occipital mandibular immobilizer
Sono	sonogram
SONP	solid organs not palpable
SOP	standard operating procedure
SOS	may be repeated once if urgently required
SOT	stream of thought
SP	suprapubic; sequential pulse; sacrum to pubis; speech pathologist
S/P	status post
SPA	albumin human; stimulation produced analgesia
SPAG	small particle aerosol generator
SPBI	serum protein bound iodine
SPBT	suprapubic bladder tap
SPE	serum protein electrolytes
spec	specimen
SPECT	single photon emission computer tomography
Spec Ed	special education
SPEP	serum protein electrophoresis
SPF	sun protective factor
sp fl	spinal fluid
sp gr	specific gravity
SPK	superficial punctate keratitis
SPMA	spinal progressive muscle atrophy
SPMSQ	Short Portable Mental Status Questionnaire
SPN	solitary pulmonary nodule
SPP	suprapubic prostatectomy
SPROM	spontaneous premature rupture of membrane
SPT	skin prick test
SP TAP	spinal tap
SPU	short procedure unit
SPVR	systemic peripheral vascular resistance
SQ	subcutaneous

Sq CCa	squamous cell carcinoma
SR	sedimentation rate; sustained release; side rails; system review; sinus rhythm
SRBC	sickle/sheep red blood cells
SRBOW	spontaneous rupture of bag of waters
SRC	scleroderma renal crisis
Sr Cr	serum creatinine
SRF	somatotropin releasing factor
SRF-A	slow releasing factor of anaphylaxis
SRIF	somatotropin-release-inhibiting factor
SRMD	stress-related mucosal damage
SR/NE	sinus rhythm, no ectopy
SRNS	steroid responsive nephrotic syndrome
SROM	spontaneous rupture of membrane
SRS-A	slow reacting substance of anaphylaxis
SRT	speech reception threshold; sedimentation rate test
SRU	side rails up
SS	saline solution; salt substitute; sickle cell; social security/service; slip sent; symmetrical strength
S & S	signs and symptoms
SSCA	single shoulder contrast arthrography
SSD	social security disability; source to skin distance
SSDI	social security disability income
SSE	saline solution/soapsuds enema; systemic side effects
SSEPs	somatosensory evoked potentials
SSM	superficial spreading melanoma
SSOP	Second Surgical Opinion Program
SSPE	subacute sclerosing panencephalitis
SSS	sick sinus syndrome; sterile saline soak
SSSS	staphylococcal scalded skin syndrome
ST	speech therapist; sinus tachycardia; split thickness
STA	superficial temporal artery
stab	polymorphonuclear leukocytes in nonmature form
staph	*Staphylococcus aureus*
stat	immediately
STB	stillborn
ST BY	standby
STD	sexually transmitted disease; skin test dose
STD TF	standard tube feeding
STET	submaximal treadmill exercise test
STF	special tube feeding
STG	short-term goals
STH	soft tissue hemorrhage; somatotrophic hormone
STJ	subtalar joint
STM	short-term memory
sTNM	surgical-evaluative staging of cancer
STNR	symmetrical tonic neck reflex
STORCH	syphilis, toxoplasmosis, other agents, rubella, cytomegalovirus, and herpes
STPD	standard temperature and pressure-dry
strep	streptococcus
STS	serologic test for syphilis
STSG	split thickness skin graft
STU	shock trauma unit

S & U	supine and upright
SU	sensory urgency; Somogyi units
SUB	Skene's urethra and Bartholin's glands
sub q	subcutaneous
SUD	sudden unexpected death
SUID	sudden unexplained infant death
SUNDS	sudden unexpected nocturnal death syndrome
SUP	supinator; superior
supp	suppository
SUR	surgery; surgical
SV	single ventricle; stock volume; sigmoid volvulus
SVC	superior vena cava
SVCO	superior vena cava obstruction
SVD	spontaneous vaginal delivery
SVE	sterile vaginal examination
SVPB	supraventricular premature beat
SVR	supraventricular rhythm; systemic vascular resistance
SVRI	systemic vascular resistance index
SVT	supraventricular tachycardia
SW	social worker
SWD	short wave diathermy
SWFI	sterile water for injection
SWI	sterile water for injection
SWOG	Southwest Oncology Group
SWS	slow wave sleep; Sturge-Weber syndrome; student ward secretary
SWT	stab wound of the throat
Sx	symptom; signs; surgery
SZ	seizure; suction; schizophrenic
T	temperature
T1/2	half-life
T1	tricuspid first sound; first thoracic vertebra
T3	triiodothyronine
4	thyroxine
T-7	free thyroxine factor
TA	therapeutic abortion; temperature axillary; tricuspid atresia
Ta	tonometry applanation
T & A	tonsillectomy and adenoidectomy
T(A)	axillary temperature
TAA	total ankle arthroplasty; thoracic aortic aneurysm; tumor-associated antigen (antibodies); transverse aortic arch
TAB	therapeutic abortion; triple antibiotic; tablet
TAD	transverse abdominal diameter
TAE	transcatheter arterial embolization
TAF	tissue angiogenesis factor
TAH	total abdominal hysterectomy; total artificial heart
TAL	tendon Achilles lengthening
TANI	total axial node irradiation
TAO	thromboangiitis obliterans
TAPVC	total anomalous pulmonary venous connection
TAPVD	total anomalous pulmonary venous drainage
TAPVR	total anomalous pulmonary venous return

TAR	thrombocytopenia with absent radius
TARA	total articular replacement arthroplasty
TAS	therapeutics activities specialist
TAT	tetanus antitoxin; till all taken; Thematic Apperception Test
TB	tuberculosis
TBA	to be admitted; to be absorbed
TBB	transbronchial biopsy
tbc	tuberculosis
TBE	tick-borne encephalitis
TBG	thyroxine-binding globulin
TBI	total body irradiation
T bili	total bilirubin
tbl	tablespoon (15 mL)
TBM	tubule basement membrane
TBNA	treated but not admitted
TBPA	thyroxine-binding prealbumin
TBR	total bed rest
TBSA	total burn surface area
tbsp	tablespoon (15 mL)
TBV	total blood volume; transluminal balloon valvuloplasty
TBW	total body water
T/C	to consider
TC	throat culture; true conjugate
T & C	type and crossmatch; turn and cough
TCA	tricuspid atresia; terminal cancer
TCABG	triple coronary artery bypass graft
TCBS agar	thiosulfate-citrate-bile salt-sucrose agar
TCCB	transitional cell carcinoma of bladder
TCDB	turn, cough, and deep breathe
T-cell	small lymphocyte
TCH	turn, cough, hyperventilate
TCID50	median tissue culture doses
TCM	transcutaneous monitor; tissue culture media
TCMH	tumor-direct cell-mediated hypersensitivity
TCT	thrombin clotting
TCVA	thromboembolic cerebral vascular accident
TD	tardive dyskinesia; travelers diarrhea; Takayasu's disease; transverse diameter; tidal volume; treatment discontinued; tetanus-diphtheria toxoid
Td	tetanus-diphtheria toxoid
TDD	thoracic duct drainage
TDE	total daily energy (requirement)
TDF	tumor dose fractionation
TDK	tardive dyskinesia
TDM	therapeutic drug monitoring
TdP	torsades de pointes
TDT	tentative discharge tomorrow
TE	tracheoesophageal; trace elements; thromboembolism
T & E	trial and error
TEA	total elbow arthroplasty; thromboendarterectomy
TEC	total eosinophil count
TEDS®	anti-embolism stockings
TEE	transesophageal echocardiography

TEF	tracheoesophageal fistula
TEG	thromboelastogram
tele	telemetry
TEM	transmission electron microscopy
TEN	toxic epidermal necrolysis
TEN®	total enteral nutrition
TENS	transcutaneous electrical nerve stimulation
tert	tertiary
TES	treatment emergent symptoms; trace element solution
TET	treadmill exercise test
TF	tetralogy of Fallot; tactile fremitus; tube feeding; to follow
TFB	trifascicular block
TFTs	thyroid function tests
TG	triglycerides
TGA	transient global amnesia; transposition of the great arteries
TGF	tissue/transforming growth factor
TGFA	triglyceride fatty acid
TGS	tincture of green soap
TGT	thromboplastin generation test
TH	total hysterectomy; thyroid hormone; thrill
THA	total hip arthroplasty; transient hemispheric attack
THC	transhepatic cholangiogram
TH-CULT	throat culture
THE	transhepatic embolization
Ther Ex	therapeutic exercise
THI	transient hypogammaglobulinemia of infancy
THR	total hip replacement
TI	tricuspid insufficiency
TIA	transient ischemic attack
tib	tibia
TIBC	total iron binding capacity
TIE	transient ischemia episode
TIG	tetanus immune globulin
TIN	tubulointerstitial nephritis
tinct	tincture
TJ	triceps jerk
TJN	twin jet nebulizer
TKA	total knee arthroplasty
TKNO	to keep needle open
TKP	thermokeratoplasty
TKO	to keep open
TKR	total knee replacement
TL	tubal ligation; team leader; trial leave
TLC	triple lumen catheter; thin layer chromatography; total lung capacity; total lymphocyte count; tender loving care
TLI	total lymphoid irradiation
TLS	tumor lysis syndrome
TLV	total lung volume
TM	tympanic membrane; trabecular meshwork
TMA	transmetatarsal amputation
TMB	transient monocular blindness
TMC	transmural colitis

TMET	treadmill exercise test
TMI	threatened myocardial infarction
TMJ	temporomandibular joint
TMP	trimethoprim; thallium myocardial perfusion
TMS	trace metal solution
TMTC	too many to count
Tn	normal intraocular tension
TNF	tumor necrosis factor
TNI	total nodal irradiation
TNM	tumor node metastasis
TNTC	too numerous to count
TO	telephone order
T(O)	oral temperature
TOA	tubo-ovarian abscess; time of arrival
TOF	tetralogy of Fallot
TOGV	transposition of the great vessels
TOL	trial of labor
tomo	tomography
TOP	termination of pregnancy
TOPP	a drug combination protocol
TOPV	trivalent oral polio vaccine
TORCH	toxoplasmosis, other (syphilis, hepatitis, Zoster), rubella, cytomegalovirus, and herpes simplex
TORP	total ossicular replacement prosthesis
TOS	thoracic outlet syndrome
TP	total protein; Todd's paralysis
TPA	tissue plasminogen activator; tissue polypeptide antigen; total parenteral alimentation
TPC	total patient care
TPD	tropical pancreatic diabetes
TPE	total protective environment
TPH	thromboembolic pulmonary hypertension
TPI	Treponema pallidum immobilization test
TPM	temporary pacemaker
TPN	total parenteral nutrition
TP & P	time, place, and person
TPPE	time, person, place, and event
TPPN	total peripheral parenteral nutrition
TPR	temperature, pulse and respiration; temperature; total peripheral resistance
TPT	time to peak tension
TPVR	total peripheral vascular resistance
Tr	trace; tremor; treatment; tincture
T(R)	rectal temperature
TRA	therapeutic recreation associate
trach	tracheal; tracheostomy
Trans D	transverse diameter
TRC	tanned red cells
TRD	traction retinal detachment
Tren	Trendelenberg
TRH	thyrotropin-releasing hormone
TRIG	triglycerides
tRNA	transfer ribonucleic acid

TRNG	tetracycline resistant Neisseria gonorrhea
TRP	tubular reabsorption of phosphate
TRT	thermoradiotherapy
T3RU	triiodothyroxine resin uptake
TS	test solution; Tourette's syndrome
TSA	total shoulder arthroplasty
TSAR®	tape surrounded Appli-rulers®
TSBB	transtracheal selective bronchial brushing
TSD	Tay-Sachs disease; target to skin distance
T set	tracheotomy set
TSF	triceps skin fold
TSH	thyroid stimulating hormone
tsp	teaspoon (5 mL)
TSP	total serum protein
TSR	total shoulder replacement
TSS	toxic shock syndrome
TST	titmus stereocuity test
T & T	touch and tone
TT	thrombin time; thymol turbidity; twitch tension; transtracheal; tilt table
TT3	total serum triiodothyronine
TT4	total thyroxine
TTA	total toe arthroplasty
TTN	transient tachypnea of the newborn
TTNB	transient tachypnea of the newborn
TTP	thrombotic thrombocytopenic purpura
TTS	through the skin
TTVP	temporary transvenous pacemaker
TTY-TDD	teletypewriter for the deaf
TU	tuberculin units
TUN	total urinary nitrogen
TUR	transurethral resection
T3UR	triiodothyronine uptake ratio
TURB	turbidity
TURBN	transurethral resection bladder tumor
TURP	transurethral resection of prostate
TURV	transurethral resection valves
TV	tidal volume; trial visit; *Trichomonas vaginalis*
TVC	triple voiding cystogram; true vocal cord
TVH	total vaginal hysterectomy
TVP	transvenous pacemaker
TW	test weight
TWD	total white and differential count
TWE	tapwater enema
TWETC	tapwater enema till clear
TWWD	tapwater wet dressing
Tx	treatment; therapy; traction; transfuse; transplant
TxA2	thromboxane A2
Tyl	tyloma
U	units; urine
U/1	1 finger breadth below umbilicus
1/U	1 finger over umbilicus

U/	at umbilicus
UA	uric acid; urinalysis; unauthorized absence; uncertain about
UAC	umbilical artery
UAE	urinary albumin excretion
UAL	umbilical artery line
UAO	upper airway obstruction
UAT	up as tolerated
UAVC	univentricular atrioventricular connection
UBF	unknown black female
UBI	ultraviolet blood irradiation
UBM	unknown black male
UC	urine culture; urethral catheter; uterine contraction; ulcerative colitis
U & C	urethral and cervical
UCD	usual childhood diseases
UCG	urinary chorionic-gonadotropins
UCHD	usual childhood diseases
UCI	urethral catheter in
UCO	urethral catheter out
UCX	urine culture
UD	urethral discharge
UDC	usual diseases of childhood
UE	upper extremity
UES	upper esophageal sphincter
UFO	unflagged order
UFR	uroflowmetry
UG	urogenital
UGDP	University Group Diabetes Program
UGH	uveitis, glaucoma, hyphema
UGI	upper gastrointestinal series
UHBI	upper hemibody irradiation
UHDDS	Uniform Hospital Discharge Data Set
UID	once daily
UIQ	upper inner quadrant
U/L	upper and lower
ULN	upper limits of normal
ULQ	upper left quadrant
UK	urokinase; unknown
UN	urinary nitrogen
UNA	urinary nitrogen appearance; urine sodium
ung	ointment
UNK	unknown
UOQ	upper outer quadrant
UPEP	urine protein electrophoresis
UPJ	ureteropelvic junction
U/P ratio	urine to plasma ratio
UPP	urethral pressure profile studies
UPT	urine pregnancy test
UR	utilization review
URI	upper respiratory infection
urol	urology
US	ultrasonography; unit secretary
USA	unit services assistant

USB	upper sternal border
USG	ultrasonography
USI	urinary stress incontinence
USN	ultrasonic nebulizer
USP	*United States Pharmacopeia*
USRDS	United States Renal Data System
UTD	up to date
ut dict	as directed
UTF	usual throat flora
UTI	urinary tract infection
UTO	upper tibial osteotomy
UTZ	ultrasound
UUN	urine urea nitrogen
UV	ultraviolet
UVA	ultraviolet A light; ureterovesical angle
UVB	ultraviolet B light
UVC	umbilical vein catheter
UVJ	ureterovesical junction
UVL	ultraviolet light
UVR	ultraviolet rays
UWF	unknown white female
UWM	unknown white male
V	vomiting; vein; vagina; five
VA	Veterans Administration; visual acuity; vacuum aspiration
VAC	ventriculoarterial connections
VAD	vascular/venous access device
vag	vagina
VAG HYST	vaginal hysterectomy
VAH	Veterans Administration Hospital
VAMC	Veterans Administration Medical Center
VAPA	a drug combination protocol
VAR	variant
VAS	vascular; visual analogue scale
VASC	Visual-Auditory Screen Test for Children
VAS RAD	vascular radiology
VB	VanBuren (catheter)
VBAC	vaginal birth after cesarean
VBI	vertebrobasilar insufficiency
VBS	vertebral-basilar system
VC	vital capacity; vena cava; vocal cords; color vision; vomiting center
VCG	vectorcardiography
VCT	venous clotting time
VCU	voiding cystourethrogram
VCUG	vesicoureterogram; voiding cystourethrogram
VD	venereal disease; volume of distribution; voided
VDA	visual discriminatory acuity; venous digital angiogram
VDG	venereal disease—gonorrhea
VDH	valvular disease of the heart
VDRL	Venereal Disease Research Laboratory (test for syphilis)
VDRR	vitamin D-resistant rickets
VDS	venereal disease—syphilis

VDT	video display terminal
VE	vaginal examination; vertex; volume of expired gas
VEB	ventricular ectopic beat
VEE	Venezuelan equine encephalitis
vent	ventricular; ventral
VEP	visual evoked potential
VER	visual evoked response; ventricular escape rhythm
VF	ventricular fibrillation; vision field; vocal fremitus
V fib	ventricular fibrillation
VFP	vitreous fluorophotometry
VG	vein graft; ventricular gallop; very good
VH	vaginal hysterectomy; viral hepatitis; vitreous hemorrhage; Veterans Hospital
VI	volume index; six
vib	vibration
VID	videodensitometry
VIG	vaccinia immune globulin
VIP	voluntary interruption of pregnancy; vasoactive intestinal peptide
VISC	vitreous infusion suction cutter
VIT	vitamin; vital; venom immunotherapy
vit cap	vital capacity
VKC	vernal keratoconjunctivitis
VLBW	very low birth weight
VLDL	very low density lipoprotein
VLH	ventrolateral nucleus of the hypothalamus
VMH	ventromedial hypothalamus
VNA	Visiting Nurses Association
VO	verbal order
VOCTOR	void on call to operating room
VOD	vision right eye; venocclusive disease
VOL	voluntary
VOR	vestibular ocular reflex
VOS	vision left eye
VOU	vision both eyes
VP	venous pressure; variegate porphyria; ventriculoperitoneal; ventricular-peritoneal
V & P	ventilation and perfusion; vagotomy and pyloroplasty
VPB	ventricular premature beat
VPC	ventricular premature contractions
VPDs	ventricular premature depolarizations
VPL	vento-posterolateral
V/Q	ventilation/perfusion (scan)
VR	ventricular rhythm; verbal reprimand
VRA	visual reinforcement audiometry
VS	vital signs; versus
VSD	venous stasis retinopathy
VSS	vital signs stable
VT	ventricular tachycardia; tidal volume
v tach	ventricular tachycardia
VTE	venous thromboembolism
VTX	vertex
VV	varicose veins
V & V	vulva and vagina
V/V	volume to volume ratio

VVFR	vesicovaginal fistula repair
VVOR	visual-vestibulo-ocular-reflex
VW	vessel wall
VWM	ventricular wall motion
VZ	varicella zoster
VZIG	varicella zoster immune globulin
VZV	varicella zoster virus
w	white; with; widowed
WA	while awake; when awake
WAIS	Wechsler Adult Intelligence Scale
WAIS-R	Wechsler Adult Intelligence Scale—Revised
WAP	wandering atrial pacemaker
WAS	Wiskott-Aldrich syndrome
WASS	Wasserman test
WB	whole blood; weight bearing
WBAT	weight bearing as tolerated
WBC	white blood cell/count
WBH	whole-body hyperthermia
WBN	wellborn nursery
WC	wheelchair; white count; ward clerk; whooping cough
W/D	warm and dry; withdrawal
W-D	wet to dry
WDHA	watery diarrhea, hypokalemia, and achlorhydria
WDL	well-differentiated lymphocyte
WDLL	well-differentiated lymphocytic lymphoma
WDWN-BF	well-developed, well-nourished black female
WDWN-BM	well-developed, well-nourished black male
WDWN-WF	well-developed, well-nourished white female
WDWN-WM	well-developed, well-nourished white male
WE	weekend
WEE	western equine encephalitis
WEP	weekend pass
WF	white female
WFI	water for injection
WFL	within functional limits
WFR	wheel-and-flare reaction
WHO	World Health Organization
WHV	woodchuck hepatitis virus
WHVP	wedged hepatic venous pressure
WIA	wounded in action
WIC	women, infants, and children
WID	widow; widower
WISC	Wechsler Intelligence Scale for Children
WLS	wet lung syndrome
WLT	waterload test
WKS	Wernicke-Korsakoff syndrome
WM	white male
WMA	wall motion abnormality
WN	well-nourished
WND	wound
WNL	within normal limits

W/O	without
WO	written order; weeks old
WP	whirlpool
WPFM	Wright peak flow meter
WPPSI	Wechsler Preschool Primary Scale of Intelligence
WPW	Wolff-Parkinson-White
WR	Wasserman reaction; wrist
WS	ward secretary; watt seconds
wt	weight
WWAC	walk with aid of cane
W/U	workup
W/V	weight-to-volume ratio
W/W	weight-to-weight ratio
X	cross-match; start of anesthesia; except; times; ten; break
X3	orientation as to person, place, and time
X & D	examination and diagnosis
XM	cross-match
X-mat	cross-match
XMM	xeromammography
XRT	radiotherapy
XS-LIM	exceeds limits of procedure
XT	exotropia
XX	normal female sex chromosome type
XY	normal male sex chromosome type
YACP	young adult chronic patient
YAG	yttrium aluminum garnert (laser)
YF	yellow fever
YJV	yellow jacket venom
YLC	youngest living child
YO	years old
YORA	younger-onset rheumatoid arthritis
YSC	yolk sac carcinoma
ZEEP	zero end-expiratory pressure
ZES	Zollinger-Ellison syndrome
Z-ESR	zeta erythrocyte sedimentation rate
ZIFT	zygote intrafallopian transfer
ZIG	zoster serum immune globulin
ZIP	zoster immune plasma
ZIZ	zoster serum immune globulin
ZMC	zygomatic
Zn	zinc

Study Examinations

Readers who study the text may wish to review what they have learned, testing themselves on specific chapters to discover how much they recall before they proceed to the next unit. As a result, these self-tests were designed to provide a means of examining what a reader has learned and a sample of potential questions a teacher might use in examining students. Although these study examinations are limited in nature, they test the reader on a wide range of the terminology in each chapter, giving an overview of how much was learned. Answer keys are provided at the end of the appendix.

Most readers will not be able to answer all the questions correctly, even after a careful reading of the text; after all, medical terminology is so vast that a person may be able to communicate quite effectively and still not recall all the terms studied. Those unable to answer a number of questions in a recently completed chapter, however, may wish to review further.

Self-Tests

Chapter 1: Fundamentals of Medical Terms

Prefixes

1. Define these terms containing prefixes related to *without*:
   apnea—
   anemia—

2. Define these terms containing prefixes related to *away from*:
   decapitate—
   abductor—

3. Define these terms containing prefixes related to *before*:
   prognosis—
   antepartum—

4. Define these terms containing prefixes related to *against*:
   antipyretic—
   contraceptive—

5. Define these terms containing prefixes related to *outside*:
   ectoderm—
   exogenous—

6. Define these terms containing prefixes related to *within*:
   endocarditis—
   intraocular—

7. Define these terms containing prefixes related to *below/under*:
   hypotension—
   subcostal—

8. Define these terms containing prefixes related to above/excessive:
   suprarenal—
   supernatant—

9. Define the following terms containing prefixes related to number/measurement:
   hyporeflexia—
   octose—
   monophasia—

10. Define the following terms containing prefixes related to color:
    cyanosis—
    xanthoma—

Roots

For each of the medical terms listed below, (a) indicate the root in each word and (b) give the meaning of the root:

1. ankylosis—

2. blastoma—

3. cytolysis—

4. hyperglycemia—

5. thermolysis—

6. blennorrhea—

7. stenosis—

8. aerocele—

9. ergotherapy—

10. pedionalgia—

Suffixes

1. In the words *septicemia* and *hypokalemia,* the suffix is _____, meaning _____.

2. In the word *adenopathy,* the suffix is _____, meaning _____.

3. The words *cardiorrhexis* and *angiorrhexis* both contain the suffix _____, meaning _____.

4. The suffix in the word *quadriplegia* is _____, meaning _____.

5. Surgical terms ending in the suffix ''-rrhaphy'' denote a procedure involving _____.

6. Surgical terms ending in the suffix ''-ectomy'' denote a procedure involving _____.

7. Two suffixes that denote ''pain'' are _____ and _____.

8. Words ending in the suffix ''-phagia'' refer to _____, while those ending in ''-phasia'' denote involvement of _____.

9. Any word ending with the suffix ''-itis'' denotes some form of _____ is involved.

10. In the words *carcinoma* and *lymphoma*, the suffix is _____, meaning _____.

Chapter 2: The Health Care System and Its Structure

1. Certifying boards for physicians come under the general jurisdiction of the _____.

2. Determinations of major diagnostic categories for Medicare reimbursement are made by the _____.

3. Among the abbreviations denoting specific health care professions are ''PT,'' denoting a _____, and ''SP,'' denoting a _____.

4. The abbreviation commonly used to denote the accrediting agency for most hospitals is _____, referring to the _____.

5. The medical specialty dealing with diagnosis and treatment of disorders of the foot may be designated as either _____ or _____.

6. The Medicare prospective reimbursement system is based on categorization of patients into _____.

7. Two examples of medical specialties established to treat a particular organ system are _____ and _____.

8. _____ is the medical specialty dealing with diseases of children, while _____ specializes in diseases associated with aging.

9. Three abbreviations pertaining to quality control programs performed by the hospital pharmacy are _____, _____, and _____.

10. A managed care system that controls a patient's access to care by relying on employed and contracted providers is known as a(n) _____.

Chapter 3: Translating the Medical Record

1. The notation ''FCSNVD'' on a medical record would indicate that the patient was experiencing _____, _____, _____, _____, _____, and _____.

2. A chronological description of signs and symptoms relating to a patient's presenting problem is known as the _____.

3. Pathogens (disease-producing organisms) would be detected in the patient through the use of _____ laboratory studies.

4. Immunodiagnostic studies, also called _____ tests, study _____ reactions within the body.

5. The use of X rays is called _____.

6. The term *sigmoidoscopy* would denote a diagnostic procedure involving the _____.

7. Two combining forms or roots that denote the presence of pus are _____ and _____.

8. The designation used for recurrent episodes of rapid breathing followed by cessation of breathing is _____.

9. The procedure utilizing radioactive chemicals and antibiotics to detect the presence of drugs and hormones in a blood specimen is known as _____.

10. A patient admitted to the hospital with symptoms of a heart attack could be treated in a location designated as _____ (CCU), _____ (CICU), _____ (ICCU), or _____ (CSU).

Chapter 4: Abbreviations, Eponyms, and Lay Terms

Lay Terms

1. The commonly used lay term for the tympanic membrane is _____. The patella is the correct medical term for the _____.

2. The correct medical term for "bedsore" is _____.

3. A child who wets the bed at night would have a condition known as _____.

4. A patient who reports a (a) boil, (b) fever blister, and a (c) wart would be referring to the medical terms: (a) _____; (b) _____; and (c) _____.

5. Commonly used slang terms for barbiturates include _____, _____, _____, and _____.

6. A patient who reports having "done a Space Base" should be considered to have administered the combination of _____ and _____.

7. The commonly used lay term for head cold is _____. Pyrosis is more commonly referred to as _____.

8. The correct medical term for fever is _____. A patient described as having "food poisoning" would probably be diagnosed with _____.

9. Reference to the carpus denotes the area of the _____. The thigh bone is correctly termed the _____.

10. A child with pink eye would have the medical diagnosis of _____, while one with the mumps would have _____.

Eponyms

1. The eponym for the condition involving a general mental deterioration is _____.

2. Eponyms involving disorders of the gastrointestinal tract include _____ and _____.

3. Paralysis of the facial nerve is known as _____.

4. The eponym for a condition involving wasting of muscles in the leg is _____.

5. Eponyms may be found in a standard medical dictionary most often under the headings of _____ or _____.

6. Two eponyms involving fractures of bones in the arm or leg are _____ and _____.

7. Give the medical term for the following eponyms: Buerger's disease _____

8. Down's syndrome _____

9. Fanconi's syndrome _____

10. Hodgkin's disease _____

Chapter 5: The Cardiovascular System and Its Disorders

1. The large artery emerging from the top of the heart and leading to the systemic circulation is the _____; the segment closest to the heart is called the _____ because of its position and the direction of blood flow.

2. The openings between the atria and ventricles are called _____ orifices. The right orifice is covered by the _____ valve, so named because of the number of flaps it incorporates; within the left orifice is the _____ valve, also called the _____ valve because of the shape of its flaps.

3. The Greek word for heart is the source of the root appearing in the words _____, an inflammation of the lining and valves of the heart, and _____, an inflammation of the heart muscle.

4. The Latin word for crown refers to the heart because of the location of the _____ arteries, the vessels that supply blood to the heart.

5. The word indicating an inflammation within a vessel or duct is _____, from the root meaning ''vessel'' and the suffix indicating an inflammation.

6. Pulse-reflected ultrasound can be used to produce line tracings to allow evaluation of cardiac structure, but multiple scans can be integrated into a more complete visualization called a(n) _____ _____, which produces a real-time "picture" of the internal structures of the heart.

7. Depression of the _____ segment on an electrocardiogram during a treadmill stress test is often indicative of _____.

8. The transfer of gasses and the elimination of volatile waste takes place in the _____ of the pulmonary circuit. Similarly, supply of nutrients and oxygen to tissues takes place in the same structures of the systemic circulation, endothelial tubes between the microscopic _____ of the arterial side and _____ of the venous side.

9. The basic cause of angina pectoris is _____ _____, a relative lack of oxygen supply to heart muscle. If angina does not respond adequately to initial therapy, the patient may require a procedure to visualize the arteries of the heart, called _____ _____, to evaluate the specific areas and degree of arterial occlusion.

10. Depolarizations of the ventricle before the next expected beat are called _____ _____ _____, often referred to as _____, and may be precipitated by diseases causing myocardial inflammation, myocardial stretching, ischemia, or other factors.

Chapter 6: The Digestive System and Its Disorders

1. The digestive process begins with the secretion of _____ in the mouth. Its function is to _____.

2. Food is moved by the tongue to the _____, at which time swallowing becomes involuntary. It is then moved down the _____ by a process known as _____.

3. The four regions of the stomach are _____, _____, _____, and _____. Their primary secretions are _____.

4. The three portions of the small intestine are the _____, _____, and _____.

5. In addition to _____ processed by the small intestine, secretions from the _____ and _____ also enter here.

6. The portions of the large intestine are _____, _____, _____, _____, _____, and _____.

7. Bleeding from the gastrointestinal tract may present as _____, _____, or _____.

8. _____ and _____ are the most commonly observed causes of jaundice.

9. Three clinical symptoms of esophageal disease are _____, _____, and _____.

10. The three areas of a tooth are the _____, _____, and the _____. The tooth is composed of _____, _____, _____, and _____.

Chapter 7: The Musculoskeletal System and Its Disorders

1. The primary components of the musculoskeletal system are the _____, _____, _____, _____, and _____.

2. The three bones of the leg are the _____, _____, and _____. The bones comprising the arm are the _____, _____, and _____.

3. The flexible tissue that forms the connecting structures of the skeleton, acting as a shock absorber, is the _____.

4. A long bone consists of the shaft or main body, known as the _____, and the end or _____.

5. Three types of inflammatory muscle disorders are _____, _____, and _____.

6. Inflammation of the bursa is called bursitis, while the term for inflammation of the tendon and tendon sheath is _____.

7. The most common type of hernia is _____. Four other types of hernias are _____, _____, _____, and _____.

8. A(n) _____ is a specialist in correction of bone and joint deformities.

9. Gout, ankylosing spondylitis and systemic lupus erythematosus are considered to be diseases of the _____.

10. A herniated disk would involve bones located in the _____.

Chapter 8: The Integumentary System and Its Disorders

1. The parts of the body included in the integumentary system are the _____, _____, _____, and _____.

2. The term that denotes study of the integumentary system is _____; a _____ is a specialist in the diagnosis and treatment of skin disorders.

3. List six of the twelve types of skin lesions: _____, _____, _____, _____, _____, and _____.

4. The medical term for itching is _____; _____ is a chronic skin disorder characterized by exacerbation of thick, scaly lesions.

5. The primary disease of the oil or _____ glands in humans is _____.

6. Three types of superficial skin infections are _____, _____, and _____.

7. Skin lesions appearing in patches that have thickened layers are described as being _____.

8. Give the medical equivalent of the following lay terms: freckles _____; moles _____; blackheads _____.

9. Two disorders of melanin pigmentation are overproduction or _____ and underproduction or _____.

10. Two roots meaning "skin" are _____ and _____.

Chapter 9: The Respiratory System and Its Disorders

1. Organs that function in the respiratory process include the _____, _____, _____, _____, _____, and _____.

2. In the lung, the bronchi branch into minute tubes called _____, which terminate in tiny air sacs called _____.

3. Oxygen passes into the bloodstream from the _____ in the lungs.

4. The protein molecule that carries oxygen in the blood is called _____.

5. The lungs rest upon a large muscle called the _____, which _____ during inspiration and _____ during expiration.

6. Two terms that denote chest pain are _____ and _____.

7. The term for collection of gas in the pleural space is _____, while the term _____ refers to presence of blood in the pleural cavity.

8. An increase in the level of carbon dioxide in the blood is called _____. This produces a deficiency of oxygen, which is termed _____.

9. Three types of procedures performed on the respiratory tract with an endoscope are _____, _____, and _____.

10. Two terms that denote incision into the chest wall are _____ and _____.

Chapter 10: The Reproductive System and Its Disorders

1. In the male, sperm production takes place within the _____ _____ _____, so named because they are literally "twisted, seed-producing small tubes."

2. The broadened portions of both the ductus deferens and the uterine tube are called the _____, a name indicating their shape; in fact, the term is the Latin word for "bottle." Similarly, the narrowing of the uterine tube and the narrowing of the uterus are both referred to as the _____, a term that indicates a narrow connection between two larger bodies and is even applied to the geographical connection between land masses.

3. Developing ova can be called _____ or _____, words derived from Latin and Greek terms for "egg" and a root meaning "cell."

4. Infection and inflammation of the fallopian tube may be referred to by three names: _____, a combination of the root meaning uterine tube and a suffix indicating inflammation; _____, which is actually an English description of the disorder; and the commonly used acronym _____.

5. Menstrual disorders are frequently described by a combination of the root for menstruation and a prefix denoting the abnormality. For example, painful menstruation is called _____; lack of menstrual flow is _____; reduced flow is _____; excessive flow is _____; abnormally frequent flow is _____ or _____; and occluded flow that causes retention of the menstrual products is _____.

6. Many infectious diseases must be reported to the appropriate public health authorities, which are called _____; although such infectious diseases as rubella and measles are included, a large proportion of these infections are _____, what were formerly more frequently called venereal diseases.

7. Literally meaning "cave-like body," the term _____ _____ refers to erectile tissue in either the penis or the clitoris.

8. Of the possible presentations of the fetus at birth, most of the terms describe the part of the fetus that is toward the cervix—the face, head (cephalic), buttocks (breech), and so on. One of the terms, however, refers to the position of the axis of the fetal body, which is across the axis of the maternal body; such a _____ presentation may place the fetal torso, arm, or shoulder closest to the cervix.

9. In a pregnant woman's medical record, she may be listed as _____ or _____ if this is her third pregnancy. However, she may also be classified as _____ if none of the previous two pregnancies produced a birth of a viable offspring.

10. A Class IV Papanicolaou test indicates the presence of carcinoma cells, so the lesion should be biopsied by _____ biopsy and endocervical curettage or by _____ biopsy, which may remove enough of the tissue to effectively treat the lesion.

Chapter 11: The Urinary System and Its Disorders

1. A knot of capillaries that filters the blood in the kidneys, beginning the formation of urine, is called the _____; the filtrate then passes from the Bowman's capsule into the _____.

2. The funnel-shaped collecting structure in the kidney that drains into the ureter is the _____. The urine entering this structure comes from the major and minor _____ in the renal medulla.

3. Named for its ability to "push down" on the bladder contents and evacuate the bladder, the _____ is the term applied to the muscles of the bladder.

4. Abnormal urinary output volume is a common symptom of renal disease, although usually nonspecific. For example, _____ (excessive urinary output) may suggest diabetes mellitus, but it is not diagnostic. Similarly, _____ (decreased output) can result from numerous renal disorders.

5. The procedure for removing urinary calculi from the bladder without surgery has two names: _____ is named for the process in which sound waves "rub" the stone to pieces, and _____ is derived from the second part of the procedure involving washing the pieces out through the urethra.

6. Imaging of the bladder by roentgenography after injecting or infusing a radiopaque medium is referred to as _____; similarly, imaging of the entire urinary system is called _____.

7. After centrifugation of the urine from a patient with glomerulonephritis, microscopic examination of the sediment will almost always reveal the presence of _____, caused by damage to the glomerulus, which causes the "leakage" of red blood cells into the filtrate.

8. Inflammation of the renal pelvis caused by bacterial infection is called _____ _____, a condition that is diagnosed by the laboratory finding of bacterial casts and bacteriuria, and the clinical symptoms of dysuria with abrupt onset and decreased urinary output.

9. Severe proteinuria and increased serum albumin are symptoms that form the complex known as _____, often leading to hyperlipidemia and edema.

10. Fiber optic examination of the lumen of the urethra, a procedure known as _____, is helpful in diagnosing inflammatory, malignant, and structural disorders of the urethra.

Chapter 12: The Nervous System and Its Disorders

1. Multiple sclerosis is caused by degeneration of the _____ surrounding sensory and motor nerves, causing a loss in _____ conduction and a resultant muscular weakness or paralysis.

2. Viral or bacterial infection, particularly of the arachnoid or pia mater, is the most common cause of _____, an inflammation of the _____.

3. The terms for procedures performed on the same part of the anatomy may use the same root but different suffixes. For example, _____ denotes an incision into the skull, while _____ denotes removal of part of the skull.

4. The two-word term that literally means "mass of blood under the dura mater" is _____, an accumulation of blood that responds well to surgical drainage; similarly, bleeding within the brain itself would cause an accumulation of blood known as an intracranial hematoma.

5. Several drugs can be used in surgery to cause paralysis by blocking the transmission of an impulse from a nerve to the muscle it innervates at the point where they meet, called the _____.

6. If the body's immune system produces antibodies to the acetylcholine receptors, the receptors become less responsive to acetylcholine, resulting in a paralysis called _____, a severe muscle weakness treated with cholinesterase inhibitors.

7. The term for the accumulation of fluid within the brain causing increased intracranial pressure is _____, literally meaning ''water in the head.''

8. Phenothiazines are known for their _____ side effects, which refers to effects on nerve transmission through the nerve tracts of the lower medulla, which are outside the ridges known as _____.

9. In an afferent nerve, impulses are carried toward the _____; an efferent nerve carries impulses toward _____. In both, however, the impulse arrives at the cell body from the shorter processes called _____ and is transmitted away from the cell body through the _____.

10. To analyze the white cell and glucose content of cerebrospinal fluid in a patient suspected of viral or bacterial meningitis, a physician would collect a sample of the CSF through a procedure known as a _____.

Chapter 13: The Special Sense Organs and Their Disorders

1. The five special senses are _____, _____, _____, _____, and _____.

2. Three terms used to denote the sense of smell are _____, _____, and _____.

3. The primary receptors for equilibrium in the inner ear are the _____, _____, and _____.

4. Three accessory structures of the eye that function as supportive and protective devices are the _____, _____, and _____.

5. Inflammation of the middle ear is called _____.

6. List five terms that denote inflammation of various parts of the optic system: _____, _____, _____, _____, and _____.

7. Two terms that describe pain in the ear are _____, and _____.

8. A physician who specializes in treating eye disorders is an _____ or _____.

9. A specialist in treating disorders of the ear is an _____.

10. List four terms that describe surgical procedures utilized to correct disorders of vision: _____, _____, _____, and _____.

Chapter 14: Psychiatric Disorders

1. In a patient with a(n) _____, the psychological and physical reactions to stress differ quantitatively from the reactions of normal individuals, being more intense and of longer

duration; in a patient with a(n) _____, the reactions differ qualitatively and the perception of reality is usually disturbed.

2. A person with abnormal recurrent thoughts and feelings on a specific theme is said to have a(n) _____; when the person is driven to express those thoughts through repetitive acts, the acts are called a(n) _____; such a person suffers from a neurosis classified as a(n) _____ disorder.

3. In response to a precipitating stressful event, a patient may develop a paralysis, deafness, blindness, nervous tic, or other physical anomaly as a means of avoiding or dealing with the stress. The development of such a symptom is called a(n) _____ reaction, which is classified as a(n) _____ neurosis.

4. Multiple personality is often termed by the lay public as schizophrenia, although it is actually a(n) _____ state, which is more accurately classified as a(n) _____ neurosis.

5. A feeling of anxiety that is both inappropriate and long-lasting, even if the initial trigger really is an external stressful event, is called _____ and may be accompanied by hallucinations and other symptoms.

6. The patient exhibiting a(n) _____ personality tends to project his positive, egocentric self-perception on others, manipulating others and blaming them for his own misfortunes and failures; conversely, the _____ personality tends to project his negative self-perception, aggression, and hostility onto others.

7. The depressive state that lacks a realistic external reference and seems to arise from conflicts within the patient is called _____ depression, hence its name.

8. The psychosurgical technique most commonly employed in a leukotomy is _____, a term derived from the Greek words for "solid" and "arrangement."

9. Currently modified by the administration of anesthetics and muscle relaxants (to reduce physical trauma) and by unilateral treatment of the nondominant hemisphere (to reduce memory loss, confusion, and headache), _____ is often helpful in treating severe depression.

10. Rejection of reality and withdrawal into the patient's own world is called _____, which is also the term applied to children who fail to respond to external stimuli and instead seem to respond to their own reality, essentially the same symptom.

Chapter 15: The Endocrine System and Its Disorders

1. Glands of the endocrine system function primarily to regulate the body's _____ processes.

2. More than _____ hormones are found in the human body. These are categorized as _____, _____ and _____.

3. Adrenocorticotropic hormone is one of those secreted by the _____.

4. The thyroid gland secretes the hormone _____ that contains _____. This stimulates the _____ of body cells.

5. The principal sites of action of the parathyroid hormone are the _____ and the _____.

6. Hormones secreted by the adrenal cortex are referred to as _____.

7. The endocrine functions of the pancreas are performed by the _____, which secrete the hormone _____.

8. Male and female sex glands are referred to as _____. The most important hormone produced in the male is _____; in the female it is _____ and _____.

9. Two diseases resulting from overproduction of the pituitary gland are _____ and _____. Insufficient secretion by this gland results in _____.

10. A metabolic disease resulting from lack of sufficient insulin production by the pancreas is known as _____.

Chapter 16: The Hematologic System and Its Disorders

1. Red blood cells are called _____ because of their color; the molecule that provides that color and that binds with the oxygen for transport is _____.

2. Initiating the production of red blood cells, oxygen depletion stimulates production of _____ by the kidneys, which stimulates the production of _____, so named because they are "cells that form blood cells."

3. Several of the white blood cells move toward areas of tissue damage in response to chemotactic substances such as leukotaxine, but _____ and _____ are the primary scavengers and exhibit the greatest degree or ameboid movement.

4. The white blood cells involved in coagulation are called _____ because they are small, disc-shaped structures; they are also known as _____, so named for their role in clot formation.

5. The extrinsic system of blood coagulation is based on the initial actions of _____, and the intrinsic system depends on the activity of _____ to begin the cascade.

6. A normocytic normochromic anemia would most likely be posthemorrhagic because the disorder arises from the rapid loss of red blood cells with no change in production; a microcytic hypochromic anemia, however, is usually caused by a deficiency of _____ or chronic loss of _____.

7. A reduction in the number of platelets is known as _____, which can cause bleeding into the skin, a condition known as _____.

8. If an Rh positive father and an Rh negative mother produce an Rh positive fetus, the fetus is at risk for developing _____, so named because of the increased number of immature red blood cells produced by the fetus. Without the appropriate treatment for the

mother, the risk of this usually fatal disease increases significantly during subsequent pregnancies.

9. Red blood cell indices, which are useful in determining if the red blood cells are microcytic, macrocytic, and/or hypochromic, are actually calculated rather than measured in the laboratory. The three indices are _____, _____, and _____.

10. Sickle cell anemia requires a _____ for diagnosis since that is the main procedure by which abnormally shaped red blood cells are documented.

Chapter 17: The Lymphatic/Immune System and Its Disorders

1. Negative fluid pressure is maintained in the tissues by the drainage of _____, a fluid with a composition similar to the interstitial fluid and whose name is derived from the Latin word for water. This fluid initially enters the lymphatic system through the walls of the _____, also called _____.

2. Contraction of the lymphatic vessels, called _____, as well as pressure on them by muscles and blood vessels, creates unidirectional flow because of the presence of _____ in all the vessels.

3. Removal of bacteria, tissue debris, and other particles from the lymph is carried out in enlarged areas of the vessels called _____, which filter the lymph and pass it over large numbers of _____ cells that phagocytize the particles.

4. B-lymphocytes or B-cells are also named _____ lymphocytes for the analogous avian cell; B-lymphocytes are involved in humoral immunity, so called because sensitized B-cells mature into _____ cells, which produce _____ that are carried in the circulation.

5. The process by which immunoglobulins attach to the surface of bacterial cells, coat the cell through a complement reaction, and allow it to be phagocytized is called _____.

6. Cellular immunity relies on the activity of _____ lymphocytes, also called T-lymphocytes or T-cells. Two subsets of these cells are the T-_____ cells and the T-_____ cells, so called because they assist or inhibit the production of antibodies.

7. Monocytes are formed in lymphoid tissue and serve a protective function in the body. When they are mature, they become _____, which are highly mobile cells that scavenge bacterial cells and tissue debris. The mature cells may also exhibit very little ameboid motion and remain relatively fixed, in which case they are called _____.

8. Failure of the lymphatic system to maintain a negative interstitial fluid pressure results in _____, a swelling of the tissues with an accumulation of fluid. If the accumulation is in the abdominal space, the resulting effusion is referred to as _____.

9. A direct skin test is used to detect a type I or _____ hypersensitivity. A positive response to a direct skin test is indicated by a _____ reaction, resulting in a raised erythematous area at the site.

10. Lack of an allergic reaction to antigenic skin tests (patch or direct) is called _____ and indicates severe immunosuppression, such as in the patient with AIDS.

Chapter 18: Oncology

1. The term denoting the branch of medicine devoted to the study of tumors is _____. Physicians specializing in this area are _____.

2. The term denoting abnormal growth of new tissue is _____.

3. The process by which a tumor spreads to other locations is known as _____.

4. The TNM method of classifying oncologic diseases refers to evaluation of _____, _____, and _____.

5. The use of drugs in treatment of oncologic disorders is known as _____.

6. Surgical excision of an organ as a method of treating tumors is denoted by the suffix-ectomy. Two examples of such procedures would be _____ and _____.

7. Neoplastic disorders of the blood-forming cells of the bone marrow are known as the _____.

8. A melanoma is a malignant neoplasm of the _____ that spreads through the body via the _____ and _____.

9. Two radiographic procedures used in diagnosis of breast cancer are _____ and _____.

10. A method of treatment that utilizes a substance injected into an artery to stop blood flow in the tumor and produce ischemia is known as _____.

Chapter 19: Trauma and Poisoning

1. Fractures are often described by the way the bone breaks; for example, a _____ fracture results when the bone is crushed, and the most common fracture of the wrist is called a _____ fracture and frequently results from a fall.

2. Although most frequently applied to the brain, the term _____ actually refers to any generalized violent force or shock.

3. Failure to respond to the vasodilatory effects of heat causes _____; a more severe condition is the loss of the body's heat regulatory mechanism known _____, also called _____.

4. Third degree burns, also called _____ burns, destroy both the _____ and _____, thus precluding tissue regeneration, except from the wound margin where less tissue damage has occurred.

5. Asphyxiation by near-drowning causes loss of surfactant in the lungs and collapse of the lung, a condition called _____.

6. With any severe trauma, pain, fear, and anxiety can cause vasodilation severe enough to cause the hypoperfusive state known as _____, also called _____.

7. Hypovolemic shock, also known as _____, can lead to cardiac and respiratory arrest; therefore, a primary therapeutic measure in first aid of the shock victim should be _____.

8. Although technically synonymous with the word *poison,* the term _____ is usually applied specifically to toxic proteins produced by some higher plants and animals.

9. Derived from a term denoting the stomach and the French word for "washing," _____ is most frequently performed by the use of a large-bore Ewald tube.

10. Another word for poisoning, _____ is applied by the public specifically to poisoning with alcohol, although medical usage is usually much broader.

Chapter 20: Nutritional Disorders and Alternative Medicine

1. The general term used to denote a vitamin deficiency is _____. Vitamin excess is known as _____.

2. A deficiency of vitamin B, or _____, results in the clinical syndrome affecting the nervous system called _____.

3. The nutritional standard that specifies the type and amount of nutrients required to maintain health is the _____.

4. The two types of primary malnutrition are _____ and _____.

5. The term _____ refers to the type of measurements taken of skin fold and muscle circumference.

6. _____ denotes an approach to treatment that views the mind and body as a continually interacting, living, integrated system.

7. The medical specialty that focuses on adjustment of the spinal vertebra as a basis for treatment is known as _____.

8. Use of individual muscle functions to provide information about overall health of an individual is called _____.

9. _____ is the form of treatment that considers symptoms as a part of the curative process rather than a manifestation of the disease itself.

10. Two terms that can be used to indicate botanical medicines are _____ and _____.

Answer Keys

Chapter 1: Fundamentals of Medical Terms

Prefixes

1. apnea—absence of breathing
   anemia—deficiency of red blood cells, hemoglobin, and packed cells
2. decapitate—to remove the head
   abductor—muscle that draws a part away from the median
3. prognosis—prediction of the outcome of a disease
   antepartum—period before childbirth
4. antipyretic—reducing fever
   contraceptive—preventing conception/impregnation
5. ectoderm—outer layer of cells in the embryo
   exogenous—originating outside of the organism
6. endocarditis—inflammation of the heart muscle
   intraocular—within the eyeball
7. hypotension—low blood pressure
   subcostal—located below the ribs
8. suprarenal—above the kidney
   superacidity—excess of acid
9. hyporeflexia—condition of weakened reflexes
   octose—sugar containing eight carbon atoms
   monophasia—able to speak only a single word or sentence
10. cyanosis—dark bluish or purple coloration of the skin
    xanthoma—yellow nodule or plaque

Roots

1. ankyl—stiffening or fixation of a joint
2. blast—a neoplasm composed of immature, undifferentiated cells
3. cyt—the dissolution of a cell
4. hyper—elevated level of glucose in the blood
5. therm—loss of body heat by evaporation, radiation, etc.
6. blenn—any mucus discharge
7. steno—a stricture or narrowing of any canal
8. aer—distention of a small natural cavity with gas
9. ergo—treatment of disease by muscular exercise
10. ped—pain in the foot

Suffixes

1. ''-emia''; blood
2. ''-pathy''; disease
3. ''-rrhexis''; rupture
4. ''-plegia''; paralysis
5. suture
6. excision
7. ''-dynia''; ''-algia''
8. eating/swallowing; speech

9. inflammation
10. "-oma"; tumor

Chapter 2: The Health Care System and Its Structure

1. American Medical Association (AMA)
2. Health Care Financing Administration (HCFA)
3. physical therapist; speech pathologist
4. JCAHO; Joint Commission on Accreditation of Healthcare Organizations
5. chiropody; podiatry
6. diagnostic related groups (DRGs)
7. dermatology; neurology (or ophthalmology, urology)
8. Pediatrics; geriatrics
9. DUE; DUR; DRR
10. health maintenance organization

Chapter 3: Translating the Medical Record

1. fever, chills, sweating, nausea, vomiting, diarrhea
2. history of present illness
3. microbiologic
4. serodiagnostic; antigen-antibody
5. roentgenography/radiology
6. colon/intestines
7. puri-; pyo-
8. Cheyne-Stokes respiration
9. radioimmunoassay
10. coronary care unit; cardiac intensive care unit; intensive coronary care unit; cardiac surveillance unit

Chapter 4: Abbreviations, Eponyms, and Lay Terms

Lay Terms

1. eardrum; kneecap
2. decubitus ulcer
3. enuresis
4. furuncle; herpes simplex; verruca
5. barbs, candy, goofballs, sleeping pills, downs
6. cocaine and phencyclidine
7. coryza; heartburn
8. pyrexia; botulism
9. wrist; femur
10. conjunctivitis; epidemic parotitis

Eponyms

1. Alzheimer's disease
2. Barrett's syndrome; Crohn's disease
3. Bell's palsy
4. Charcot-Marie-Tooth disease

5. disease or syndrome
6. Colle's; Pott's
7. thromboangiitis obliterans
8. mongolism
9. renal tubular dysfunction
10. anemia lymphatica; lymphoma

Chapter 5: The Cardiovascular System and Its Disorders

1. aorta; ascending aorta
2. atrioventricular; bicuspid; tricuspid; mitral
3. endocarditis; myocarditis
4. coronary
5. vasculitis
6. two-dimensional echocardiogram (2-d echo)
7. S-T; angina pectoris
8. capillaries; arterioles; venules
9. myocardial ischemia; coronary arteriography
10. premature ventricular contractions (or ventricular premature beats); PVCs (or VPBs)

Chapter 6: The Digestive System and Its Disorders

1. saliva, facilitate swallowing/break down carbohydrate
2. pharynx, esophagus, peristalsis
3. cardiac, fundus, antrum, pylorus; hydrochloric acid, pepsin, mucus
4. duodenum, jejunum, ileum
5. chyme; liver, pancreas
6. cecum, ascending colon, transverse colon, descending colon, sigmoid colon, appendix
7. hematemesis, melena, hematochezia
8. viral hepatitis, cirrhosis
9. dysphagia, pyrosis, odynophagia
10. root, crown, neck; enamel, dentin, pulp, cement

Chapter 7: The Musculoskeletal System and Its Disorders

1. muscles, tendons, ligaments, joints, bone
2. femur, tibia, fibula—humerus, radius, ulna
3. cartilage
4. diaphysis, epiphysis
5. myositis, polymyositis, dermatomyositis
6. bursitis, tendonitis
7. inguinal, hiatal, femoral, incisional, umbilical
8. orthopedist
9. joints
10. spine/vertebra

Chapter 8: The Integumentary System and Its Disorders

1. skin, glands, nails, hair
2. dermatology; dermatologist
3. bulla, crust, cyst, macule, nodule, papule, plaque, pustule, scale, ulcer, vesicle, wheal
4. pruritus; psoriasis

5. sebaceous; acne vulgaris
6. folliculitis, erysipelas, impetigo
7. lichenified
8. ephelides; nevi; comedones
9. hypermelanosis; hypomelanosis
10. cutis, dermis

Chapter 9: The Respiratory System and Its Disorders

1. nostrils, pharynx, epiglottis, trachea, bronchi, lungs
2. bronchioles; alveoli
3. alveoli
4. hemoglobin
5. diaphragm; contracts; relaxes
6. thoracodynia, thoracalgia
7. pneumothorax; hemothorax
8. hypercapnia/hypercarbia; hypoxemia
9. bronchoscopy, mediastinoscopy, laryngoscopy, thoracoscopy
10. thoracotomy, pleurotomy

Chapter 10: The Reproductive System and Its Disorders

1. convoluted seminiferous tubules
2. ampulla; isthmus
3. oocytes, ovocytes
4. salpingitis; pelvic inflammatory disease; PID
5. dysmenorrhea; amenorrhea; oligomenorrhea; hypermenorrhea; epimenorrhea, polymenorrhea; cryptomenorrhea
6. reportable; sexually transmitted diseases (or STDs)
7. corpus cavernosum
8. transverse
9. trigravida, gravida III; nulliparous
10. cervical punch; cold knife cone

Chapter 11: The Urinary System and Its Disorders

1. glomerulus; tubule (proximal convoluted tubule)
2. renal pelvis; calyces
3. detrusor uniae
4. polyuria; oliguria
5. lithotripsy; litholapaxy
6. cystography; urography
7. RBC casts
8. acute pyelonephritis or bacterial pyelonephritis
9. nephrotic syndrome
10. urethroscopy

Chapter 12: The Nervous System and Its Disorders

1. myelin sheath; saltatory
2. spinal meningitis; meninges

3. craniotomy; craniectomy
4. subdural hematoma
5. neuromuscular junction
6. myasthenia gravis
7. hydrocephalus
8. extrapyramidal; pyramids
9. central nervous system; muscles; dendrites; axon
10. lumbar puncture

Chapter 13: The Special Sense Organs and Their Disorders

1. taste, smell, hearing, equilibrium, vision
2. osmesis, osphresis, olfaction
3. utricle, saccule, semicircular ducts
4. eyelids, eyelashes, eyebrows, conjunctiva, bony orbits, ocular muscle, tear ducts
5. otitis media
6. retinitis, scleritis, keratitis, uveitis, iritis, blepharitis
7. otalgia, otodynia
8. oculist, ophthalmologist
9. otologist
10. iridectomy, goniotomy, goniopuncture, trabeculectomy, iridencleisis, cyclodialysis, cyclodiathermy, cyclocryosurgery, sclerectomy, cryosurgery, photocoagulation

Chapter 14: Psychiatric Disorders

1. neurosis; psychosis
2. obsession; compulsion; obsessive-compulsive
3. conversion; hysterical
4. dissociative; hysterical
5. anxiety neurosis
6. hysterical (histrionic); paranoid
7. endogenous (psychotic)
8. stereotaxy
9. electroconvulsive therapy (ECT)
10. autism

Chapter 15: The Endocrine System and Its Disorders

1. metabolic/metabolism
2. fifty; peptides, steroids, amines
3. pituitary gland
4. thyroxin; iodine; metabolism
5. bones, kidneys
6. corticosteroids
7. Islands of Langerhans; insulin
8. gonads; testosterone; progesterone and estrogen
9. giantism, acromegaly; dwarfism
10. diabetes mellitus

Chapter 16: The Hematologic System and Its Disorders

1. erythrocytes; hemoglobin
2. erythropoietin; hemocytoblasts
3. neutrophils; monocytes (or macrophages)
4. platelets; thrombocytes
5. thromboplastin; platelets (platelet factor 3)
6. iron; blood
7. thrombocytopenia; purpura
8. erythroblastosis fetalis
9. mean corpuscular volume (MCV); mean corpuscular hemoglobin (MCH); mean corpuscular hemoglobin concentration (MCHC)
10. peripheral blood smear

Chapter 17: The Lymphatic/Immune System and Its Disorders

1. lymph; initial lymphatics; lymphatic capillaries
2. lymphoducts; lymphatic valves (valvulae lymphaticum)
3. lymph nodes (lymphaden); reticuloendothelial
4. bursa-equivalent (bursal); plasma; antibodies (immunoglobulins)
5. opsonization
6. thymic; helper; suppressor
7. macrophages; histiocytes
8. edema; ascites
9. immediate or IgE-mediated; wheal-and-flare
10. anergy

Chapter 18: Oncology

1. oncology; oncologists
2. neoplasm
3. metastasis
4. tumor, lymph nodes, metastasis
5. chemotherapy
6. colectomy, gastrectomy, hysterectomy, lobectomy, lymphadenectomy, mastectomy
7. leukemias
8. skin; blood, lymphatics
9. mammography, thermography
10. chemoembolization

Chapter 19: Trauma and Poisoning

1. comminuted; Colles'
2. concussion
3. heat prostration; heat hyperpyrexia; heatstroke
4. full-thickness; epidermis; dermis
5. atelectasis
6. primary shock; neurogenic shock
7. secondary shock; cardiopulmonary resuscitation (CPR)
8. toxin

9. gastric lavage
10. intoxication

Chapter 20: Nutritional Disorders and Alternative Medicine

1. hypovitaminosis; hypervitaminosis
2. thiamine; Wernicke-Korsakoff syndrome, dry beriberi
3. recommended dietary allowance
4. marasmus, kwashiorkor
5. anthropometric
6. holistic
7. chiropractic
8. kinesiology
9. homeopathy
10. phytopharmaceuticals, herbal medicines

BIBLIOGRAPHY

American Medical Association. *Physician's Current Procedural Terminology*. Chicago, Illinois, 1996

Balch, James F. and Balch, Phyllis A. *Prescriptions for Nutritional Healing*. Avery Publishing Group Inc., Garden City Park, NY, 1990

Dorland's Illustrated Medical Dictionary. 28th edition. W. B. Saunders Publishing Company, Philadelphia PA, 1994

Eisenberg, Myron G. *Dictionary of Rehabilitation*. Springer Publishing Company, Inc., New York NY, 1995

Firkin, Barry G. and Whitworth, J. A. *Dictionary of Medical Eponyms,* 2nd edition. Parthenon Publishing Group, New York NY, 1995

Harrison's Principles of Internal Medicine, 12th edition. McGraw-Hill Book Company, New York NY, 1991

Holt, Robert J. and Stanaszek, Walter F. *The Medical WordBook.* H & S Scientific Publishers, Oklahoma City, Oklahoma, 1994

Marti, James E. *Alternative Health and Medicine Encyclopedia*. Visible Ink Press, Detroit, Michigan, 1995

Taber's Cyclopedic Medical Dictionary. 18th edition. F. A. Davis Company, Philadelphia, Pennsylvania, 1997

Thibodeau, Gary A. *Anatomy and Physiology*. C. V. Mosby Company, St. Louis MO, 1993

Young, Lloyd Y. and Koda-Kimble, Mary A. *Applied Therapeutics: The Clinical Use of Drugs.* 6th edition. Applied Therapeutics, Inc., Vancouver, WA, 1995.

INDEX

2-D echo 74
abbreviations 41
abdominal pregnancy 151
abdominal surgery 22
abortifacient 160
abortion 157, 158, 159, 160–161
abortion, artificial 160
abortion, induced 160
abortion, spontaneous 160
abortion, therapeutic 160, 161
ABR 36
abrasion 281, 282, 285
abruptio placentae 157, 162
abscess 121, 126, 154, 158, 185, 188
absence seizure 185
absence seizure, atypical 185
absence seizure, complex 185
absence seizure, simple 185
absorptiometry 88, 106, 114
accommodation 203, 206
acetylcholine 179, 190
achalasia 84, 93
achlorhydria 84, 93
achromatopsia 198, 206
acid-base disorder 291–292
acidosis 134, 141
acne 123, 126
acne vulgaris 123
acoustic 193, 206
acquired immune deficiency syndrome 256, 258
acromegaly 104, 229, 236
acrophobia 214, 221
actinic keratoses 282, 285
acupressure 297
acupuncture 297, 300
AD 186, 189
addiction medicine 23
Addison's disease 230
adenocarcinoma 157, 273–275, 277
adenohypophysis 227
adenoma 236, 274, 277
adenovirus 135, 141
adiposis 294
adiposity 294, 300
adipostat 294
adrenal 165, 227–228, 236
adrenalectomy 273
adrenaline 179

adrenergic 179, 180
adrenocorticotropic hormone 226–227
adrenogenital syndrome 236
adsorbent 284–285
adult respiratory distress syndrome 136
adynamia 104, 114
aeroallergens 142
affect 213, 221
afferent 183
afterload 66
ageusia 196, 206
agglutination 254, 257, 260
agglutinin 254, 260
agglutinogen 242, 248
aggregation, platelet 242
agonist 102
agoraphobia 214, 221
agranulocytosis 244, 248
AIDS 256, 258
air concussion 282, 285
albinism 123
aldosterone 227, 236
aldosteronism 66, 236
alimentary 79, 93
alimentary canal 79
alkalosis 134, 142
allergen 257
allergic purpura 246
allergy 256, 258
allergy & immunology 23
allogenic 267, 272
allopathic 296, 300
alpha-fetoprotein 161
alternative medicine 296
alveolalgia 83
alveolar bone 88
alveoli 130
alveolitis 88
alveoloplasty 90, 93
alveolus 83, 93
Alzheimer's disease 186, 187, 188, 189, 212
amalgam restorations 90
amaurosis 198, 206
amblyopia 199, 206
ameboid 241
amenorrhea 154–155
amenorrhea, relative 155
American Medical Association 19